ANTIOXIDANT-ANTIDIABETIC AGENTS AND HUMAN HEALTH

Edited by **Oluwafemi Oguntibeju**

Antioxidant-Antidiabetic Agents and Human Health
http://dx.doi.org/10.5772/57029
Edited by Oluwafemi Oguntibeju

Contributors
Elizabeth Anamenechukwu Udenta, Oluwafemi O. Oguntibeju, Ikemefuna C. Obizoba, Afolabi Clement Akinmoladun, Oluwafemi Omoniyi Oguntibeju, Ebenezer Farombi, Victoria Jideani, Claudine Diedericks, Ademola Oyagbemi, E. Olatunde Farombi, Charles Nnadi, Akachukwu Ibezim, Chika Mbah, Ngozi Nwodo, Rotimi Arise, Aderounmu Ganiyu, Stefan S Du Plessis, Bongikele Skosana, Yapo Aboua, Guillaume Aboua, Omolola Ayepola, Olatogni Berenice L Alinde, Wongama Given Pantsi, Dirk Bester, A. J. Esterhuyse, Afam I. O. Jideani, Thakhani Takalani, Henry Silungwe, Tonna Anyasi, Adewale Omolola, Henry Udeh, Adeolu Adedapo, Sunday Ofuegbe

Published by InTech
Janeza Trdine 9, 51000 Rijeka, Croatia

Publishing Process Manager Iva Lipovic
Technical Editor InTech DTP team
Cover InTech Design team

First published February, 2014
Printed in Croatia

Additional hard copies can be obtained from orders@intechopen.com

Antioxidant-Antidiabetic Agents and Human Health, Edited by Oluwafemi Oguntibeju
p. cm.
ISBN 978-953-51-1215-0

For EU product safety concerns:
IN TECH d.o.o., Prolaz Marije Krucifikse Kozulić 3, 51000 Rijeka, Croatia,
info@intechopen.com or visit our website at intechopen.com.

Meet the editor

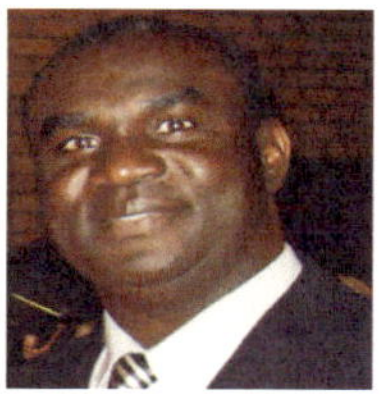

Prof Oluwafemi.O Oguntibeju is Associate Professor and Group Leader (Nutrition and Chronic Disease Research Group) at the Oxidative Stress Research Centre, Department of Biomedical Sciences, Cape Peninsula University of Technology, South Africa. He lectures and supervises postgraduate students and collaborates with national and international scientists. Over the years, he has been involved in the field of nutrition, HIV and AIDS but more recently on natural products and health (Phytomedicine). He has successfully supervised 17 master's and 2 doctoral students and is currently supervising 4 doctoral and two master's students at various stages of their programmes. Prof Oguntibeju has published over 90 scientific papers in peer-reviewed journals, 16 book chapters, acted as editor of three books on diabetes, and presented over 36 papers at international conferences. He reviews manuscripts for over 30 international scientific journals and has received various awards such as the Platinum Research Excellence Award at his current university. He is National Research Foundation-South Africa (NRF) C-rated researcher. He holds a master's degree in Biochemistry from the University of Ibadan, Nigeria and a doctoral degree in Biomedical Science from the Central University of Technology, Bloemfontein, South Africa. He completed his postdoctoral research fellowship at the Cape Peninsula University of Technology, South Africa. He is Chartered Scientist (CSci, UK) and Fellow of the Institute of Biomedical Science (FIBMS), London. He is registered with the South African Council for Scientific Professions as Professional Natural Scientist (Pri.Sc.Nat).

Contents

Preface

The book "Antioxidant-Antidiabetic Agents and Human Health" is divided into five sections covering specific chapters. The book containing 15 chapters primarily addresses the health benefits of antioxidant-rich natural products and medicinal plants in management and treatment of diabetes and other chronic diseases. Each chapter draws on the scientific and educational expertise of the authors presenting unique content, style of communication and scientific background, making it an excellent book in the field of medicinal plants and human health. It provides historical and scientific evidence on the usefulness of antioxidant-rich natural products and plants with therapeutic potentials in management and treatment of diabetes mellitus and other chronic diseases. Scientists, professional health workers, academics and students of different backgrounds would undoubtedly appreciate and value its deeply educative contents. The book pointedly adds to the pool of scientific and professional knowledge in the field, but further provides better understanding on the topics covered. The carefully selected references provided in each chapter would act as catalyst for further information on the diverse topics treated in the book.

Oluwafemi Oguntibeju
Nutrition & Chronic Disease Research Unit, Oxidative Stress Research Centre,
Department of Biomedical Sciences
Faculty of Health & Wellness Sciences
Cape Peninsula University of Technology
Bellville, South Africa

Section 1

Antidiabetic Agents

Chapter 1

Lipid Profile, Antidiabetic and Antioxidant Activity of *Acacia ataxacantha* Bark Extract in Streptozotocin-Induced Diabetic Rats

Rotimi O. Arise, Aderounmu I. Ganiyu and
Oluwafemi O. Oguntibeju

Additional information is available at the end of the chapter

http://dx.doi.org/10.5772/57151

1. Introduction

Diabetes mellitus is a heterogeneous primary disorder of carbohydrate metabolism which exists everywhere in the world and interests approximately 371 million people worldwide. The prevalence of diabetes mellitus is increasing with ageing of the population and lifestyle changes associated with rapid urbanization and westernization. The disease is found in all parts of the world and is rapidly increasing in its coverage [1, 2]. WHO projects that diabetes will be the 7th leading cause of death in 2030 [2, 3]. It is a metabolic disorder initially characterized by a loss of glucose homeostasis with disturbances of carbohydrate, fat and protein metabolism resulting from defects in insulin secretion, insulin action, or both [4]. Without enough insulin, the cells of the body cannot absorb sufficient glucose from the blood; hence blood glucose levels increase, which is termed as hyperglycemia. If the glucose level in the blood remains high over a long period of time, this can result in long-term damage to organs, such as the kidneys, liver, eyes, nerves, heart and blood vessels. Complications in some of these organs can lead to death [5]

The roles of certain organs such as the pancreas, liver and kidney in diabetes mellitus are very important.The pancreas plays a primary role in the metabolism of glucose by secreting the hormones insulin and glucagon (Figure 1). The islets of Langerhans secrete insulin and glucagon directly into the blood. Insulin is a protein that is essential for proper regulation of glucose and for maintenance of proper blood glucose levels [6]. Glucagon is a hormone that opposes the action of insulin. It is secreted when blood glucose level falls. It increases blood glucose concentration partly by breaking down stored glycogen in the liver by a pathway known as glycogenolysis. Gluconeogenesis is the production of glucose in the liver from non-carbohydrate precursors such as glycogenic amino acids [7].

WHO classification of diabetes introduced in 1980 and revised in 1985 was based on clinical characteristics. The two most common types of diabetes were insulin-dependent diabetes mellitus (IDDM) or (type I) and non-insulin-dependent diabetes mellitus (NIDDM) or (type II). WHO classification also recognized malnutrition-related diabetes mellitus and gestational diabetes. Malnutrition-related diabetes was omitted from the new classification because its etiology is uncertain, and it is unclear whether it is a separate type of diabetes [8, 9, and 10].

International Diabetes Federation [11] reported that one in 10 adults will have diabetes by 2030, posing a huge challenge to health care systems around the world. According to the report, the number of people living with diabetes worldwide will increase to 552 million by 2030 from 366 million in 2011 unless action is taken. Over 80 percent of its related deaths occur in low- and middle-income countries. It has been predicted that the number of cases may jump by 90 percent even in Africa, where infectious diseases have previously been the top killer [11].

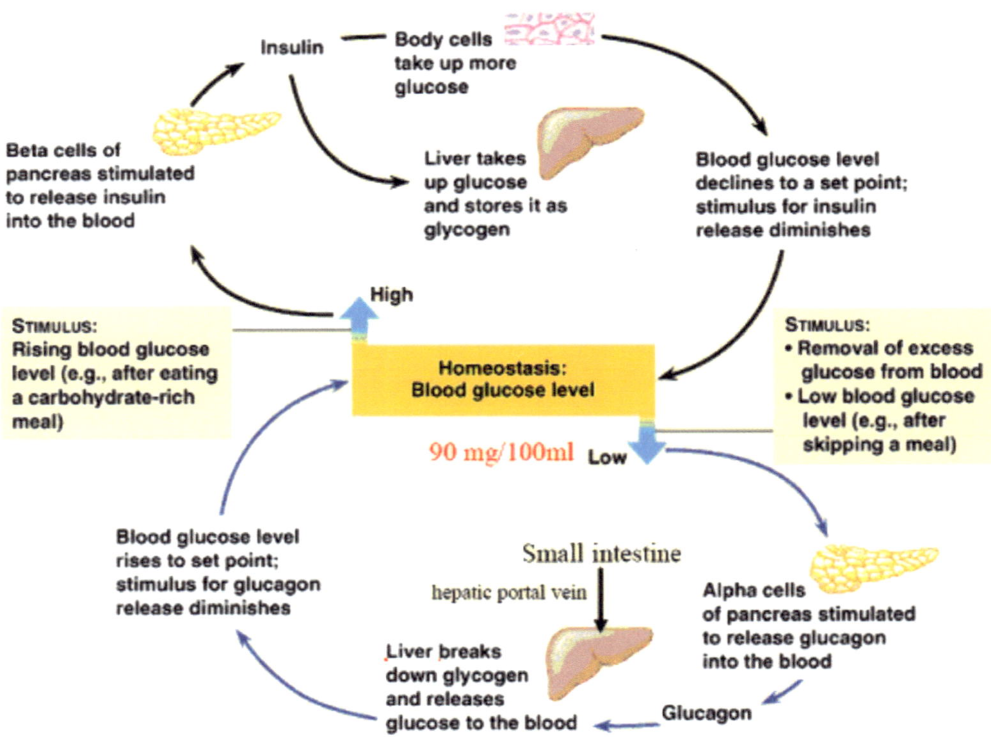

Source: Worthley [6]

Figure 1. The role of pancreas in the body

The conventional treatment for diabetes mellitus is oral hypoglycemic agents/insulin therapy [12]. However these have been shown to have prominent side effects and they do not modify the course of diabetic complications [13, 14]. The need to develop new antidiabetic drugs has led to studies that have attempted to screen some indigenous plants for antidiabetic activity [15, 16]. Traditional preparations of plant sources are widely used almost everywhere in the world to treat this disease. Therefore plant materials are considered to be the alternative sources for finding out new leads for antihyperglycemic agents. The plant drugs are frequently considered to be less toxic when compared to synthetic drugs [17]. More than 1,123 plant species have been used to treat diabetes and more than 200 pure compounds have been shown to possess characteristics of lowering blood glucose activity [18]. *Acacia ataxacantha* or *Flame Thorn* is an African tree species with conspicuous red pods and numerous hooked prickles. It is wide-spread in sub-Saharan Africa from Senegal in the west to Sudan in the east, Namibia, Botswana, Zimbabwe, and in the Transvaal and KwaZulu-Natal. In arid regions it prefers low-lying sites near streams, water courses and in valleys, but in higher rainfall areas it is a common member of the vegetation, often favouring forest margins. The flaking bark is light grey, splitting longitudinally and transversely, and revealing a buff under-colour. The persistent prickles are profuse on young twigs, but can also be found on older wood. Unlike most Acacias, the prickles are not in pairs, but scattered along young twigs ('ataxacantha' i.e orderless prickles).

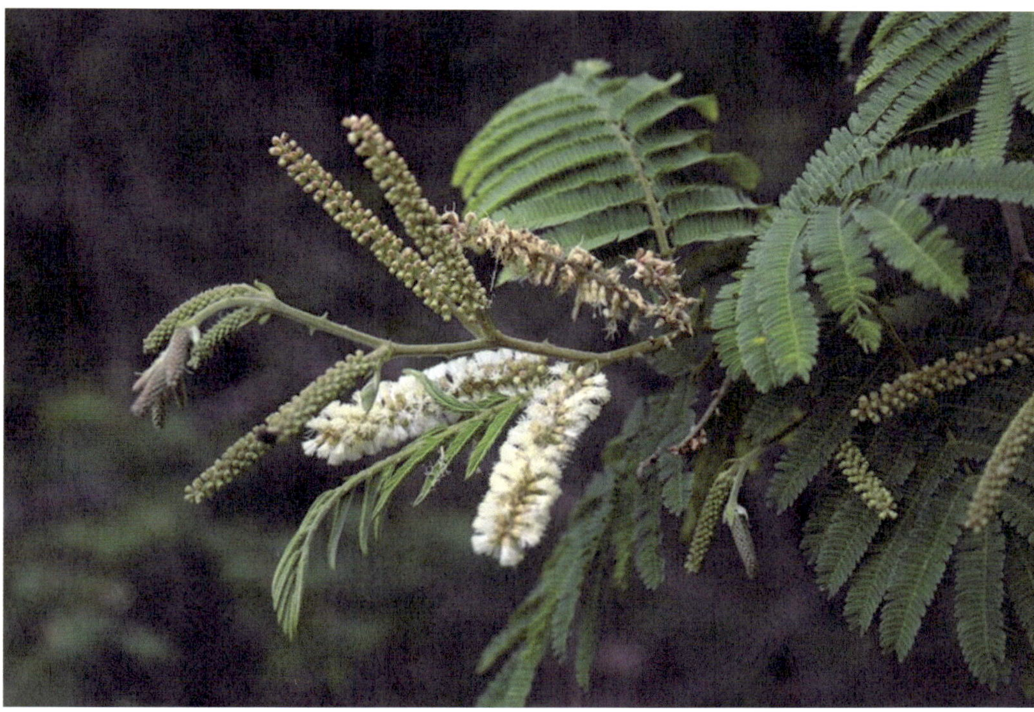

Source : Davidson and Jeppe [19]

Figure 2. *Acacia ataxacantha*

Hence, the aim of this study is to investigate the anti-diabetic potential and safety evaluation of ethanolic extract of *Acacia ataxacantha* bark in streptozotocin-induced diabetic rats. The results were compared with standard anti-diabetic drug, metformin.

2. Materials and methods

2.1. Experimental animals and reagents

36 Albino rats (*Rattus norvegicus*) with an average weight of 132.5 g were obtained from the Animal Holding Unit of the Department of Biochemistry, University of Ilorin, Ilorin, Kwara State, Nigeria. Animal husbandry and experimentation were consistent with Guiding Principles in the use of Animals in Toxicology [20]. All the reagents used for this study were of analytical grade and were prepared in all glass-distilled water.

2.2. Plant extract preparation

The bark of *Acacia ataxacantha* was obtained from Akure, Ondo State, Nigeria. Identification was carried out at the University Ilorin Herbarium, Department of Plant Biology, Ilorin, Nigeria where voucher number 872 was deposited. The bark was air-dried under shade and pulverized into fine powder. 200 g of the fine powder was percolated in 500 ml of absolute ethanol (60-80 °C) for 24h. The percolated mixture was filtered and evaporated at room temperature according to the method of Majekodunmi *et al.* [21]. A homogenous aqueous suspension of the extract was made before administration to the experimental animals [21].

2.3. Induction of experimental diabetes

The animals were fasted overnight and diabetes was induced by a single intra-peritoneal injection of freshly-prepared STZ (55 mg/kg body weight of rats) in 0.1 M citrate buffer (pH 4.5) [22]. The animals were allowed to drink 5% glucose solution overnight to overcome the drug-induced hypoglycaemia. Control rats were injected with citrate buffer alone. The animals were considered as diabetic, if their blood glucose values were above 250 mg/dL on the third day after the STZ injection. The treatment was started on the fourth day after the STZ injection and this was considered the first day of treatment.

2.4. Animals grouping

All rats were maintained under standard laboratory conditions (12 h light/dark cycle, 25 ± 2 °C). The rats were acclimatized for a week in the laboratory. They were fed with standard rodent diet and tap water *ad libitum*. The animals were then randomly divided into 6 groups-

Group 1: Received distilled water (Control)

Group 2: Diabetic untreated rats

Group 3: Diabetic and treated with125 mg/kg b.w of ethanolic extract of *Acacia ataxacantha* bark

Group 4: Diabetic and treated with 250 mg/kg b.w of ethanolic extract of *Acacia ataxacantha* bark.

Group 5: Diabetic and treated with 500 mg/kg b.w of ethanolic extract of *Acacia ataxacantha* bark

Group 6: Diabetic and treated with standard drug (Metformin)

2.5. Sample preparation

At the end of the experimental period, venous blood was collected from the experimental animals and serum was prepared by centrifuging the blood samples at 3000 rpm for 5 minutes [23] and serum collected by pippeting. The animals were thereafter quickly dissected and the liver and pancreas removed. The pancreas and liver were suspended in ice-cold 0.25 M sucrose solution (1:5 w/v) and homogenized. The homogenates were kept frozen overnight to ensure maximum release of enzymes [24].

2.6. Estimation of hepatic glucose and glycogen

Hepatic glucose and glycogen were estimated using the method of Barham and Trinder [25] and Passoneau and Lauderdale [26] respectively.

2.7. Determination of liver enzyme activities

The method described by Reitman and Frankel [27] was used for assaying the activity of alanine aminotransferase and aspartate aminotransferase.

2.8. Lipids profile analysis

Total cholesterol, triglyceride, high density lipoprotein cholesterol, low density lipoprotein cholesterol were assayed using the method of Zlakis *et al.* [28], Foster and Dunn [29], Burstein *et al.*[30] and Friedwald *et al.* [31] respectively.

2.9. Determination of liver function indices

The procedure described by Doumas *et al.* [32] and Sherlock [33] was used for the determination of albumin and bilirubin concentrations respectively.

The method of Tietz *et al.* [34] was used to determine the levels of serum urea and creatinine.

2.10. Determination of superoxide dismutase activity and malondialdehyde concentration

The pancreatic superoxide dismutase activity was determined by the method of Misra and Fridovich [35] while malondialdehyde concentration was assayed using the method described by Varshney and Kale [36].

2.11. Statistical analysis

All data are expressed as the mean of sixth replicates ± standard error of mean (S.E.M). Statistical evaluation of data was performed by SPSS version 16 using one way analysis of variance (ANOVA), followed by Dunett's posthoc test for multiple comparism. Values were considered statistically significant at $p<0.05$ (confidence level = 95%).

3. Results

3.1. Phytochemical constituents of ethanolic extract of *Acacia ataxacantha* bark

Table 1 shows the phytochemical constituents of ethanolic extract of *Acacia ataxacantha* bark. In the analysis carried out, alkaloids, polyphenols, flavonoids, saponins, tannins, terpernoids were present while glycoside was not detected.

3.2. Glycemic effects of ethanolic extract of *Acacia ataxacantha* bark in streptozotocin-induced diabetic rats

Figure 3 presents the glycemic effects of ethanolic extract of *Acacia ataxacantha* bark in streptozotocin-induced diabetic rats. There was continuous increase in the fasting blood glucose level of diabetic control rats from the first day of treatment till the sixth day. While, upon oral administration of ethanolic extract of *Acacia ataxacantha* bark, there was a significant reduction ($p<0.05$) in the fasting blood glucose level, of rats administered 125 mg/kg body weight of the extract, decline in the fasting blood glucose concentration began on day 3 and continued till day 6. Whereas, continuous reduction was recorded for fasting blood glucose concentration from day 2 upon oral administration of 250 mg/kg and 500 mg/kg body weight of the extract and standard drug (metformin).

3.3. Effects of ethanolic extract of *Acacia ataxacantha* bark on hepatic glucose and glycogen concentration

Figures 4 and 5 depict the effects of ethanolic extract of *Acacia ataxacantha* bark on the hepatic glucose and glycogen levels of STZ – induced diabetic rats. There was a significant difference ($p>0.05$) in the hepatic glucose and glycogen levels in all the treatment groups compared to the normal control. However, highest hepatic glucose and least glycogen concentrations were recorded in the diabetic control when compared to the control.

Phytochemicals	Extract
Alkaloids	+
Polyphenols	+
Flavonoids	+
Saponin	+
Glycoside	_
Tannins	+
Terpenoid	+

Keys: Presence of constituents (+); Absence of constituents (-)

Table 1. Phytochemical screening of ethanolic extract of *Acacia ataxacantha* bark

http://dx.doi.org/10.5772/57151

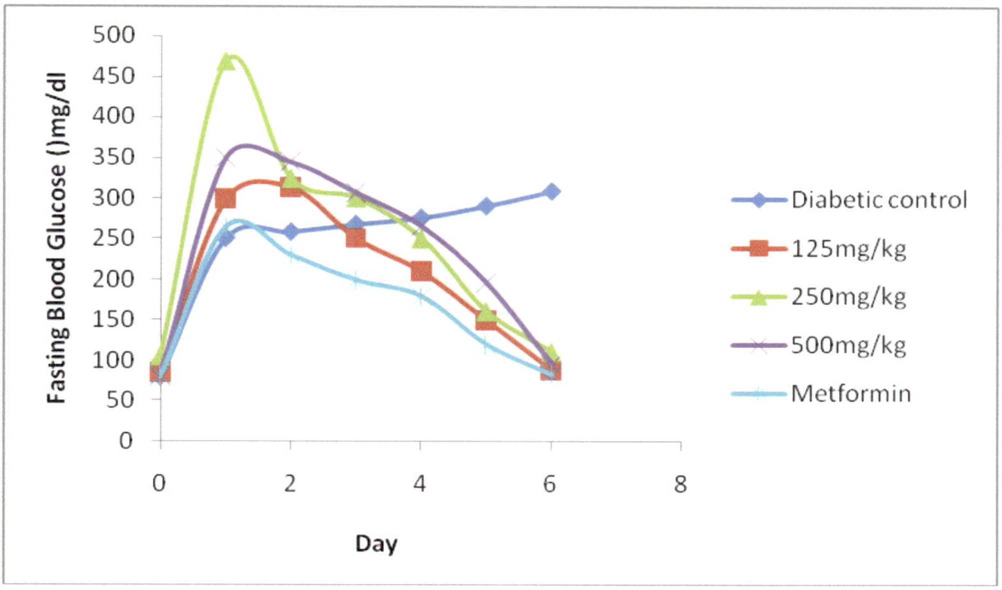

Figure 3. Effects of ethanolic extract of *Acacia ataxacantha* bark on the fasting blood level of STZ-induced diabetic rats

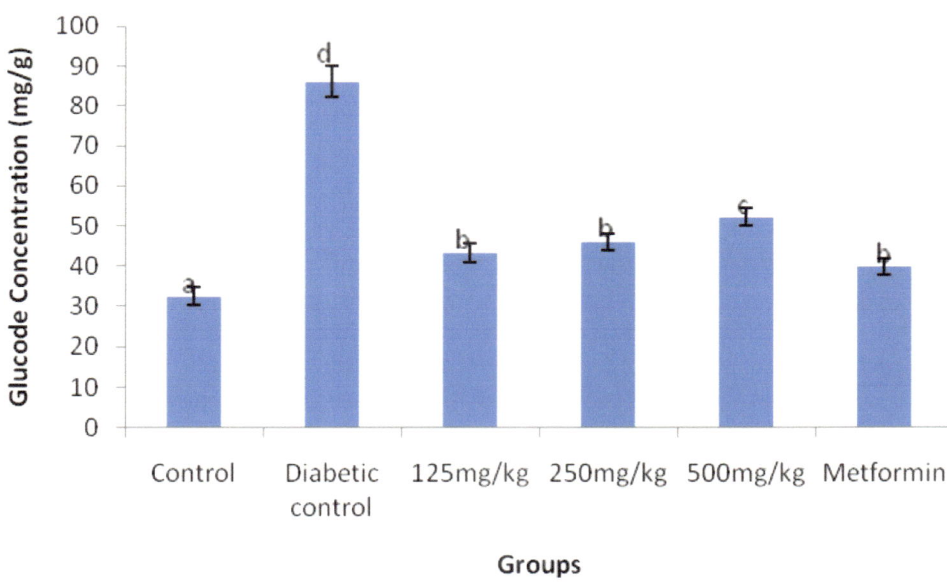

Values are means (n=6) ± S.D (bars with different superscripts are significantly different at $p<0.05$).

Figure 4. Effects of ethanolic extract of *Acacia ataxacantha* bark on the hepatic glucose concentration of STZ-induced diabetic rats

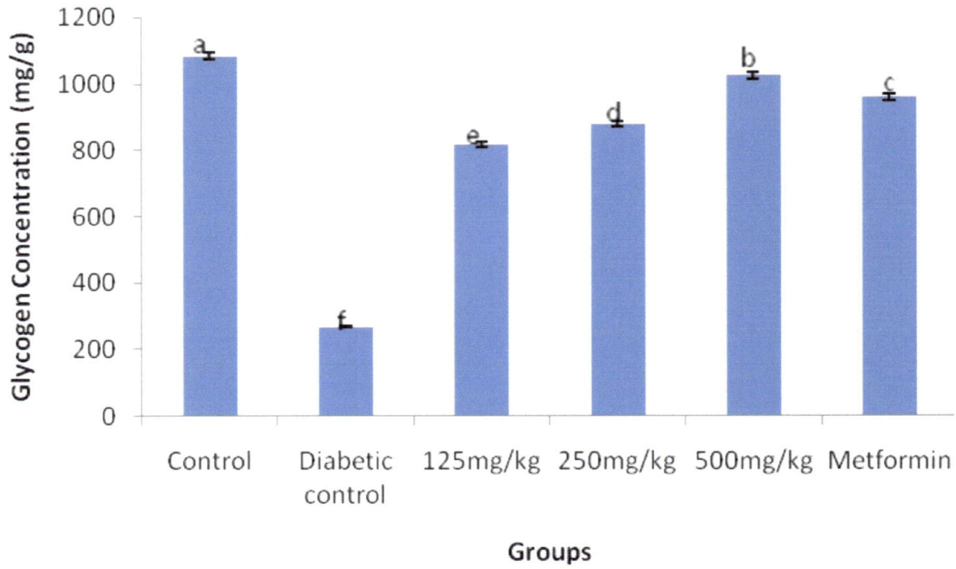

Values are means (n=6) ± S.D (bars with different superscripts are significantly different at $p<0.05$).

Figure 5. Effects of ethanolic extract of *Acacia ataxacantha* bark on the hepatic glycogen concentration of STZ-induced diabetic rats

3.4. Effect of administration of ethanolic extract of *Acacia ataxacantha* bark on serum parameters of streptozotocin-induced diabetic rats

The influence of administration of ethanolic extract of *Acacia ataxacantha* bark on serum parameters is shown in Table 2. There was a significant difference ($p<0.05$) in the urea level in all the treatment groups when compared to the control except that 250 mg/kg body weight and metformin displayed a similar pattern to the control. Also, there was no significant difference ($p>0.05$) in the creatinine level in all the treatment groups when compared to the control but a significant increase ($p<0.05$) was observed in diabetic control compared to the normal control. There were significant differences ($p<0.05$) in albumin level of all groups compared to the control except that 250 mg/kg b.w and metformin were similar in pattern to the control.

3.5. Effect of administration of ethanolic extract of *Acacia ataxacantha* bark on the lipids profile of streptozotocin-induced diabetic rats

Figure 6 shows the effect of ethanolic extract of *Acacia ataxacantha* bark on serum total cholesterol (TC), high density lipoprotein cholesterol (HDL-C), low density lipoprotein cholesterol (LDL-C) and triglyceride. The serum total cholesterol (TC), low density lipoprotein cholesterol (LDL-C) and triglyceride concentrations were significantly reduced ($p<0.05$) upon administration of ethanolic extract of *Acacia ataxacantha* bark and metformin.

Parameters	Control	Diabetic control	125mg/kg	250mg/kg	500mg/kg	Metformin
Urea	29.67±0.3[a]	40.23±0.10[c]	23.49±1.19[b]	29.82±0.59[a]	21.04±1.22[b]	30.29±0.5[a]
Creatinine	0.47±0.14[a]	0.57±0.12[b]	0.48±0.15[a]	0.48±0.01[a]	0.50±0.13[a]	0.49±0.10[a]
Albumin	18.67±0.33[a]	27.01±0.61[c]	22.00±1.15[b]	21.33±0.33[c]	25.33±0.88[c]	20.00±1.2[ab]

Values are expressed as mean of six determinations ± SEM

Row values with different superscripts are significantly (p<0.05) different

Table 2. Effects of ethanolic extract of *Acacia ataxacantha* bark on the concentration of some serum parameters of STZ-induced diabetic rats

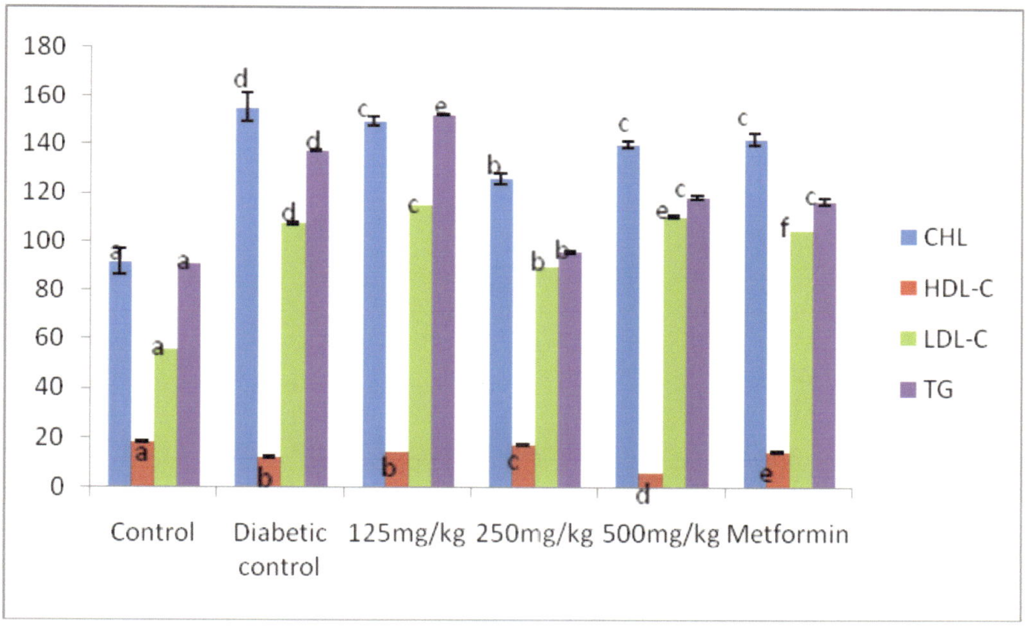

Values are means (n=6) ± S.D (bars with different superscripts are significantly different at p<0.05).

Figure 6. Effects of ethanolic extract of *Acacia ataxacantha* bark on the serum lipid profile of STZ-induced diabetic rats

Figure 7 shows the effect of administration of ethanolic extract of *Acacia ataxacantha* bark on the total bilirubin and conjugated bilirubin level in streptozotocin induced diabetic rats. Both total biliribin and conjugated bilirubin were significantly higher (p<0.05) in diabetic untreated compared to the control, but it was significantly decreased (p<0.05) upon administration of ethanolic extract of *Acacia ataxacantha* bark and metformin.

3.6. Effect of the administration of ethanolic extract of *Acacia ataxacantha* bark on aspartate and alanine aminotransferase activities in streptozotocin induced diabetic rats

Tables 3 and 4 show the effect of administration of ethanolic extract of *Acacia ataxacantha* bark on alanine and aspartate aminotransferase activities in the liver and serum respectively. There was a significant reduction ($p<0.05$) in the activity of ALT in the groups administered 500mg/kg b.w when compared to the control while there was no significant difference in the remaining treatment groups. However, in the serum, there was no significant difference ($p>0.05$) in ALT activity except in the groups administered 500mg/kg b.w and metformin when compared to the normal control. There were significant alterations ($p<0.05$) in the activity of AST in the liver of all the groups compared to the normal control. However, significant elevations ($p<0.05$) were observed in the activity of AST in the serum of all treatment groups when compared to the control.

3.7. Effects of ethanolic extract of *Acacia ataxacantha* bark on pancreatic lipid peroxidation of streptozotocin-induced diabetic rats

Figure 8 depicts the effects of ethanolic extract of *Acacia ataxacantha* bark on the pancreatic lipid peroxidation in STZ - induced diabetic rats. There were no significant differences ($p>0.05$) in malondialdehyde concentration in the pancreas of rats administered 125mg/kg body weight and metformin when compared to the control. However, there was a significant elevation ($p<0.05$) in the concentration of thiobarbituric acid (TBA) reacting substance in the pancreas of rats administered 250 mg/kg b.w, 500 mg/kg b.w and diabetic but not treated rats when compared to the normal control.

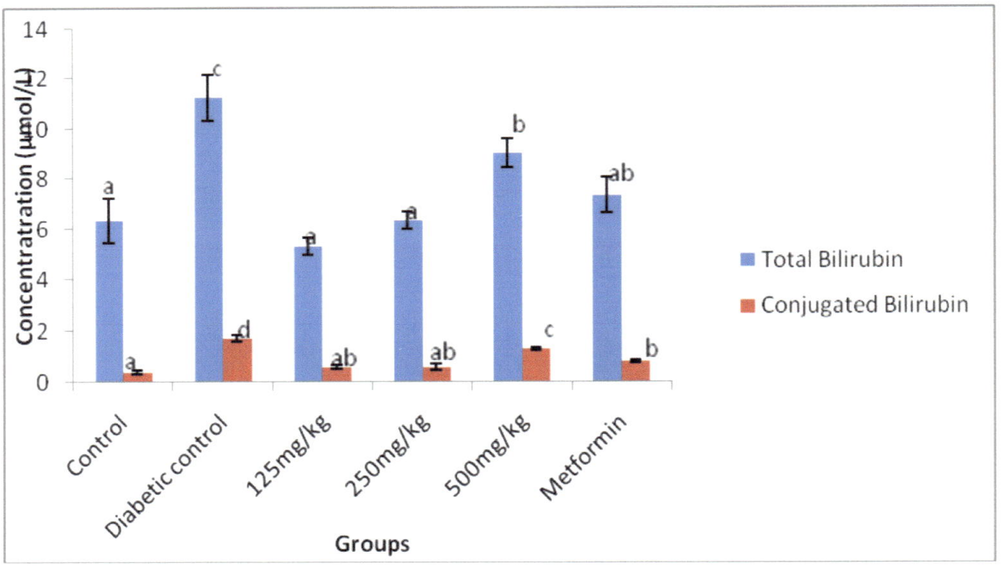

Values are means ($n=6$) ± S.D (bars with different superscripts are significantly different at $p<0.05$).

Figure 7. Effects of ethanolic extract of *Acacia ataxacantha* bark on the bilirubin levels of STZ-induced diabetic rats

Parameters	Control	Diabetic control	125mg/kg	250mg/kg	500mg/kg	Metformin
Liver	0.48±0.00[a]	0.14±0.00[b]	0.45±0.01[a]	0.46±0.00[a]	0.14±0.00[b]	0.57±0.00[a]
Serum	0.15±0.01[a]	0.46±0.00[c]	0.43±0.22[b]	0.17±0.00[a]	0.26±0.00[b]	0.15±0.20[a]

Values are expressed as mean of six determinations ± SEM

Row values with different superscripts are significantly ($p<0.05$) different

Table 3. Effect of the administration of ethanolic extract of *Acacia ataxacantha* bark on the alanine aminotransferase activities in streptozotocin-induced diabetic rats

Parameters	Control	Diabetic control	125mg/kg	250mg/kg	500mg/kg	Metformin
Liver	0.36±0.03[a]	0.14±0.00[b]	0.68±0.00[c]	0.67±0.01[c]	0.13±0.02[b]	0.65±0.01[c]
Serum	0.24±0.08[a]	0.72±0.01[d]	0.48±0.00[b]	0.62±0.00[c]	0.60±0.01[c]	0.52±0.01[b]

Values are expressed as mean of six determinations ± SEM

Row values with different superscripts are significantly ($p<0.05$) different.

Table 4. Effect of the administration of ethanolic extract of *Acacia ataxacantha* bark on aspartate aminotransferase activity in streptozotocin-induced diabetic rats

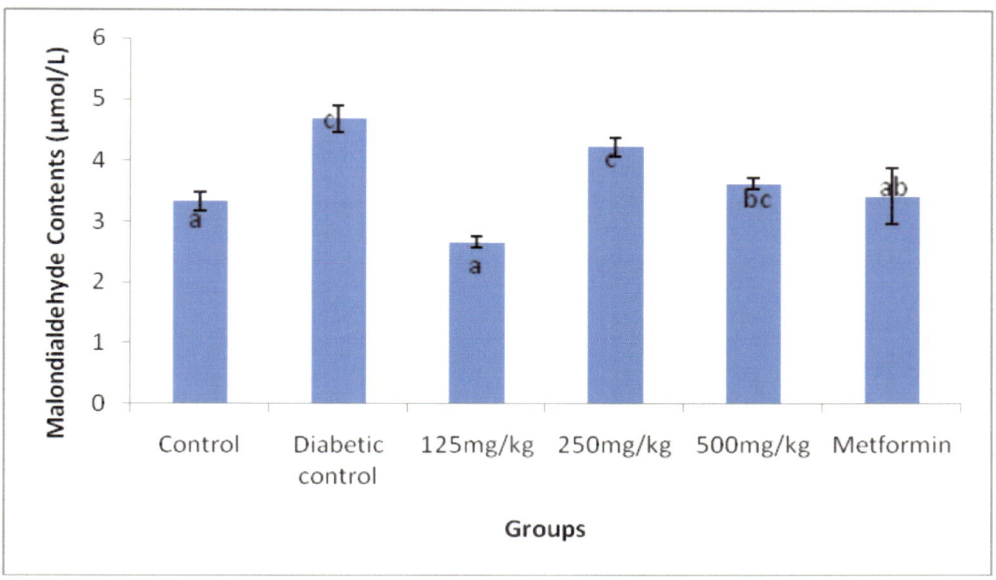

Values are means (n=6) ± S.D (bars with different superscripts are significantly different at $p<0.05$)

Figure 8. Effects of ethanolic extract of *Acacia ataxacantha* bark on the lipid peroxidation in STZ-induced diabetic rats

3.8. Effects of ethanolic extract of *Acacia ataxacantha* bark on pancreatic superoxide dismutase activities of streptozotocin-induced diabetic rats

Figure 9 shows the effects of ethanolic extract of *Acacia ataxacantha* bark on the activity of pancreatic superoxide dismutase. There were significant alterations ($p<0.05$) in the superoxide dismutase activity in the pancreas of all the tretment groups except the groups administered 500 mg/kg b.w of the extract and metformin, which compared favourably with the control.

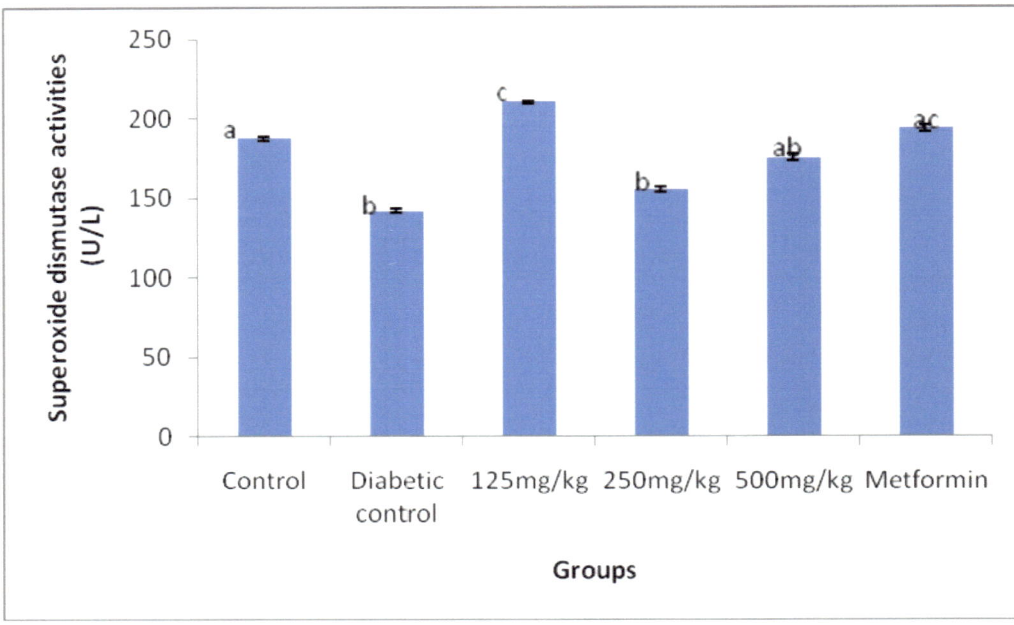

Values are means (n=6) ± S.D (bars with different superscripts are significantly different at $p<0.05$).

Figure 9. Effects of ethanolic extract of *Acacia ataxacantha* bark on the superoxide dismutase activity of STZ-induced diabetic rats

4. Discussion

Diabetes mellitus is a metabolic disorder that has arguably achieved epidemic proportions. It is known to affect more than 371 million persons globally, and is projected to affect 522 million people by the year 2030 [1, 2 and 11]. Phytotherapy for some decades has played an important role in the management of the disease especially in resource-poor countries. Clearly, the identification of plant materials that can manage diabetes and its complications would save millions of people, especially in developing countries, from untimely death.

The presence of secondary metabolites such as alkaloids, polyphenols, flavonoid, saponins, tannins, and terpenoid in the ethanolic extract of *Acacia ataxacantha* bark may contribute to its hypoglyceamic activity and medicinal value. These compounds have been shown to be responsible for hypoglyceamic activity in *Momordica charantia* [37]. The activities of flavonoids and polyphenol have been ascribed to the structural relationship between different parts of their chemical structures [38].

STZ is a broad spectrum antibiotic extracted from *Streptomyces acromogenes*. The STZ-induced diabetes causes the destruction of pancreatic β cells of islets, which leads to a reduction of insulin release and increase in blood glucose. STZ – induced diabetes has been described as a useful experimental model to study the antidiabetic activity of several agents [39]. STZ is well known for its selective pancreatic islet β-cell cytotoxicity used to induce diabetes mellitus in animals. It interferes with cellular metabolic oxidative mechanisms [39]. Significant elevation was observed in fasting blood glucose in diabetic rats. This observed hyperglycemia may be due to induced gluconeogenesis in the absence of insulin [40]. However, marked reductions observed after 2 days and the progressive decrease till the 6th day which was highest in 125 mg/kg and 250 mg/kg b.w of the extract compared well with the standard drug (metformin). These decreases could be due to the direct stimulation of the secretion of insulin thus promoting glucose uptake metabolism by inhibiting hepatic gluconeogenesis through the stimulation of a regeneration process and revitalization of the remaining beta cells [41].

The increased levels of hepatic glucose in streptozotocin - induced diabetic rats were reduced following the administration of ethanolic extract of *Acacia ataxacantha* bark. The reduced glucose levels suggests that ethanolic extract of *Acacia ataxacantha* bark may have exerted insulin-like effect on peripheral tissues by either promoting glucose uptake metabolism by inhibiting hepatic gluconeogenesis [42] or by absorption of glucose into the muscle and adipose tissues [43] through the stimulation of a regeneration process and revitalization of the remaining beta cells [42,43].

Glycogen is the primary intracellular storable form of glucose in various tissues and its level in such tissues especially the liver is a direct reflection of insulin activity [44]. The glycogen content was decreased in the liver of diabetic rats in this study. But upon oral administration of ethanolic extract of *Acacia ataxacantha* bark, glycogen content were increased significantly which is comparable to that of metformin, thus confirming its insulin potentiating action to a marked extent. This may be due to the activation of glycogen synthase system and inhibition of glycogen phosphorylase [45] by the extract. It may also be due to decreased enzymatic activities of hexokinase and phosphofructokinase resulting in depletion of liver and muscle glycogen [46].

The concentrations of total protein, bilirubin and albumin may indicate state of the liver and type of damage [47]. Bilirubin is formed by the breakdown of hemoglobin in the liver, spleen and bone marrow [48]. An increase in tissue or serum albumin concentrations results in jaundice. Jaundice occurs in toxic or infectious diseases of the liver [49]. The significant increase in the total bilirubin, conjugated bilirubin and albumin levels in the diabetic control rats and reduction following oral administration of ethanolic extract of *Acacia ataxacantha* bark are indicative of amelioration of the adverse effects caused by diabetes.

The kidneys remove metabolic wastes such as urea, uric acid, creatinine and ions and thus optimum chemical composition of body fluids is maintained. The concentrations of these metabolites increase in blood during renal diseases or renal damage associated with uncontrolled diabetes mellitus. Blood urea and creatinine are considered as significant markers of renal dysfunction [50]. Observed increase in urea and creatinine level in the diabetic control were reduced following the administration of ethanolic extract of *Acacia ataxacantha* bark to a level close to the value obtained for the normal control. Due to continuous catabolism of amino acid during diabetic state, high quantity of urea will be formed from urea cycle. On the other hand, it may be as a result of repression of glycolytic enzymes, thus glucose is channeled into pentose phosphate pathway resulting in the increased availability of ribose-5-phosphate which may lead to increased formation of phosphoribosyl pyrophosphate (PRPP) and ultimately resulting in high concentration of uric acid in the blood [51].

Lipids play a vital role in the pathogenesis of diabetic mellitus. Diabetic is associated with profound alterations in the plasma lipid, triglycerides and lipoprotein profile and with an increased risk of coronary heart disease [52]. The most common lipid abnormalities in diabetes are hypertriglyceridemia and hypercholesterolemia. The increase in the levels of serum lipids such as cholesterol and triglycerides in the diabetic rats may be due to the fact that under normal circumstances, insulin activates lipoprotein lipase and hydrolyses triglycerides. Insulin increases uptake of fatty acids into adipose tissue and increases triglyceride synthesis. Moreover, insulin inhibits lipolysis. In case of insulin deficiency, lipolysis is not inhibited but an increased lipolysis which finally leads to hyperlipidemia. In diabetic condition, the concentration of serum free acids is elevated as a result of free fatty acid outflow from fat deposited, where the balance of the free fatty acid esterification-triglyceride lipolysis cycle is displaced in favour of lipolysis [53].

HDL is an anti-atherogenic lipoprotein. It transports cholesterol from peripheral tissues into the liver and thereby acts as a protective factor against coronary heart disease. The level of HDL-cholesterol slightly increased after administration of ethanolic extract of *Acacia ataxacantha* bark at 250 mg/kg and 500 mg/kg b.w. This might be due to increase in the activity of lecithin cholesterol acyl transferase (LCAT), which may contribute to the regulation of blood lipids [54]. Administration of ethanolic extract of *Acacia ataxacantha* bark lowered cholesterol level at all doses while 250 mg/kg and 500 mg/kg b.w were able to reduce triglycerides and LDL-cholesterol levels. Significant lowering of total cholesterol, triglycerides, LDL-cholesterol and rise in HDL-cholesterol is a very desirable biochemical state for prevention of atherosclerosis and ischaemic conditions [55].

Liver is the vital organ of metabolism, detoxification, storage and excretion of xenobiotic and their metabolites [56]. Aspartate aminotransferase, alanine aminotransferase, albumin and bilirubin are considered as part of liver toxicity markers [57]. In streptozotocin-induced diabetic animals, change in the serum enzymes is directly related to change in the metabolic functions of aspartate aminotransferase, alanine aminotransferase, albumin and bilirubin [58, 59]. It has been reported that the increased aminotransferase activities under insulin deficiency [60] were responsible for the increased gluconeogenesis and ketogenesis during diabetic. Aspartate aminotransferase is an enzyme found mainly in the cell of the liver, heart, skeletal muscles, kidney, and pancreas and to a lesser amount in red blood cells. Its serum concentration is proportional to the amount of cellular leakage or damage and it is released into the serum in larger quantities when any one of these tissues is damaged and its increase is usually associated with heart attack or liver disease. While on the other hand, alanine aminotransferase is an enzyme found mainly in the liver and elevated levels in serum usually indicates liver damage [61]. The mechanism by which the serum aspartate and alanine aminotransferases are raised in diabetic untreated may involve increased liberation of these enzymes from tissues (mainly liver), owing to oxidative stress or the formation of advanced glycosylation end product [57]. The increase in the activities of these enzymes in serum of diabetic control might be induced due to liver dysfunction. Ohaeri [62] reported that liver was necrotized in STZ-induced diabetic rats. Therefore an increase in the activities of ALT and AST in the serum might be mainly due to the leakage of these enzymes from the liver cytosol into the blood stream [63] which gives an indication of hepatotoxic effect of STZ. Reduction in the activities of ALT and AST in the serum might consequently be due to alleviation of liver damage caused by STZ–induced diabetic mellitus [64], while 500mg/kg body weight might be toxic.

Malondialdehyde is used as a biomarker to measure level of oxidative stress in an organism [65]. Malondialdehyde participate in a variety of chemical and biological reactions including covalent binding to protein, RNA, and DNA. The significant increase ($p<0.05$) in pancreatic malondialdehyde concentration in the diabetic but treated groups was reduced upon oral administration of the ethanolic extract of *Acacia ataxacantha* bark. These may be due to the presence of antioxidant phytochemicals in the extract which reduced the oxidative stress that caused lipid peroxidation thereby reducing the generation of free radicals and thus may have prevented the damage of cellular organelles either by decreasing localized oxygen concentration, presenting first chain initiation by scavenging initial radicals and binding metals or by decomposing peroxide. Antioxidant enzymes have been shown to play important role in maintaining physiological levels of oxygen and hydrogen peroxide by hastening the dismutation of oxygen radicals and eliminating organic peroxide and hydro-peroxides generated from inadvertent exposure to STZ [66]. In the enzymatic antioxidant defense system, SOD is one of the important enzymes that scavenge the superoxide radicals by converting them to hydrogen peroxides and molecular oxygen [67]. The observed decrease in the pancreatic SOD activity in diabetic control rats could result from inactivation by H_2O_2 or by glycosylation of the enzymes, which has been reported to occur in diabetes [68, 69]. However, the increased SOD activity following oral administration of ethanolic extract of *Acacia ataxacantha* bark might be due to presence of antioxidant phytochemicals which scavenge the superoxide radical by converting them to hydrogen peroxides and molecular oxygen [67].

5. Conlusion

Overall, it may be concluded that ethanolic extract of *Acacia ataxacantha bark* at 125 mg/kg b.w exhibited promising antidiabetic activity in streptozotocin-induced diabetic rats. Thus, the antihyperglyceamic and anti-dyslipidemic activity of ethanolic extract of *Acacia ataxacantha* bark could represent a protective mechanism against the development of atherosclerosis, especially in diabetic condition and may prove to be of clinical importance in the management of type 2 diabetes. However, this may not be safe at higher doses.

Author details

Rotimi O. Arise[1*], Aderounmu I. Ganiyu[1] and Oluwafemi O. Oguntibeju[2]

*Address all correspondence to: arisedshine@yahoo.com

1 Department of Biochemistry, Faculty of Science, University of Ilorin, Ilorin, Nigeria

2 Department of Biomedical Sciences, Faculty of Health & Wellness Sciences, Cape Peninsula University of Technology, South Africa

References

[1] Basu, S., Yoffe, P., Hills, N and Lustig, R.H (2013). The Relationship of Sugar to Population- Level Diabetes Prevalence: An Econometric Analysis of Repeated Cross-Sectional Data. *PLoS ONE* 8(2): e57873.

[2] Oputa, R.N and Chinenye, S. (2012). Diabetes mellitus: A global epidemic with potential solution. *African Journal of Diabetes Medicine* 20(2); 33-35.

[3] Wild, S.G., Roglie, A., Green, R., Sicree, E., King, H. (2004). Global prevalence of diabetes. Estimates for the year 2000 and projections for 2030. *Diabet. Care*, 27: 1047-1054

[4] Barcelo, A and Rajpathak, S. (2001). Incidence and prevalence of diabetes mellitus in the Americas. *American Journal of Public Health,* 10: 300-308

[5] Pari, L and Venkateswaran, S. (2003). Effect of an aqueous extract of *Phaseolus vulgaris* on the properties of tail tendon collagen of rats with streptozotocin-induced diabetes. *Brazilian Journal of Medical and Biological Research,* 36: 861-870

[6] Worthley, L.I.G. (2003).*The Australian short course on intensive care medicine,* Handbook, Gillingham printers, South Australia, PP 31-55

[7] Sowka, J. W., Gurwood, A. S. and Kabat, A. G. (2001). Handbook of ocular disease management diabetes mellitus. (http://www.revoptom.com/HANDBOOK/sect59a.htm)

[8] Holt, R. I. G. (2004). Diagnosis, epidemiology and pathogenesis of diabetes mellitus: an update for psychiatrists. *British journal of Psychiatry,* 184 (suppl.4 7), s 55- s 63

[9] Tiwari, A. K. and Rao, J. M. (2002). Diabetes mellitus and multiple therapeutic approaches of phytochemicals: Present status and future prospects. *Current Science,* 83: 30-38

[10] Trachtenbarg, D. E. (2005). Diabetic ketoacidosis. *American Family Physician,* 71: 1705-1714

[11] International Diabetes Federation (2011). *Diabetes Atlas: 5th Edition.*

[12] Grover, J.K., Yadar, S. and Vats, V. (2002). Medicinal plants of India with anti-diabetic potential *J. Ethnopharmacol.* ; 81: 81-100.

[13] Rang H.P. and Dale M.M., (1991).The Endocrine System Pharmacology, (Longman, Harlow) 504.

[14] Bastaki, S. (2005). Diabetes mellitus and its treatment. *Int. J. Diabetes and Metabolism.* 13: 111-134.

[15] Kofi, N., Edouard, K.K and Kouassi, K (2009). Ethnobotanical Study of Plants Used to Treat Diabetes, in Traditional Medicine, by Abbey and Krobou People of Agboville (Côte- d'Ivoire) *Am. J. Sci. Res.* 4: 45-58.

[16] Oyedemi, S.O, Yakubu, M.T and Afolayan, A.J. (2011). Antidiabetic activities of aqueous leaves extract of *Leonotis leonurus* in streptozotocin induced diabetic Rats. *Journal of Medicinal Plants Research,* 5(1):119-125.

[17] Pari, L. and Uma Maheswari, J. (2000). Antihyperglycemic activity of *Musa sapientum* flowers. Effects on lipid peroxidation in alloxan diabetic rats. *J. Ethnopharmacol.,* 14, 1-3

[18] Grover, J.K., Yadav, S. and Vats V. (2002). Medicinal plants of Indian with antidiabetic potential. *J. Ethnopharmacol.,* 81, 81-100.

[19] Davidson, L and Jeppe, B (1981). Acacias: A field guide to the Acacias of southern Africa. 1st ed. Johannesburg: Centaur, Johannesburg.

[20] Derelanko M.J. Guiding Principles in the use of Animals in Toxicology In: Toxicologist's pocket handbook. CRC Press Boca Raton, London.2000; pp 1-7.

[21] Majekodunmi OF, Zany I, Ohanyaga IE, Shi LE, Mclanghin JL, (1996).Selective cytotoxic diterpene from Euphorbia poisonic. *J. Med.Chem.,* 39: 1005-1008

[22] Sekar N, Kanthasamy S, William S, Subramanian S, Govindasamy S. Insulinic actions of vanadate in diabetic rats. *Pharmacol Res* 1990; 22:207-17.

[23] Ogbu SI, Okechukwu EI (2001). The effect of storage temperature prior to separation on plasma and serum potassium. *J.Med. Lab. Sci.,* 10:1-4.

[24] Ngaha EO, Akanji MA, Madusolomo MA (1989). Studies on correlation between chloroquine-induced tissue damage and serum changes in rats. *Experimentia,* 45: 143.

[25] Barham, D. and P. Trinder, (1972). An improved colour reagent for the determination of blood glucose by the oxidase system. *The Analyst*, 97:142-145.

[26] Passonneau J. V. and Lauderdale V. R. (1974) A comparison of three methods of glycogen measurement in tissues. *Anal. Biochem.* 60, 405–412

[27] Reitman, S. and Frankel, S. (1957). A colourimetric method for determination of serum glutamate-oxaloacetate and pyruvate transaminase. Am. J. Clinpath. 28:56-59. *Research Service, 25-30.*

[28] Zlakis, A., B. Zak and A.Boyle, (1953). A new method for the direct determination of serum cholesterol. *J Lab. Clin. Medic.*, 4: 486-492.

[29] Foster C.S, Dunn O (1973). Stable reagents for determination of serum triglycerides by a colorimetric Hantzsch condensation method. *Clin Chim Acta*, 19, 338–340.

[30] Burstein, M., Scholnick, H. R. and Morfin, R. (1970) Rapid method for the isolation of lipoproteins from human serum by precipitation with polyanions. *J. Lipid Res.* 11, 583-595.

[31] Friedewald, W.T., Levi, R.I., Fredrickson, D.S. (1972). Estimation of the Concentration of Low-Density Lipoprotein Cholesterol in Plasma, Without Use of the Preparative Ultracentrifuge *Clin. Chem.*, 18: 499.

[32] Doumas, B.T., Watson, W.A., Biggs, H.G. (1971). Albumin standards and measurement of serum albumin with bromocresol green. *Clin. Chim. Acta.* 31: 87-92.

[33] Sherlock, S. (1951). In Liver Disease. Chuchill London. p. 204.

[34] Tietz, N.W., Prude, E.L. and Sirgard- Anderson, O (1994). Tietz Textbook of clinical chemistry. 2nd edition,W.B. Saunders Company, London, pp. 1354-1374.

[35] Misra, H.P. and Fridovich, I. (1972). The role of superoxide anion in the autooxidation of epinephrine and a simple assay for superoxide dismutase. J Biol chem. 247: 3170-3175.

[36] Varshey, R., Kale, R.K. (1990). Effect of calmodulin antagonist on radiation induced lipid peroxidation in microsome. *Int. J. Rad. Biol. 58, 733–743.*

[37] Akhtar, M.S., Athar, M.A and Yaqub, M. (1981). Effect of Momordica charantia on blood glucose level of normal and alloxan-diabetic rabbits. *Planta Med.*, 42: 205-212.

[38] Rice-Evans, C., Miller, N.J and Paganga, G. (1996). Structure-antioxidant activity relationship of flavonoids and phenolic acids. *Free Radical Biology and Medicine*, 20:933-956.

[39] Papaccio, G., Eposito, V., Latronico, M.V and Pisanti, F.A.(1995). Administration of a nitric oxide synthase inhibitor does not suppress low-dose streptozotocin-induced diabetes in mice. *Int.J. Pancreatol.* 17:63-68.

[40] Gao Z, Hwang D, Bataille F, Lefevre M, York D, Quon MJ, Ye J. 2002. Serine phosphorylation of insulin receptor substrate 1 by inhibitor kappa B kinase complex. *J. Biol. Chem.* 277: 48115-48121.

[41] Rokeya, B. (1993): Studies on the hypoglycemic effects of fruits pulp, seed and whole plant of *Momordica charantia* on normal and diabetic model rats, *Planta Med.* 59: 408-412.

[42] Ali, L., Azad Khan, A. K., Mamun, M.I.R., Mosihuzzaman, M., Nahar, N., Alan, M.N.E. Anderson, O.M. and Markham, K.R. (2006). Flavonoids: Chemistry, Biochemistry and Applications. CRC Press.

[43] Kamanyi, A., Dajmen, D. and Nkeh, B. (1994): Hypoglycemic properties of the aqueous root extract of *Morinda lucida* (Rubiacea) study in the mouse, *Phytoter Res.* 8: 369-371.

[44] Sharma, A.K. (1993). Diabetes mellitus and its complications: An update, 1ed. Macmillan India Ltd, New Delhi: Sharma AK (ed), pp 92- 205.

[45] Bansal, R., Ahmad, N and Kidwai, J.R. (1981). Effect of oral administration of *Eugenia jambolana* seeds and chloropropamide on blood glucose level and pancreatic cathepsin B in rats, *Indian J. Biochem. Biophys.* 18: 377-381.

[46] Grover, J.K., Vats, V. and Rathi, S.S. (2000). Antihyperglycemic effect of *Eugenia jambolana* and *Tinospora cordifolia* in experimental diabetes and their effects on key metabolic enzymes involved in carbohydrate metabolism. *J. Ethnopharmacol.* 73: 461-470.

[47] Yakubu, M.T., Akanji, M.A. and Oladiji, A.T. (2005). Aphrodisiac potentials of the aqueous extract of *Fadogia agrestis* (Schweinf. Ex Heirn) stem in male albino rats. *Asian J. Androl.* 7: 399-404.

[48] Vasudevan, D.M. and S. Sreekumari, (2005). Textbook of Biochemistry (For Medical Students). 4th Edn., Jaypee Brothers Medical Publishers (P) Ltd., New Delhi, India, pp: 502-503.

[49] Edem, D.O. and Usoh, I.F. (2009). Biochemical Changes in Wistar Rats on Oral Doses of Mistletoe (*Loranthus micranthus*). *American Journal of Pharmacology and Toxicology*, 4 (3):94-97.

[50] Almdal, T.P, Vilstrup, H. (1988). Strict insulin treat-ment normalizes the organic nitrogen contents and the capacity of urea–N synthesis in experimental diabetes in rats. *Diabetologia*; 31:114-118.

[51] Lal, S.S., Sukla, Y., Singh, U. (1991). Treating insulin resistance in hypertension with metformin reduces both blood pressure and metabolic risk factors. *J. Intern. Med.* 229:181-187.

[52] Maghrain, M. Lemhadri, A., Zeggwagh, N. A., El-Amraoui, M., Haloui, M., Jouad, H. and Eddouks, M. (2004): Effects of an aqueos extract of Triticum repens on lipid metabolism in normal and recent-onset diabetic rats. *J. Ethnopharmacol.* 90:331-336.

[53] Sirwalkar, A., Rajendran, K., Kumar, C.D. and Bodla, R. (2004): Antidiabetic activities of aqueous leaf extract of Annona squamosa in streptozotocin-nicotonamide type 2 diabetic rats. *J. Ethnopharmacol.* 91: 171-175.

[54] Patil, U. K., Saraf, S. and Dixit, V.K. (2004): Hypolipidemic activity of seeds of *Cassia tora* Linn. *J. Ethnopharmacol.* 90:249-252.

[55] Luc, G. and Fruchart, J.C. (1991): Oxidation of lipoproteins and atherosclerosis. *American Journal of Clinial Nutrition* 53: 2065-2095.

[56] Rej, R. (1978): Aspartate aminotransferase activity and isoenzymes proportions in human liver tissues, *Clin. Chem.* 24 (11): 1971-1979.

[57] Mori, d. M., Baviera, A.M., Ramallo, L.T.D.O., Vendramini, R.C., Brunetti, I. L. and Pepato, M.T. (2003): Temporal response pattern of biochemical analytes in experimental diabetes, *Biotechnol. Appl. Biochem.* 38, 183-191.

[58] Asayama, K., Nakane, T., Uchida, N., Hayashihe, H., Dobashi, K., Nakazawa, S. (1994); Serum antioxidant status in streptozotocin-induced diabetic rat. *Horm. Metab. Res.* 26: 313- 315.

[59] Junad, A., Lambery, a. e., Orci, L., Pictet, R., Gonet, A.E. and Ronald, A.E. (1967): Studies of diabetogenic action of streptozotocin. *Proc. Soc. Exp. Biol. Med.* 126:201-205.

[60] Fleig, P., Marliss, E., Ohman, J. and Cahill, J. F. (1970): Plasma amino acid levels in diabetic keto *acidosis*. Diabetes 19: 727-729.

[61] Kesari, A.N., Kesari, S., Singh, S. K., Gupta, R.K. and Watal, G. (2007): Studies on the glycemic and lipidemic effect of *Murraya koenigii* in experimental animals. *J. Ethnopharmacol.* 112:305-311.

[62] Ohaeri, O.C. (2001): Effect of garlic oil on the levels of various enzymes in the serum and tissue of streptozotocin diabetic rats, *Biosci. Rep.* 21:19-24.

[63] Navarro, C.M., Montilla, P.M., Martin, A., Jimenez, J. and Utrilla, P. M. (1993): Free radical scanvenger and antihepatotoxic activity of Rosmarinus, *Plant Med.* 59:312-314.

[64] El-demerdash, F.M., Yousef, M. I. and Abou El-Naga N. I. (2005): Biochemical study on the hypoglycemic effects of onion and garlic in alloxan-induced diabetic rats, *Food Chem. Toxicol.* 43: 57-63.

[65] Moore, K.L. and Dalley, A.F. (1999). Clinical Oriented Anatomy (4th Edition). Lippincot Williams and Williams; a Woller klumner Corporation, Philadelphia. pp. 263-271.

[66] Pari, L. and Uma Maheswari, J. (2000). Antihyperglycemic activity of *Musa sapientum* flowers. Effects on lipid peroxidation in alloxan diabetic rats. *J. Ethnopharmacol.*, 14, 1-3 67.

[67] Vincent, A.M., Russell, J.W., Low, P. and Feldman, E. L. (2004): Oxidative stress in the pathogenesis of diabetic neuropathy. *Endocr Rev* 25:612-628.

[68] Ravi, K., Ramanchandran, B and Subramanian, S. (2004): Protective effect of *Eugenia jambolana* seed kernel on tissue antioxidants in streptozotocin-induced diabetic rats. *Biol Pharm Bull* 27: 1212-1217.

[69] Soon, Y.Y. and Tan, B.K. (2002): Evaluation of the hypoglycemic and antioxidant activities of *Morinda officinalis* in streptozotocin-induced diabetic rats. *Singapore Med J* 3: 77-85

Chapter 2

Oxidative Stress and Diabetic Complications: The Role of Antioxidant Vitamins and Flavonoids

Omolola R. Ayepola, Nicole L. Brooks and Oluwafemi O. Oguntibeju

Additional information is available at the end of the chapter

http://dx.doi.org/10.5772/57282

1. Introduction

Diabetes mellitus is a group of disorders of multiple aetiologies resulting from a defect in insulin secretion, insulin action, or both. Insulin deficiency in turn leads to chronic hyperglycemia (very high blood glucose levels) with disturbances in carbohydrate, fat and protein metabolism [1]. The two major types of diabetes mellitus (DM) are insulin dependent (IDDM) - type 1 and non -insulin dependent (NIDDM) -type 2. Type 1 DM is characterized by a specific destruction of the pancreatic β cells commonly associated with immune-mediated damage [2]. Individuals with type 2 DM display a gradual change in glucose homeostasis due to insulin resistance and/or decreased insulin secretion [3].

Sustained hyperglycemia leads to the progressive development of long-term microvascular and macrovascular complications which causes morbidity and mortality among those affected [4, 5]. Although glycemic control has long been the mainstay for preventing the progression of diabetic complications, there is far less evidence that these interventions reverse diabetic complications [6]. Also, limitations in intensive glycemic treatment such as difficulty in achieving and/or maintaining tight glycemic control [7], incidence of hypoglycemia and increased mortality [8, 9] suggest an urgent need for alternative and/or complementary therapies to this disorder.

Hyperglycemia-induced oxidative stress is now recognized as the driving force for the development of diabetic complications [10]. Oxidative stress in diabetes results in stimulation of the polyol pathway, formation of advanced glycation end products (AGE), activation of protein kinase C (PKC) and subsequent formation of reactive oxygen radicals [11, 12]. Hyperglycemia, not only generates more reactive oxygen species (ROS), but also attenuates antioxidative mechanisms by scavenging enzymes and substances [13].

2. The complications of diabetes mellitus (DM)

The injurious effects of hyperglycemia are separated into microvascular (involving small vessels such as capillaries) and macrovascular complications (involving large vessels, such as arteries and veins). Microvascular complications include diabetic nephropathy, neuropathy and retinopathy while macrovascular complications include coronary artery disease, peripheral arterial disease and stroke [5].

Diabetic nephropathy is a major cause of end-stage renal disease worldwide. It is a progressive decline in the glomerular filtration rate, characterized by glomerular hyperfiltration, glomerular and tubular epithelial hypertrophy, increased urinary albumin excretion, increased basement membrane thickness and mesangial expansion with the accumulation of extracellular matrix proteins (ECM) [14]. Alteration of the permeability characteristics of the glomerular capillary wall manifests clinically as abnormal albuminuria [15]. Microalbuminuria progresses to end-stage renal disease through a number of stages including normoalbuminuria, microalbuminuria and macroalbuminuria [16].

Diabetic retinopathy results from the damage of the small vasculature of the retina, multi cellular and the light sensitive tissue at the back of the eye. It is a major cause of visual impairment worldwide [17, 18]. The retina capillaries are lined with endothelial cells responsible for maintaining the blood retinal barrier, and are surrounded by smooth muscle cells, pericytes, which provide tone to the vessels [18]. The vascular lesions that are identified at the early stage of diabetic retinopathy include pericytes disappearance from capillaries resulting in pericyte ghosts, obliteration of capillaries and small arterioles, gradual thickening of vascular basement membrane, increased permeability of endothelial cells, and formation of microaneurysms (i.e. weakening of vessel walls that results in the projection of a balloonlike sac), vessel leakage, exudate, and hemorrhage [19, 20].

Neuropathies are characterized by a progressive loss of nerve fiber function. A widely accepted definition of diabetic neuropathy is "the presence of symptoms and/or signs of peripheral nerve dysfunction in people with mellitus after exclusion of other causes" [21]. In the peripheral nervous system, diabetes causes a progressive deterioration of sensory nerves and damage to motor nerves [22]. Diabetic neuropathy is ultimately the leading cause of lower extremity amputation [23]. Peripheral neuropathy is thought to develop because of cellular damage to endothelial cells, affecting nerve blood flow and also damage to the neurons affecting conductivity of impulses [23]. Signs and symptoms of diabetic neuropathy include decrease or no sweating, numbness, or tingling, and some sort of burning sensation, weakness and loss of reflexes [24].

http://dx.doi.org/10.5772/57282

Both type I and type II diabetes are powerful and independent risk factors for coronary artery disease (CAD), stroke, and peripheral arterial disease [25, 26, 27]. Diabetics have a 2- to 4-fold higher risk for cardiovascular events [28] and nearly 80% of diabetes-associated deaths are caused by cardiovascular disease (CVD) [29]. Atherosclerosis, (excessive accumulation of lipids, cholesterol, inflammatory cells, and connective tissue in the vessel wall) accounts for more than 80% of the CVD-associated death and disability [30, 31]. Formation of atherosclerotic plaques can result in occlusion of vessel lumen and a rapid cessation in blood flow to target tissue [32]. Hyperglycemia, increased free fatty acids, and insulin resistance induce a large number of alterations at the cellular level that contribute to vascular dysfunction and accelerate the atherosclerotic process. These include increased oxidative stress, decreased bioavailability of NO, disturbances of intracellular signal transduction and increased production of several prothrombotic factors [32, 33].

3. Role of oxidative stress in diabetic complications

Reactive oxygen species (ROS) and reactive nitrogen species (RNS) are the terms collectively describing free radicals and other non-radical reactive derivatives also called oxidants. Biological free radicals are highly unstable molecules which are products of normal cellular metabolism. They have electrons available to react with various organic substrates such as lipids, proteins and deoxyribonucleic acid (DNA). Free radicals are well recognized for playing a dual role as both deleterious and beneficial species, since they can be either harmful or beneficial to living systems [34]. At low or moderate levels free radicals (ROS and RNS) exerts beneficial effects such as defence against infectious agents, induction of a mitogenic response and the maturation process of cellular structures [35-37]. ROS include superoxide anion ($O_2^{\cdot-}$), hydroxyl ($^{\cdot}OH$), hydrogen peroxide (H_2O_2) and hypochlorous acid (HOCl) while RNS include nitric oxide ($^{\cdot}NO$), nitrogen dioxide ($NO_2^{\cdot-}$) and peroxynitrite ($OONO^-$) [38, 39]. High concentrations of free radicals on the other hand result in deleterious processes that can damage cell structures due to oxidative stress [40, 41].

Free radicals produced under physiological conditions are maintained at steady state levels by endogenous or exogenous antioxidants (externally supplied through foods or supplements) which act as free radical scavengers. However, oxidative stress occurs when the production of free radicals overwhelms the detoxification capacity of cellular antioxidant system causing biological damage [42-44]. The endogenous antioxidants (Table 1) comprise of the enzymatic antioxidants such as superoxide dismutase (SOD), glutathione peroxidase (GPx), glutathione reductase (GR), catalase (CAT), and non-enzymatic antioxidants including glutathione (GSH), α lipoic acid, vitamins C and E [39, 45, 46]. On the other hand, the exogenous antioxidants include micronutrients and other exogenously administered compounds such as vitamin E, vitamin C, trace metals (selenium, manganese, zinc), carotenoids and flavonoids [39, 44, 47].

Antioxidants	Cellular location	Role	Reference
Enzymatic Antioxidants			
(A) Catalase	Peroxisomes	Decomposition of H_2O_2 to water and oxygen	[48]
(B) Glutathione peroxidase	Cytoplasm, mitochondria, and nucleus	Detoxifies H_2O_2 and lipid peroxides with simultaneous oxidation of GSH and generation of GSSG	[49]
(C) Glutathione reductase	Cytoplasm, mitochondria, and nucleus	Recycles Glutathione disulfide back to glutathione using the cofactor NADPH	[50]
(D) Superoxide dismutase	Cytoplasm, nucleus lysosomes, mitochondria	Conversion of superoxide radical to H_2O_2	[51]
Non enzymatic antioxidants			
(A) GSH	Cytoplasm, mitochondria and nucleus	Acts as a cofactor for antioxidant enzymes (GPx, GST), regenerates other antioxidants such as Vitamins C and E to their active forms	[52]
(B) Vitamin-E	Membrane	Directly scavenge singlet oxygen, peroxyl and superoxide radicals , protects against peroxidation of membrane lipids	[34]
(C) Vitamin-C	Cytosol	Acts synergistically with vitamin E to terminate radical inducedlipid peroxidation	[34, 53]
(D) α-Lipoic acid	Cell membrane and cytoplasm	Increases glutathione and vitamin C levels	[54]

Table 1. Role of antioxidants in the protection against free radical damage

Numerous experimental evidences have highlighted a direct link between oxidative stress and diabetes through the measurement of oxidative stress biomarkers in both diabetic patient and rodents. As shown in Table 2, a hyperglycemic state can lead to an increase in the levels of oxidative DNA damage markers such as 8-hydroxy-2'-deoxyguanosine (8-OHdG) and 8-oxo-7, 8-dihydro-2'-deoxyguanosine (8-oxodG); lipid-peroxidation products measured as thiobarbituric acid-reactive substances (TBARS); protein oxidation products such as nitrotyrosine and carbonyl levels and also lower the activity of antioxidant enzymes. Cell culture studies using pancreatic beta cells, aortic smooth muscle cells and endothelial cells have also provided evidence for an increase in ROS production in diabetes [55, 56].

Due to their ability to directly oxidize and damage DNA, proteins, and lipids, free radicals are believed to play a key role in the onset and progression of late-diabetic complications [57]. In the absence of an appropriate condensation by antioxidant defense network, increased oxidative stress leads to activation of stress-sensitive intracellular signaling pathways and the formation of gene products that cause cellular damage and contribute to late diabetic complications [58-61].

http://dx.doi.org/10.5772/57282

	Antioxidants and macromolecules	Evidence of oxidative stress	Target tissue/organ	References
Animals	Enzymatic antioxidants	↓ SOD,CAT,GR, GPX	Liver, Pancreas, Liver, kidney	[62-64]
	Non-enzymatic antioxidant	↓ Vit E and C	Liver, kidney	[64]
		↓ GSH /GSSG,GSH	Kidney, hippocampus. Retina, Heart	[65] [66] [67] [68]
	Lipids	↑ TBARS, lipid peroxides, MDA	Kidney	[69-70]
	DNA	↑ 8-OHdG, 8-OHG	Plasma, Liver, Kidney	[71-72]
	Protein	↑ Nitrotyrosine	kidney Retina	[73] [67]
	Reactive oxygen species	↑ ROS	Hippocampus	[66]
Humans	Enzymatic antioxidants	↑ SOD,CAT, GPX	Erythrocyte	[74]
	Non enzymatic antioxidants	↓ GSH	Erythrocyte	[75]
	Lipid	↑ F2-Isoprostanes ↑ MDA	Urine Erythrocyte	[76] [77]
	DNA	↑ 8-OHdG	Urine	[78-79]
	Protein	↑ Nitrotyrosine Protein carbonyl	Plasma	[80, 81]

Table 2. Experimental evidence supporting the involvement of oxidative stress

4. Pathways of free radical generation in diabetes mellitus and its associated complications

In diabetes, ROS is thought to be generated through increased polyol pathway [82], increased formation of advanced-glycation end products (AGEs) [83] and protein kinase C (PKC) activation [84].

4.1. Aldose reductase pathway and ROS generation

Aldose reductase is the rate limiting enzyme of the polyol pathway. The nicotinamide adenine dinucleotide phosphate (NAD(P)H)-requiring aldose reductase, catalyses the reduction of glucose to sorbitol followed by the oxidation of sorbitol to fructose by NAD+ dependent sorbitol dehydrogenase. At normal blood glucose concentration (5.5 mM), aldose reductase catalyzed reaction represents less than 3% of total glucose utilization [85]. However, hyperglycemia results in saturation of hexokinase and more than 30% of glucose is directed into the polyol pathway [86]. In a diabetic state, polyol pathway increases in tissues that do not require insulin for cellular glucose uptake, such as retina, kidney, peripheral nerves and blood vessels [87].

The overall reaction of the polyol pathway leads to a shortage of intracellular NAD(P)H and a surplus of NADH, i.e, a reductive imbalance. Increased NADH generation during conversion of sorbitol to fructose provides substrate for NADH oxidase to generate ROS [88]. NADH serves as a source of electrons in complex 1 of the electron transport chain resulting in increased mitochondrial generation of superoxide radical. In diabetic cells, oxidative phosphorylation in mitochondria is enhanced due to increase flux of electron donors into the electron transport chain. This drives the inner mitochondrial membrane potential upward causing blockage of electron transfer inside complex III [89]. Electrons back up to coenzyme Q results and electrons are transferred one at a time to molecular oxygen, generating superoxide. DNA damage by superoxide and peroxynitrite results in the activation of poly (ADP-ribose) polymerase (PARP), a DNA repair enzyme. PARP reduces the activity of glyceraldehyde-3- phosphate dehydrogenase (GAPDH) (an enzyme of the glycolytic pathway which catalyses the conversion of glyceraldehydes -3 phosphate to 1, 3 biphosphoglycerate) by ADP- ribosylation [90, 91]. A consequence of GAPDH inhibition by PARP is an increase in triose phosphate pool, upstream of GAPDH and increase flux of intermediates into the damaging pathways of diabetic complications.

The polyol pathway also results in reduction in the bioavailability of NAD(P)H. The reduced bioavailability of NAD(P)H negatively affects the antioxidant defence system by depleting glutathione (GSH) a very important antioxidant. This is because the activity of GSH reductase, an antioxidant enzyme that generates GSH from its oxidized form (GSSH) depends on NAD(P)H. Depletion of NAD(P)H also decreases the synthesis of nitric oxide (NO), a vaculo-protective agent. NAD(P)H serves as a cofactor for nitric oxide synthase (NOS) which synthesizes NO from L-arginine. If endothelial nitric oxide synthase (eNOS) lack its substrate, L-arginine or one of its co-factor, it may produce superoxide radical ($\cdot O_2^{\cdot-}$) instead of NO and this is referred to as "uncoupled state of nitric oxide"[92]. Nitric oxide performs several physiological roles such as inhibition of platelet activation, vascular relaxation [93] and acts as an anti-inflammatory agent by reducing platelet aggregation and adhesion [94]. These properties inhibit atherogenesis and protect the blood vessel. Reduced bioavailability of NO level will therefore increase inflammation, enhance thrombosis and disrupt the integrity of endothelial cells. Reduction in NO has been documented in diabetes subjects with nephropathy [95]. Superoxide anion directly quenches NO by forming highly reactive peroxynitrite ($ONOO^-$) which initiates lipid peroxidation, oxidizes sulfhydryl group in protein and nitrates amino acids such as tyrosine, thereby affecting many signal transduction pathways. The polyol pathway serves as a main source of ROS generation in the retina [96]. In addition, sorbitol accumulation has been implicated in osmotic swelling of the eye lens and cataractogenesis [97].

4.2. Advanced glycation end product (AGEs) formation and ROS generation in diabetic complications

Glucose can react spontaneously with free amino groups of protein to form Schiff bases. These Schiff bases through complex reactions such as amadori rearrangement, dehydration and condensation forms cross-linked heterogeneous fluorescent derivatives called advanced glycation end products (AGEs). Advanced glycation end products constitute a heterogeneous group of molecules formed by non-enzymatic reactions of reducing sugars, ascorbate and other carbohydrates with amino acids, lipids and nucleic acids [98, 99]. Glycation end product's adducts such as pyraline, pentosidine and N- Carboxy- methyl lysine (CML) are found to be elevated in diabetic tissues [100 - 102].

Once formed, AGEs can cause tissue damage by two main pathways which are: (1) formation of cross links that alter protein structure and function and, (2) interaction of AGE with AGE-cell surface receptors on the surfaces of various cells such as endothelial cells, macrophages, neurons, and smooth-muscle cells resulting in activation of cell signaling and gene expression that induces oxidative stress and inflammation [98, 99; 102-105]. Oxidative stress can accelerate AGE formation while AGE formation can also amplify the production of more ROS resulting in a vicious cycle of AGE formation and oxidative stress.

AGE's mediate some of their effect via interaction with some receptors that have been shown to bind to these chemical moieties. Among these receptors, Receptor for Advanced Glycation End products (RAGE) is the most extensively studied [106]. Evidence from numerous studies suggest that AGE's are involved in a vicious cycle of inflammation, generation of ROS and increased production of AGE's. Ligand RAGE interaction results in activation of pathways such as p21ras, erk1/2 (p44/p42), MAP kinases, p38 and SAPK/JNK MAP kinases [107-109]. A consequence of the activation of these pathways is the nuclear translocation of transcription factor, Nuclear Factor Kappa B (NF-KB). Translocation of NF-KB to the nucleus increases the transcription of a number of proteins such as, vascular endothelial growth factor (VEGF), monocyte chemoattractant protein-1 (MCP-1), vascular cell adhesion molecule-1 (VCAM-1) and intracellular adhesion molecule-1 (ICAM-1) and pro-inflammatory cytokines such as interleukin (IL)-1β, IL-6, 1L-18 and tumour necrosis factor (TNF)-α which are centrally involved in the endothelial recruitment of neutrophil and subsequent development or progression of atherosclerotic plaque [109-112].

The gene regions of NF-KB are located at the promoter region of RAGE. Moreover, binding of NF-KB to the promoter region of RAGE results in up-regulation of RAGE itsel. Interaction of AGE with RAGE generates more oxidative stress and this further potentiates the formation of AGE's [109, 113]. Generation of ROS by ligand stimulated RAGE activation is mediated at least in part via activation of NADPH oxidase [114]. Other mechanisms by which AGE's may be linked to increased generation of ROS is by reducing the activities of enzymatic antioxidant such as SOD and CAT, lowering of glutathione stores, and activation of PKC [107, 115, 116].

Increased renal AGE in diabetic animals and patients have been linked to structural abnormality observed in diabetic nephropathy such as mesangial expansion, glomerular basement membrane thickening and tubulointerstitial fibrosis [117]. Advanced Glycation End Product's level is increased with decreased renal function in type 1 diabetic patients [118]. Evidence from clinical studies indicates a correlation between progression of diabetic retinopathy and the level of AGE in serum and retinal blood vessels of diabetic patients [100, 119]. In diabetes, increased AGE's are observed within retinal capillary cells and causes pericyte loss in diabetic retinopathy [120]. AGE's induce toxic effects on retinal pericytes by causing oxidative stress and subsequent apoptosis [121].

High levels of serum AGE's have been documented in patients with type 2 diabetes mellitus and coronary heart disease [122]. Glycation increases susceptibility of low density lipoprotein (LDL) to oxidative modification which is considered a critical step in its atherogenicity [123]. Glycation end products can also enhance atherosclerosis by trapping LDL in the subendothelium and decrease the recognition of AGE-modified LDL by LDL receptor [124]. Modification of LDL and its increased localization in vessels increases foam cell production and accelerates atherosclerosis development [125]. Oxidative stress induces AGE's formation on collagen leading to cross-linking which is considered to play a role in diabetic cardiomyopathy [126]. The intermolecular collagen cross-linking caused by AGE increases vascular stiffness and interferes with arterial blood flow [127, 128] and this partly explains the diastolic dysfunction and systolic hypertension seen in diabetic subjects.

4.3. Protein kinase C (PKC) activation and ROS generation in diabetic complications

PKC activation is related to vasoconstriction, proliferation and overgrowth of smooth muscle cells as well as accelerated synthesis of extracellular matrix proteins, and thus plays significant roles in the onset and progression of vascular cell dysfunction in diabetes mellitus [129-131]. Two major pathways have been implicated in the activation of PKC in hyperglycemia. Persistent and excessive activation of several PKC isoforms result primarily from enhanced *de novo* synthesis of diacylglycerol (DAG) from glucose via increase in triose phosphate availability [90, 105, 132, 133]. There is also evidence that the interaction between AGE's and their cell-surface receptors can result in enhanced activity of PKC isoforms [134, 135].

PKC likely regulates diabetic complications on multiple levels such as activation of eNOS, NAD(P)H oxidase, phospholipase A_2 (PLA_2), endothelin-1 (ET-1), Vascular endothelial growth factor (VEGF), Transforming growth factor-β (TGF-β), and by activating NF-KB. Diacylglycerol activated PKC alters the gene expression of key proteins leading to decrease blood flow, capillary occlusion, inflammation, free radicals generation and damage to cellular macromolecule [130-132, 136, 137].

High glucose levels can stimulate ROS production via a PKC-dependent activation of NAD(P)H oxidase in cultured aortic endothelial cells, smooth muscle cells, and renal mesangial cells [84]. Nicotinamide adenine dinucleotide phosphate oxidase, which is primarily found in phagocytic cells, is the main source of ROS in non-phagocytic cells such as mesangial cells, endothelial cells [138], fibroblasts [139], podocytes [140] and smooth muscle cells [141]. The expression of NAD(P)H oxidase components is up-regulated in vascular tissues from animal models of diabetes and in patients with diabetes and coronary artery disease [142-144]. Experimental evidence indicates that NAD(P)H oxidase-dependent production of ROS may cause DNA damage in diabetic renal tissues leading to the development of nephropathy [145]. Increased activity of the NAD(P)H oxidase has also been reported in the retina of diabetic rats suggesting its involvement in the development of diabetic retinopathy [146].

5. Antioxidant as therapeutic agents in the management of diabetes mellitus

Despite efforts to control blood glucose, tissue and organ damage are cumulative over many years in most diabetic patients. Varying degrees of hyperglycemia are virtually unavoidable in subjects with diabetes mellitus and glycemic memory has been used to describe the development of diabetes-related complications in diabetic patients even after normoglycemia has been restored and initial glycemic environment is remembered in the target organs [105,147]. It is noteworthy that ROS has been implicated as a major cause of the metabolic memory after glucose normalization due to the chains of reactions leading to cell damage and loss of cellular function. Due to the implication of hyperglycemia-induced oxidative stress in diabetes, these patients should in theory benefit from antioxidant supplementation. The beneficial effect of antioxidants has been reported in animal models of diabetes and in diabetic patients [50, 148]

6. Vitamins

Vitamin E is a fat-soluble vitamin. It has been shown that plasma α-tocopherol concentrations are lower in diabetics compared to controls [58] and appear to be even lower in diabetics with complications such as microangiopathy than in diabetics without complications [81]. Administration of Vitamin E has proven to be beneficial in preventing cellular damage by inhibition of lipid peroxidation, protein oxidation, protein glycations and platelet aggregation [149-151] Vitamin E supplementation for two weeks (600 mg/day) lowered urinary F2-isoprostanes (a marker of lipid oxidation) in type 2 diabetics [152]. It was shown in a study that a decrease in plasma F2-isoprostanes was seen in type 2 diabetic patients after six weeks supplementation with Vitamin E [153].

Oxidative stress in the kidney of diabetics is usually associated with tissue damage that interferes with proper organ function, causing an increase in urinary protein excretion and blood urea nitrogen (BUN) [154]. Vitamin E supplementation (1000 IU/kg diet) to diabetic rats for 4 weeks significantly reduced urinary protein excretion and BUN suggesting a beneficial effect on kidney function [154]. Inhibitory effect of Vitamin E on glycation of hemoglobin in type I and type 2 diabetic rats has been documented [151, 155]. The ability of vitamin E to inhibit AGE's might be due to its antioxidant effect on the autoxidative pathways of AGE formation [156]. Vitamin E administration has also reduced oxidation of low density lipoprotein (LDL) and development of atherosclerosis [157].

Numerous studies have shown that vitamin E normalized parameters of oxidative stress and inhibited vascular abnormalities caused by hyperglycemia-induced production of DAG and PKC activation in the retina, glomerulus and macrophages [158-160]. Supplementation with vitamin E reduced basement membrane thickening in diabetic rat retina and reduced vascular endothelial growth factor (VEGF) and aldose reductase activity, the abnormalities associated with diabetic retinopathy [161]. Dietary supplementation of vitamin E (2000 IU/kg) to diabetic rats for 8 weeks had cardioprotective effects which was simultaneously associated with an ability of vitamin E to blunt diabetes-induced amplification of myocardial 8-*iso* PGF2 and oxidized GSSG formation [162]. Clinical trials with vitamin E provided evidence that vitamin E may improve cardiovascular function [163, 164]. However, most large studies with vitamin E have not yielded positive benefits for decreasing the development or progression of diabetic microvascular and cardiovascular pathologies or mortality [165, 166].

Vitamin C is an antioxidant vitamin which plays an important role in protecting free radical-induced damage and a decrease in basal vitamin C levels has been documented in type 2 DM. Treatment of diabetic rats with vitamin C significantly decreased renal malondialdehyde, albuminuria, proteinuria, glomerular and tubulointerstitial sclerosis, suggesting the role of vitamin C in suppressing the progression of renal injury in diabetic rats [167]. Vitamin C also improved diabetes-induced endothelial dysfunction in a rat model by enhancing NO bioavailability [168].

The beneficial effects of vitamin C supplementation in humans are controversial. A study reported that vitamin C may improve glycemic control, lowering both fasting blood glucose and glycated haemoglobin (HbA1c) [169]. Chronic oral administration of vitamin C to patients with type 2 diabetes causes a decline in plasma free radicals that is associated with improved whole body glucose disposal [170,171] and improved endothelial function [172]. Recently, another study reported a reduction in the malondialdehyde (MDA) level, a major product of oxidative damage in both fasting and postprandial states of type 2 diabetic patients after vitamin C (1000 mg day^{-1}) supplementation for 6 weeks although no effect was observed on lipid profiles [173]. Some studies have indicated that the intra-arterial infusion of vitamin c restores endothelium-dependent vasodilation in patients with type 1 or type 2 diabetes [174, 175] suggesting that hyperglycemia-induced oxidative stress mediates endothelial dysfunction in diabetic patients.

However, in contrast to these promising results, other studies showed no beneficial effect with vitamin C treatment. Chen and colleagues [176] concluded that a high oral dose of vitamin C therapy was ineffective at improving endothelial dysfunction and insulin resistance in type 2 DM. It is important to note that complete replenishment of vitamin C levels was not achieved in the subjects. This is crucial since high concentrations of vitamin C (>80 μM) has been documented as a requirement for the preservation of NO-dependent endothelial function as vitamin C only competes with NO for superoxide anion at these high concentrations [177-178]. Also, in another study, no beneficial effects of oral vitamin C supplementation (1.5 g daily for 3 weeks) was observed on blood pressure, oxidative stress, and endothelial function in type 2 diabetes [179].

7. Flavonoids

Flavonoids (bioflavonoids) are a diverse group of polyphenols (phenyl benzopyrans) which function as phytochemicals [180]. Flavonoids are well-known for their multi-directional biological activities including anti-diabetic efficacy. Experimental evidence has shown that

http://dx.doi.org/10.5772/57282

flavonoids exhibits anti-inflammatory [181], anticarcinogenic [182], antiviral [183] and antiallergic properties. These effects are generally associated with free radical scavenging activity of flavonoids. The antioxidant effects of flavonoids are enhanced by the number and position of hydroxyl groups in the molecule. The catechol structure, presence of unsaturation and 4-oxo function in the C-ring also contributes to their radical scavenging activity [184, 185]. Flavonoids may be capable of binding the transition metal ions, which play a role in glycoxidation, thus preventing metal-catalysed formation of hydroxyl radicals or related species from H_2O_2 [186].

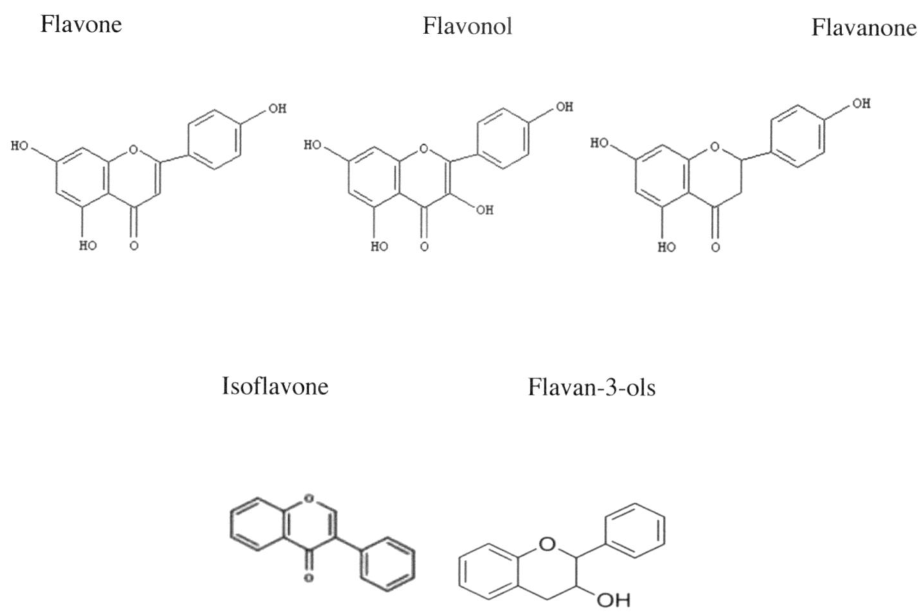

Figure 1. Classes of flavonoids [187]

The potential beneficial effects of flavonoids in the prevention of diabetes mellitus and its associated complications have been investigated both *in vitro* and *in vivo* studies (Table 3). The inhibitory effect of flavonoids on glycation has been demonstrated and it is suggested that this effect is partly due to their antioxidant properties [188]. Epigallocatechin (EGC) has a beneficial effect in a rat model of diabetic nephropathy via suppressing hyperglycemia, proteinuria and lipid peroxidation. EGC also reduced renal accumulation of AGE's and their related oxidative stress [189]. Another study demonstrated the *in vitro* inhibitory effect of different flavonoids on pentosidine formation in collagen in the presence of glucose (250 mmol/L). The decreasing inhibitiory activity was observed from myricetin, quercetin, rutin, catechin and kaempferol in a structure and concentration dependent manner [190]. Kim and colleagues [191] also investigated the effect of quercetin, isoquercitrin, hyperin and cacticin on formation of AGE's *in vitro*. At a concentration of 50 mM, the percentages of inhibition were 1.0, 89.6, 92.0 and 40.5, respectively. The inhibitory effect of hyperin on AGE formation was 6.5 times higher than that of aminoguanidine, a known AGE inhibitor which showed 14.1% inhibition at a concentration of 50 μM.

Flavonoids, in addition to their antioxidant effect, possess inhibitory activity on aldose reductase pathway and can serve as a potential multifunctional agent in the prevention of diabetic retinopathy. Goodarzi *et al.* [192] showed that oral administration of quercetin and the flavanone, naringin to streptozotocin-induced diabetic rats significantly reduced aldose reductase activity in the lenses compared to control. Oral administration of two isoflavone compounds, tectorigenin and irigenin also inhibited sorbitol accumulation in the lenses of streptozotocin induced diabetic rats [193].

Activation of PKC contributes to the loss of capillary pericytes and thickening of vascular basement membrane (BM) in diabetic retinopathy [194]. Also PKC mediated alterations in vascular permeability, blood flow, formation and response to angiogenic growth factors contribute to retinal leakage, ischemia, and neovascularisation [195]. Therefore, PKC inhibitors can be targeted for the treatment of diabetic retinopathy. Hesperetin (Hsp), a flavanone found in citrus fruits and a potent antioxidant has retina vasculo-protective properties due to its strong anti-angiogenic effect via inhibiting VEGF and PKC-β pathways [196]. Modulation of endogenous biomarkers and inhibition of diabetes induced neuropathic pain was observed in diabetic rats after naringin (4′,5,7-trihydroxy flavonone 7-rhamnoglucoside) administration [197]. In the same study, a dose dependent decrease in the levels of oxidative-nitrosative stress, inflammatory mediators as well as apoptosis was documented in neural cells. The antioxidant properties of naringin may be a factor in the inhibition of neurodegeneration.

The soy isoflavone genistein (3 and 6mg/kg), administered by a subcutaneous injection to diabetic mice relieved peripheral painful neuropathy by reverting the proinflammatory cytokine and ROS overproduction. It also restored the inducible nitric oxide synthase (iNOS) and eNOS content and increased NO production in thoracic aorta although treatment had no effect on hyperglycemia [198]. The flavonoid luteolin (200 mg/kg), when administered to rats orally, protected against the progression of diabetes-induced cardiac dysfunction by attenuation of myocardial oxidative stress probably through its antioxidant properties [199].

In a double blind placebo-controlled study, the effects of daflon 500 (made up of flavonoids diosmin (90%) and hesperidin (10%)) was investigated in a group of 28 type 1 diabetic patients. Treatment with these flavonoids resulted in a decrease in HbA_{1C} which is associated with an increase in the level and activities of thiol-containing antioxidants such as glutathione peroxidase [200]. The *in vitro* protective effect of myricetin on protein oxidation and membrane lipid peroxidation of erythrocytes from diabetic patients was reported in a study by Pandey and co-workers [201].

The treatment of diabetic rats with rutin decreased fasting plasma glucose, glycosylated haemoglobin, thiobarbituric acid reactive substances and lipid hydroperoxides while levels of non-enzymatic antioxidants were increased [202]. In another study, rutin supplementation (500 mg tablets) to diabetic patients for 60 days decreased the levels of fasting blood glucose, blood pressure and improved lipid profiles in the diabetic subjects [203]. Rutin reduced blood glucose, ameliorated oxidative stress and inhibited the accumulation of extracellular matrix

http://dx.doi.org/10.5772/57282

(ECM) component and glomerular basement membrane thickening in the renal cortex of diabetic rats suggesting its renoprotective effect in experimental diabetic nephropathy [204]. The inhibitory effect of rutin on AGE formation in STZ-induced rats has also been shown [205].

Diosmin (DS) (diosmetin 7-*O*-rutinoside) is a natural flavone glycoside which can be obtained by dehydrogenation of the corresponding flavanone glycoside, hesperidin that is abundant in the pericarp of various citrus fruits [206]. Diosmin treatment of streptozotocin-nicotinamide induced diabetic rats, ameliorated oxidative stress in plasma and tissues as evidenced by improved glycemic and antioxidant status along with decreased lipid peroxidation [207]. Experimental evidence showed the potential of rutin, a flavonol to delay glomerulosclerosis of diabetic nephropathy (DN) due to its ability to inhibit cell hypertrophy and the accumulation of ECM mediated by TGF-β1/Smads and ROS signals in mesangial cells cultured by high glucose [208] Quercetin enhances endothelium-derived NO bioavailability, reduced blood glucose levels and oxidative stress in diabetic rats suggesting its beneficial effect in vascular function [209].

Classes of Flavonoid and Food sources	**Selected examples**	**Target organ, tissue or cells**	**Mechanism of action**	**Reference**
Flavonols (Brussel sprouts, apples, onion, curly kale, leek, beans, cherries, Citrus fruits, Cranberries)	Morin	Liver	Decreased MDA levels , Increased activity of SOD and GSH concentration.	[210]
		Hepatocytes	Decreased ROS production, DNA damage and apoptosis. Modulation of antioxidant enzymes; GSH, CAT, SOD and GPX.	[211]
	Rutin	Kidney, serum, urine	Lowered blood glucose and improved renal function. Increased total antioxidant capability activities of SOD, CAT and GPX. Lowered ECM accumulation and AGE formation. Decreased renal expression of TGF-β.	[204]
	Quercetin	Pancreas, serum, erythrocyte.	Lowered MDA and NO level, increased antioxidant enzyme activity and preservation of islet cells integrity.	[212]
		Kidney , serum, urine	Lowered blood glucose and improved renal function. Reduced renal lipid peroxides and increased activity of anti-oxidative enzymes; SOD and CAT and non-enzymatic antioxidant GSH.	[213]

Classes of Flavonoid and Food sources	Selected examples	Target organ, tissue or cells	Mechanism of action	Reference
Flavanones (Citus peel, Orange juice, grape fruit juice, lemon juice)	Hesperidin & Naringin	Liver, serum	Boost antioxidant system by increasing activities of SOD, GR, GPx, CAT and levels of non-enzymatic antioxidants; GSH, VIT-C and VIT-E. Decreased lipid peroxidation product, MDA and proinflammatory markers, TNF-α, IL-6.	[214]
	Hesperidin	Retina, plasma	Decreased aldose reductase activity and levels of AGE's, VEGF, ICAM-1, TNF-α, IL-1β and MDA while increasing SOD activity.	[215]
	Naringenin	Pancreas, heamoglobin, serum, plasma	Lowered fasting blood glucose, decreased hyperglycemia, glycated haemoglobin, MDA and markers of hepatic damage. Increased levels of insulin and enzymatic and non-enzymatic antioxidants.	[216]
		Kidney, liver serum, urine,	Improved glycemic control and elevated insulin level, reduced plasma levels of kidney dysfunction markers. Lowered renal activity and expression of NF-KB and pro-inflammatory cytokine and chemokine, suppression of PKC activity.	[217]
Flavanolols (Milk thistle, red onion, Siberian larch tree)	Silymarin	Kidney	Increased expression and activity of SOD, GPX, CAT. Decreased high blood glucose	[218]
Flavones (Parsley, pepper celery, broccoli capsicum)	Luteolin	Kidney	Decreased activity of SOD, MDA content and expression of Heme Oxygenase-1 (HO-1) protein.	[219]
		Aortic ring	Aortic Vasorelaxation, decrease in ROS production, increased activity of SOD, NOS and level of NO.	[220]
	Diosmin	Liver and kidney	Decreased TBARS and hydroperoxides. Increased activity of enzymatic antioxidants ;SOD, CAT, GPx, GST and GR and non-enzymatic antioxidants; GSH, Vitamin C and Vitamin E.	[207]

Classes of Flavonoid and Food sources	Selected examples	Target organ, tissue or cells	Mechanism of action	Reference
Flavones	Chrysin and luteolin	Serum and aorta	Aortic relaxation, decreased blood pressure, decreased lipidemia and serum AGE's. Increased NO generation	[221]
	Apigenin	Serum and liver	Increased insulin levels and decreased hyperglycemia. Normalized LPO and endogeneous antioxidants, CAT, SOD, GSH in the liver.	[222]
Flavan-3-ols (Red wine and red grapes, green and black tea)	Catechin	Thoracic aorta	Decreased hyperglycemia NADPH oxidase activity and ROS production. Increased insulin level, lowered blood pressure and improved aortic relaxation.	[223]
	Epicatechin	Pancreatic Islets, plasma, haemoglobin	Increased anti-inflammatory cytokines, IL-10, IL-12. Improved glucose tolerance and insulin levels and lowered HbA1C.	[224]
Isoflavones (Soy foods and legumes)	Genistein	Kidney	Decreased MDA level and expression of PKC and pro-inflammatory proteins such as NF-KB, MCP-1 and Cox-2. Activation of antioxidant enzymes and defense against oxidative damage via increase expression of Nrf2, a transactivator of antioxidant genes.	[225]
	Daidzein	Aorta	Maintenance of endothelium dependent relaxation and attenuation of oxidative stress via decrease MDA levels and increase SOD activity	[226]

Abbreviations: Find all citations in this journal (defECM: Extracellular matrix, MDA: Malondialdehyde, NO: Nitric oxide, NOS: Nitric oxide synthase, NADPH; nicotinamide adenine dinucleotide phosphate, LPO: Lipid peroxidation, Nrf2: NF-E2-related factor-2, Cox-2: Cyclooxygenase-2, TAOC: Total antioxidative capability

Table 3. Beneficial effects of some flavonoids in diabetes mellitus

The inherent antioxidative properties of some common antidiabetic drugs such as aminoguanidine, statins, thiazolidinediones, glibenclamide and repaglinide also provides an additional support to the involvement of oxidative stress in diabetes and therefore suggest that the use of antioxidants as therapeutic agents in diabetes is a promising approach [227-231].

8. Conclusion and future perspective

Increased ROS production has been suggested as a common pathway linking diverse pathogenic mechanisms of diabetic vascular complications. There are numerous evidences from animal studies on the beneficial effect of antioxidant vitamins supplementation in diabetes mellitus, but results from clinical studies are inconclusive. The antioxidant activity of some anti-diabetic drugs has also been shown to contribute significantly to their therapeutic effect. Biflavonoids as antioxidants are promising and attractive natural substances to enrich the current therapy options against diabetes. The overall positive results from animal studies suggest that the role of antioxidants cannot be underestimated in the quest to find effective therapies for diabetic complications. A multi-therapeutic approach to the treatment of diabetic complications might increase the chance of successful therapeutic intervention. In addition to maintaining glycemic control, blockage of pathways involved in the formation of free radicals with antioxidants is a promising approach to the treatment of hyperglycemia-mediated complications in humans. The bioactivity of flavonoids *in vivo* can be greatly influenced by metabolism and bioavailability and this information is limited in many studies. Limited clinical studies have been carried out to support the beneficial effects of flavonoids in the prevention of diabetic complications. In order to achieve the goal of using flavonoids in the management of diabetes mellitus, further investigation on the long and short-term effect of the ingestion of flavonoids in humans is warranted.

Author details

Omolola R. Ayepola[1], Nicole L. Brooks[2] and Oluwafemi O. Oguntibeju[1*]

*Address all correspondence to: oguntibejuo@cput.ac.za, bejufemi@yahoo.co.uk.

1 Nutrition and Chronic Disease Research Unit, Oxidative Stress Research Centre, Department of Biomedical Sciences, Faculty of Health and Wellness Sciences, Cape Peninsula University of Technology, Bellville, South Africa

2 Department of Wellness Sciences, Faculty of Health and Wellness Sciences, Cape Peninsula University of Technology, Cape Town, South Africa

References

[1] Bastaki, A. 2005. Diabetes mellitus and its treatment. *Int J Diab and Metab* 13(3): 111.

[2] Zhao, Y. 2011. Autoimmunity and Therapeutic Challenges of Type 1 Diabetes. *Transl Med*,1: 104e

[3] Ruhe, R.C. & McDonald, R.B. 2001. Use of antioxidant nutrients in the prevention and treatment of type 2 diabetes. *J Am Coll Nutr, 20* (sup5): 363S-369S.

[4] Resnick, H.E. & Howard, B.V. 2002. Diabetes and cardiovascular disease. *Annu Rev Med,* 53(1): 245-267.

[5] Fowler, M.J. 2008. Microvascular and macrovascular complications of diabetes. *Clin Diabetes,* 26(2): 77-82.

[6] Cook, M.N., Girman, C.J., Stein, P.P., Alexander, C.M. & Holman, R.R. 2005. Glycemic control continues to deteriorate after sulfonylureas are added to metformin among patients with type 2 diabetes. *Diabetes Care,* 28(5): 995-1000.

[7] Kowluru, R.A., Abbas, S.N. & Odenbach, S. 2004. Reversal of hyperglycemia and diabetic nephropathy: effect of reinstitution of good metabolic control on oxidative stress in the kidney of diabetic rats. *J Diabetes Complication,* 18(5): 282-288.

[8] Mayor, S. 2008. Intensive glucose lowering arm of diabetes trial is stopped after excess deaths. *Br Med J,* 336(7641): 407.

[9] Ismail-Beigi, F., Craven, T., Banerji, M.A., Basile, J., Calles, J., Cohen, R.M., Cuddihy, R., Cushman, W.C., Genuth, S. & Grimm Jr, R.H. 2010. Effect of intensive treatment of hyperglycaemia on microvascular outcomes in type 2 diabetes: an analysis of the ACCORD randomised trial. *The Lancet,* 376(9739): 419-430.

[10] Kawahito, S., Kitahata, H. & Oshita, S. 2009. Problems associated with glucose toxicity: Role of hyperglycemia-induced oxidative stress. *World J Gastroenterol:* 15(33): 4137.

[11] Ceriello, A. 2003. New insights on oxidative stress and diabetic complications may lead to a "causal" antioxidant therapy. *Diabetes Care,* 26(5): 1589-1596.

[12] Giacco, F. & Brownlee, M. 2010. Oxidative stress and diabetic complications. *Circ Res,* 107(9): 1058-1070.

[13] Zhang, C., Liu, J., Pan, H., Yang, X. & Bian, K. 2011. Mitochondrial dysfunction induced by excessive ROS/RNS-metabolic cardiovascular disease and traditional Chinese medicines intervention. *China J Chinese Mat med,* 36(17): 2423.

[14] Jain, M. 2012. Histopathological changes in diabetic kidney disease. *Clin Queries: Nephrol,* 1(2): 127-133.

[15] Lewis, E.J. & Xu, X. 2008. Abnormal Glomerular Permeability Characteristics in Diabetic Nephropathy Implications for the therapeutic use of low–molecular weight heparin. *Diabetes Care,* 31(Supplement 2): S202-S207.

[16] O'Connor, A.S. & Schelling, J.R. 2005. Diabetes and the kidney. *Am J Kidney Dis,* 46(4): 766-773.

[17] Marshall, S.M.m& Flyvbjerg, A. 2006. Prevention and early detection of vascular complications of diabetes. *Br Med J,* 333(7566): 475.

[18] Santos, J.M., Mohammad, G., Zhong, Q. & Kowluru, R.A. 2011. Diabetic retinopathy, superoxide damage and antioxidants. *Curr Pharm Biotechnol* 1;12(3):352-61

[19] Engerman, R.L. 1989. Pathogenesis of diabetic retinopathy. *Diabetes,* 38 (10): 1203-1206.

[20] Hammes, H. 2005. Pericytes and the pathogenesis of diabetic retinopathy. *Horm Metab Res,* 37(S 1): 39-43.

[21] American Diabetes Association: Standards of medical care in diabetes 2007 [Position Statement]. *Diabetes Care* 30:S4–S41, 2007

[22] Pazdro, R. & Burgess, J.R. 2010. The role of vitamin E and oxidative stress in diabetes complications. *Mech Ageing Dev,* 131(4): 276-286.

[23] Obrosova, I.G. 2009. Diabetes and the peripheral nerve. *Biochim Biophys Acta,* 1792(10): 931-940.

[24] Soumya, D. 2011. Late Stage Complications of Diabetes and Insulin Resistance. *J Diabetes Metabol,* 2:167

[25] Schwartz, C.J., Valente, A.J., Sprague, E.A., Kelley, J.L., Cayatte, A.J. & Rozek, M.M. 1992. Pathogenesis of the atherosclerotic lesion: implications for diabetes mellitus. *Diabetes Care,* 15(9): 1156-1167.

[26] American Diabetes association. Consensus Statement, 1993. Role of cardiovascular risk factors in prevention and treatment of macrovascular disease in diabetes. *Diabetes Care*. 16:72-78.

[27] Orchard, T.J., Costacou, T., Kretowski, A. & Nesto, R.W. 2006. Type 1 diabetes and coronary artery disease. *Diabetes Care,* 29(11): 2528-2538.

[28] Ding, H. & Triggle, C.R. 2005. Endothelial cell dysfunction and the vascular complications associated with type 2 diabetes: assessing the health of the endothelium. *Vasc Health Risk Manag,* 1(1): 55.

[29] Winer, N. & Sowers, J.R. 2004. Epidemiology of diabetes. *J Clin Pharmacol,* 44(4): 397-405.

[30] Epstein, F.H. & Ross, R. 1999. Atherosclerosis-an inflammatory disease. *New Engl J Med,* 340(2): 115-126.

[31] Libby, P., Ridker, P.M. & Hansson, G.K. 2011. Progress and challenges in translating the biology of atherosclerosis. *Nature,* 473(7347): 317-325.

[32] Funk, S.D., Yurdagul, A. & Orr, A.W. 2012. Hyperglycemia and endothelial dysfunction in atherosclerosis: lessons from type 1 diabetes. *Int J Vasc Med,* 2012:1-19.

[33] Creager, M.A., Lüscher, T.F., Cosentino, F. & Beckman, J.A. 2003. Diabetes and vascular disease pathophysiology, clinical consequences, and medical therapy: part I. *Circulation,* 108(12): 1527-1532.

[34] Valko, M., Leibfritz, D., Moncol, J., Cronin, M.T., Mazur, M. & Telser, J. 2007. Free radicals and antioxidants in normal physiological functions and human disease. *Int J Biochem Cell Biol,* 39(1): 44-84.

[35] Dröge, W. 2002. Free radicals in the physiological control of cell function. *Physiol Rev,* 82(1): 47-95.

[36] Pacher, P., Beckman, J.S. & Liaudet, L. 2007. Nitric oxide and peroxynitrite in health and disease. *Physiol Rev,* 87(1): 315-424.

[37] Sachdev, S. & Davies, K.J. 2008. Production, detection, and adaptive responses to free radicals in exercise. *Free Radic Biol Med,* 44(2): 215-223.

[38] Sies, H. 1997. Oxidative stress: Oxidants and antioxidants. *Exp Physiol., 82,* 291–295.

[39] Halliwell, B. & Gutteridge, J. M. C., 2007. *Free Radic Biol Med.* 4th. Edn, Clarendon Press, Oxford

[40] Bahorun, T., Soobrattee, M., Luximon-Ramma, V. & Aruoma, O. 2006. Free radicals and antioxidants in cardiovascular health and disease. *Internet J Med Update,* 1(2): 25-41.

[41] Halliwell, B. 2007. Biochemistry of oxidative stress. *Biochem Soc Trans,* 35(Pt 5): 1147-1150.

[42] Abdollahi, M., Ranjbar, A., Shadnia, S., Nikfar, S. & Rezaie, A. 2004. Pesticides and oxidative stress: a review. *Medical science monitor: Int Med J Exp and Clin Res,* 10(6): RA141-7.

[43] Ridnour, L.A., Thomas, D.D., Mancardi, D., Espey, M.G., Miranda, K.M., Paolocci, N., Feelisch, M., Fukuto, J. & Wink, D.A. 2004. The chemistry of nitrosative stress induced by nitric oxide and reactive nitrogen oxide species. Putting perspective on stressful biological situations. *Biol Chem,* 385(1): 1-10.

[44] Halliwell, B. 2011. Free radicals and antioxidants. *Trends Pharmacol Sci,* 32(3): 125-130.

[45] Fukai, T. & Ushio-Fukai, M. 2011. Superoxide dismutases: role in redox signaling, vascular function, and diseases. *Antioxid Redox Signal,* 15(6): 1583-1606.

[46] Lubos, E., Loscalzo, J. & Handy, D.E. 2011. Glutathione peroxidase-1 in health and disease: from molecular mechanisms to therapeutic opportunities. *Antioxid Redox Signal,* 15(7): 1957-1997.

[47] Pham-Huy, L.A., He, H. & Pham-Huy, C. 2008. Free radicals, antioxidants in disease and health. *Int J Biomed Sc:* 4(2): 89.

[48] Winterbourn, C.C. 1993. Superoxide as an intracellular radical sink. *Free Radic Biol Med,* 14(1): 85-90.

[49] Jurkovič, S., Osredkar, J. & Marc, J. 2008. Molecular impact of glutathione peroxidases in antioxidant processes. *Biochem Med,* 18(2): 162-174.

[50] Maritim, A., Sanders, R. & Watkins, 3.J. 2003. Diabetes, oxidative stress, and antioxidants: a review. *J Biochem and Mol Tox,* 17(1): 24-38.

[51] Zelko, I.N., Mariani, T.J. & Folz, R.J. 2002. Superoxide dismutase multigene family: a comparison of the CuZn-SOD (SOD1), Mn-SOD (SOD2), and EC-SOD (SOD3) gene structures, evolution, and expression. *Free Radic Biol Med,* 33(3): 337-349.

[52] Livingstone, C. & Davis, J. 2007. Review: Targeting therapeutics against glutathione depletion in diabetes and its complications. *Br J Diabetes Vasc Dis,* 7(6): 258-265.

[53] May, J.M., Qu, Z. & Morrow, J.D. 1996. Interaction of Ascorbate and-Tocopherol in Resealed Human Erythrocyte Ghosts. Transmembrane electron transfer and protection from lipid peroxidation. *J Biol Chem,* 271(18): 10577-10582.

[54] Smith, A., Shenvi, S., Widlansky, M., Suh, J. & Hagen, T. 2004. Lipoic acid as a potential therapy for chronic diseases associated with oxidative stress. *Curr Med Chem,* 11(9): 1135-1146.

[55] Inoguchi, T., Li, P., Umeda, F., Yu, H.Y., Kakimoto, M., Imamura, M., Aoki, T., Etoh, T., Hashimoto, T. & Naruse, M. 2000. High glucose level and free fatty acid stimulate reactive oxygen species production through protein kinase C--dependent activation of NAD (P) H oxidase in cultured vascular cells. *Diabetes,* 49(11): 1939-1945.

[56] Lee JL, Suh KS, Choi MC, Chon S, Oh S, Woo JT, Kim SW,Kim JW, Kim YS (2010). Kaempferol protects HIT-15 pancreatic beta-cells from 2-deoxy-D-ribose-induced oxidative damage. *Phytother Res* 24:419-423

[57] Rösen, P., Nawroth, P., King, G., Möller, W., Tritschler, H. & Packer, L. 2001. The role of oxidative stress in the onset and progression of diabetes and its complications: asummary of a Congress Series sponsored byUNESCO-MCBN, the American Diabetes Association and the German Diabetes Society. *Diabetes Metabol Res Rev,* 17(3): 189-212.

[58] Nourooz-Zadeh, J., Rahimi, A., Tajaddini-Sarmadi, J., Tritschler, H., Rosen, P., Halliwell, B. & Betteridge, D. 1997. Relationships between plasma measures of oxidative stress and metabolic control in NIDDM. *Diabetologia,* 40(6): 647-653.

[59] Brownlee, M. 2001. Biochemistry and molecular cell biology of diabetic complications. *Nature,* 414(6865): 813-820.

[60] Evans, J.L., Goldfine, I.D., Maddux, B.A. & Grodsky, G.M. 2002. Oxidative stress and stress-activated signaling pathways: a unifying hypothesis of type 2 diabetes. *Endocr Rev,* 23(5): 599-622.

[61] Shih, C., Wu, Y. & Lin, W. 2002. Antihyperglycaemic And Anti-Oxidant Properties Of Anoectochilus Formosanus in Diabetic Rats. *Clin Exp Pharmacol Physiol,* 29(8): 684-688.

[62] Manna, P., Das, J., Ghosh, J. & Sil, P.C. 2010. Contribution of type 1 diabetes to rat liver dysfunction and cellular damage via activation of NOS, PARP, IκBα/NF-κB,

MAPKs, and mitochondria-dependent pathways: Prophylactic role of arjunolic acid. *Free Radic Biol Med,* 48(11): 1465-1484.

[63] Hamden, K., Boujbiha, M.A., Masmoudi, H., Ayadi, F.M., Jamoussi, K. & Elfeki, A. 2009. Combined vitamins (C and E) and insulin improve oxidative stress and pancreatic and hepatic injury in alloxan diabetic rats. *Biomed Pharmacother,* 63(2): 95-99.

[64] Prabakaran D, Ashokkumar N. Protective effect of esculetin on hyperglycemia-mediated oxidative damage in the hepatic and renal tissues of experimental diabetic rats. *Biochimie.* 2013 95(2):366-73.

[65] Erejuwa, O.O., Sulaiman, S.A., Wahab, M.S.A., Salam, S.K.N., Salleh, M.S.M. & Gurtu, S. 2011. Comparison of antioxidant effects of honey, glibenclamide, metformin, and their combinations in the kidneys of streptozotocin-induced diabetic rats. *Int J Mol Sci,* 12(1): 829-843.

[66] Aragno, M., Mastrocola, R., Medana, C., Restivo, F., Catalano, M.G., Pons, N., Danni, O. & Boccuzzi, G. 2005. Up-regulation of advanced glycated products receptors in the brain of diabetic rats is prevented by antioxidant treatment. *Endocrinology,* 146(12): 5561-5567.

[67] Kowluru, R.A. & Kanwar, M. 2007. Effects of curcumin on retinal oxidative stress and inflammation in diabetes. *Nutr and metabol,* 4: 8

[68] Babu, P.V.A., Sabitha, K.E. & Shyamaladevi, C.S. 2006. Therapeutic effect of green tea extract on oxidative stress in aorta and heart of streptozotocin diabetic rats. *Chem Biol Interac,* 162(2): 114-120.

[69] Ramesh, B., Viswanathan, P. & Pugalendi, K.V. 2007. Protective effect of Umbelliferone on membranous fatty acid composition in streptozotocin-induced diabetic rats. *Eur J Pharmacol,* 566(1): 231-239.

[70] Haidara, M.A., Mikhailidis, D.P., Rateb, M.A., Ahmed, Z.A., Yassin, H.Z., Ibrahim, I.M. & Rashed, L.A. 2009. Evaluation of the effect of oxidative stress and vitamin E supplementation on renal function in rats with streptozotocin-induced Type 1 diabetes. *J Diabetes and Its Complications,* 23(2): 130-136.

[71] Rajavel, V., Sattar, A., Zubaid, M., Abdulla, M.A., Kassim, N.M. & Abdullah, N.A. 2012. Chronic Administration of Oil Palm (Elaeis guineensis) Leaves Extract Attenuates Hyperglycaemic-Induced Oxidative Stress and Improves Renal Histopathology and Function in Experimental Diabetes. *Evid Base Compl Alternative Med,* doi: 10.1155/2012/195367

[72] Park, K.S., Kim, J.H., Kim, M.S., Kim, J.M., Kim, S.K., Choi, J.Y., Chung, M.H., Han, B., Kim, S.Y. & Lee, H.K. 2001. Effects of insulin and antioxidant on plasma 8-hydroxyguanine and tissue 8-hydroxydeoxyguanosine in streptozotocin-induced diabetic rats. *Diabetes,* 50(12): 2837-2841.

[73] Figarola, J., Scott, S., Loera, S., Tessler, C., Chu, P., Weiss, L. & Hardy, J. 2003. LR-90 a new advanced glycation endproduct inhibitor prevents progression of diabetic nephropathy in streptozotocin-diabetic rats. *Diabetologia,* 46(8): 1140-1152.

[74] Likidlilid A, Patchanans N, Peerapatdit T, Sriratanasathavorn C, 2010. Lipid Peroxidation and Antioxidant Enzyme Activities in Erythrocytes of Type 2 Diabetic Patients. *J Med Assoc Thai,* 93 (6): 682-93

[75] Sekhar, R.V., McKay, S.V., Patel, S.G., Guthikonda, A.P., Reddy, V.T., Balasubramanyam, A. & Jahoor, F. 2011. Glutathione synthesis is diminished in patients with uncontrolled diabetes and restored by dietary supplementation with cysteine and glycine. *Diabetes Care,* 34(1): 162-167.

[76] Flores L, Rodela S, Abian J, Clària J, Esmatjes E, 2004 F2 isoprostane is already increased at the onset of type 1 diabetes mellitus: effect of glycemic control. *Metabolism.* 2004;53(9):1118-1120.

[77] Selvaraj, N., Bobby, Z. & Sathiyapriya, V. 2006. Effect of lipid peroxides and antioxidants on glycation of hemoglobin: an in vitro study on human erythrocytes. *Clin Chim Acta,* 366(1): 190-195.

[78] Goodarzi, M.T., Navidi, A.A., Rezaei, M. & Babahmadi-Rezaei, H. 2010. Oxidative damage to DNA and lipids: correlation with protein glycation in patients with type 1 diabetes. J *Clin Lab Anal,* 24(2): 72-76.

[79] Hinokio, Y., Suzuki, S., Hirai, M., Suzuki, C., Suzuki, M. & Toyota, T. 2002. Urinary excretion of 8-oxo-7, 8-dihydro-2′-deoxyguanosine as a predictor of the development of diabetic nephropathy. *Diabetologia,* 45(6): 877-882.

[80] Ceriello, A., Mercuri, F., Quagliaro, L., Assaloni, R., Motz, E., Tonutti, L. & Taboga, C. 2001. Detection of nitrotyrosine in the diabetic plasma: evidence of oxidative stress. *Diabetologia,* 44(7): 834-838.

[81] Martín-Gallán, P., Carrascosa, A., Gussinyé, M. & Domínguez, C. 2003. Biomarkers of diabetes-associated oxidative stress and antioxidant status in young diabetic patients with or without subclinical complications. *Free Rad Biol Med,* 34(12): 1563-1574.

[82] Chung, S.S., Ho, E.C., Lam, K.S. & Chung, S.K. 2003. Contribution of polyol pathway to diabetes-induced oxidative stress. *Journal of the American Society of Nephrology,* 14(suppl 3): S233-S236.

[83] Baynes, J.W. & Thorpe, S.R. 1999. Role of oxidative stress in diabetic complications: a new perspective on an old paradigm. *Diabetes,* 48(1): 1-9.

[84] Inoguchi, T., Sonta, T., Tsubouchi, H., Etoh, T., Kakimoto, M., Sonoda, N., Sato, N., Sekiguchi, N., Kobayashi, K. & Sumimoto, H. 2003. Protein kinase C–dependent increase in reactive oxygen species (ROS) production in vascular tissues of diabetes: role of vascular NAD (P) H oxidase. *Clin J Am Soc Nephrol,* 14(suppl 3): S227-S232.

[85] Morrison, A.D., Clements Jr, R.S., Travis, S.B., Oski, F. & Winegrad, A.I. 1970. Glucose utilization by the polyol pathway in human erythrocytes. *Biochem Biophys Res Comm,* 40(1): 199-205.

[86] González, R.G., Barnett, P., Aguayo, J., Cheng, H. & Chylack, L. 1984. Direct measurement of polyol pathway activity in the ocular lens. *Diabetes,* 33(2): 196-199.

[87] Stephen S.M. Chung, Eric C.M. HO, Karen S.L. Lam, and Sookja K. Chung, 2003. Contribution of Polyol Pathway to Diabetes-Induced Oxidative Stress. *J Am Soc Nephrol* 14: S233–S236

[88] Morre, D.M., Lenaz, G. & Morre, D.J. 2000. Surface oxidase and oxidative stress propagation in aging. *J Exp Biol,* 203(10): 1513-1521.

[89] Yang, X. & Trumpower, B.L. 1988. Protonmotive Q cycle pathway of electron transfer and energy transduction in the three-subunit ubiquinol-cytochrome c oxidoreductase complex of Paracoccus denitrificans. *J Biol Chem,* 263(24): 11962-11970.

[90] Du, X., Matsumura, T., Edelstein, D., Rossetti, L., Zsengellér, Z., Szabó, C. & Brownlee, M. 2003. Inhibition of GAPDH activity by poly (ADP-ribose) polymerase activates three major pathways of hyperglycemic damage in endothelial cells. *J Clin Investig,* 112(7): 1049-1057.

[91] Soriano, F.G., Virág, L., Jagtap, P., Szabó, É., Mabley, J.G., Liaudet, L., Marton, A., Hoyt, D.G., Murthy, K.G. & Salzman, A.L. 2001. Diabetic endothelial dysfunction: the role of poly (ADP-ribose) polymerase activation. *Nature Med,* 7(1): 108-113.

[92] Vásquez-Vivar, J., Kalyanaraman, B., Martásek, P., Hogg, N., Masters, B.S.S., Karoui, H., Tordo, P. & Pritchard, K.A. 1998. Superoxide generation by endothelial nitric oxide synthase: the influence of cofactors. *Proc Natl Acad Sci,* 95(16): 9220-9225.

[93] Mehta, J.L., Rasouli, N., Sinha, A.K. & Molavi, B. 2006. Oxidative stress in diabetes: a mechanistic overview of its effects on atherogenesis and myocardial dysfunction. *Int J Biochem Cell Biol,* 38(5): 794-803.

[94] Sharma, J., Al-Omran, A. & Parvathy, S. 2007. Role of nitric oxide in inflammatory diseases. *Inflammopharmacology,* 15(6): 252-259.

[95] Tessari, P., Cecchet, D., Cosma, A., Vettore, M., Coracina, A., Millioni, R., Iori, E., Puricelli, L., Avogaro, A. & Vedovato, M. 2010. Nitric oxide synthesis is reduced in subjects with type 2 diabetes and nephropathy. *Diabetes,* 59(9): 2152-2159.

[96] Mara, L. & Oates, P.J. 2008. Diabetic Retinopathy. In *The Polyol Pathway and Diabetic Retinopathy.* : Springer: 159-186. Contemporary Diabetes 2008:159-186

[97] Patel, D., Prasad, S., Kumar, R. & Hemalatha, S. 2011. Cataract: A major secondary complication of diabetes, its epidemiology and an overview on major medicinal plants screened for anticataract activity. *Asian Pac J Tropical Dis,* 1(4): 323-329.

[98] Vlassara, H. & Palace, M. 2002. Diabetes and advanced glycation endproducts. *J Intern Medicine,* 251(2): 87-101.

[99] Peppa, M., Uribarri, J. & Vlassara, H. 2004. The role of advanced glycation end products in the development of atherosclerosis. *Curr Diabetes Rep,* 4(1): 31-36.

[100] Stitt, A.W. 2001. Advanced glycation: an important pathological event in diabetic and age related ocular disease. *Br J Ophthalmol,* 85(6): 746-753.

[101] Wautier, J. & Guillausseau, P. 2001. Advanced glycation end products, their receptors and diabetic angiopathy. *Diabetes Metabol,* 27(5; PART 1): 535-544.

[102] Ahmed, N., 2005. Advanced glycation end products-role in pathology of diabetic complications. *Diabetes Res Clin Pract* 67, 3-21.

[103] Nishikawa, T., Edelstein, D., Du, X.L., Yamagishi, S., Matsumura, T., Kaneda, Y., Yorek, M.A., Beebe, D., Oates, P.J. & Hammes, H. 2000. Normalizing mitochondrial superoxide production blocks three pathways of hyperglycaemic damage. *Nature,* 404(6779): 787-790.

[104] Sourris, K.C. & Forbes, J.M. 2009. Interactions between advanced glycation end-products (AGE) and their receptors in the development and progression of diabetic nephropathy-are these receptors valid therapeutic targets. *Curr Drug Targets,* 10(1): 42-50.

[105] Giacco, F. & Brownlee, M. 2010. Oxidative stress and diabetic complications. *Circ Res,* 107(9): 1058-1070.

[106] Ramasamy, R., Vannucci, S.J., Du Yan, S.S., Herold, K., Yan, S.F. & Schmidt, A.M. 2005. Advanced glycation end products and RAGE: a common thread in aging, diabetes, neurodegeneration, and inflammation. *Glycobiology,* 15(7): 16R-28R.

[107] Yan, S.D., Schmidt, A.M., Anderson, G.M., Zhang, J., Brett, J., Zou, Y.S., Pinsky, D. & Stern, D. 1994. Enhanced cellular oxidant stress by the interaction of advanced glycation end products with their receptors/binding proteins. *J Biol Chem,* 269(13): 9889-9897.

[108] Lander, H.M., Tauras, J.M., Ogiste, J.S., Hori, O., Moss, R.A. & Schmidt, A.M. 1997. Activation of the receptor for advanced glycation end products triggers a p21 ras-dependent mitogen-activated protein kinase pathway regulated by oxidant stress. *J Biol Chem,* 272(28): 17810-17814.

[109] Goldin, A., Beckman, J.A., Schmidt, A.M. & Creager, M.A. 2006. Advanced glycation end products sparking the development of diabetic vascular injury. *Circulation,* 114(6): 597-605.

[110] Cybulski MI, Gimbrone MA., 1991. Endothelial expression of a mononuclear leukocyte adhesion molecule during atherogenesis. *Science*. 251:788-791

[111] Rubanyi, G.M. 1993. The role of endothelium in cardiovascular homeostasis and diseases. *J Cardiovasc Pharmacol,* 22: S15-S18.

[112] Schiekofer, S., Andrassy, M., Chen, J., Rudofsky, G., Schneider, J., Wendt, T., Stefan, N., Humpert, P., Fritsche, A. & Stumvoll, M. 2003. Acute hyperglycemia causes intracellular formation of CML and activation of ras, p42/44 MAPK, and nuclear factor κB in PBMCs. *Diabetes,* 52(3): 621-633.

[113] Barbosa, J.H., Oliveira, S.L. & Seara, L.T. 2008. The role of advanced glycation end-products (AGEs) in the development of vascular diabetic complications. *Arq Bras Endocrinol Metabol,* 52(6): 940-950.

[114] Wautier, M., Chappey, O., Corda, S., Stern, D.M., Schmidt, A.M. & Wautier, J. 2001. Activation of NADPH oxidase by AGE links oxidant stress to altered gene expression via RAGE. *Am J Physiol Endocrinol Metabol,* 280(5): E685-E694.

[115] Obrosova, I.G. 2002. How does glucose generate oxidative stress in peripheral nerve? *Int Rev Neurobiol,* 50: 3-35.

[116] Jiang, J., Wang, Z. & Li, D. 2004. Effects of AGEs on oxidation stress and antioxidation abilities in cultured astrocytes. *Biomed Environ Sc,* 17(1): 79-86.

[117] Yamagishi, S. & Matsui, T. 2010. Advanced glycation end products, oxidative stress and diabetic nephropathy. *Oxid Med and Cell Longev,* 3(2): 101-108.

[118] Miura, J., Yamagishi, S., Uchigata, Y., Takeuchi, M., Yamamoto, H., Makita, Z. & Iwamoto, Y. 2003. Serum levels of non-carboxymethyllysine advanced glycation end-products are correlated to severity of microvascular complications in patients with Type 1 diabetes. *J Diabetes Complications,* 17(1): 16-21.

[119] Ono, Y., Aoki, S., Ohnishi, K., Yasuda, T., Kawano, K. & Tsukada, Y. 1998. Increased serum levels of advanced glycation end-products and diabetic complications. *Diabetes Res Clin Prac,* 41(2): 131-137.

[120] Stitt, A.W. 2003. The role of advanced glycation in the pathogenesis of diabetic retinopathy. *Exp Mol Pathol,* 75(1): 95-108.

[121] Chen, B., Jiang, D. & Tang, L. 2006. Advanced glycation end-products induce apoptosis involving the signaling pathways of oxidative stress in bovine retinal pericytes. *Life Sci,* 79(11): 1040-1048.

[122] Kilhovd, B.K., Berg, T.J., Birkeland, K.I., Thorsby, P. & Hanssen, K.F. 1999. Serum levels of advanced glycation end products are increased in patients with type 2 diabetes and coronary heart disease. *Diabetes Care,* 22(9): 1543-1548.

[123] Bowie, A., Owens, D., Collins, P., Johnson, A. & Tomkin, G.H. 1993. Glycosylated low density lipoprotein is more sensitive to oxidation: implications for the diabetic patient? *Atherosclerosis,* 102(1): 63-67.

[124] Bucala, R., Makita, Z., Vega, G., Grundy, S., Koschinsky, T., Cerami, A. & Vlassara, H. 1994. Modification of low density lipoprotein by advanced glycation end products

contributes to the dyslipidemia of diabetes and renal insufficiency. *Proc Natl Acad Sci,* 91(20): 9441-9445.

[125] Sobenin, I., Tertov, V., Koschinsky, T., Bünting, C., Slavina, E., Dedovc, I. & Orekhov, A. 1993. Modified low density lipoprotein from diabetic patients causes cholesterol accumulation in human intimal aortic cells. *Atherosclerosis,* 100(1): 41-54.

[126] Goh, S. & Cooper, M.E. 2008. The role of advanced glycation end products in progression and complications of diabetes. *J Clin Endocrinol Metabol,* 93(4): 1143-1152.

[127] Eble, A.S., Thorpe, S.R. & Baynes, J.W. 1983. Nonenzymatic glucosylation and glucose-dependent cross-linking of protein. *J Biol Chem,* 258(15): 9406-9412.

[128] Cooper, M.E., Bonnet, F., Oldfield, M. & Jandeleit-Dahm, K. 2001. Mechanisms of diabetic vasculopathy: an overview. *Am J Hypertens,* 14(5): 475-486.

[129] Koya, D. & King, G.L. 1998. Protein kinase C activation and the development of diabetic complications. *Diabetes,* 47(6): 859-866.

[130] Meier, M. & King, G.L. 2000. Protein kinase C activation and its pharmacological inhibition in vascular disease. *Vasc Med,* 5(3): 173-185.

[131] Way, K., Katai, N. & King, G. 2001. Protein kinase C and the development of diabetic vascular complications. *Diabet Med,* 18(12): 945-959.

[132] Inoguchi, T., Battan, R., Handler, E., Sportsman, J.R., Heath, W. & King, G.L. 1992. Preferential elevation of protein kinase C isoform beta II and diacylglycerol levels in the aorta and heart of diabetic rats: differential reversibility to glycemic control by islet cell transplantation. *Proc Natl Acad Sci,* 89(22): 11059-11063.

[133] Shiba, T., Inoguchi, T., Sportsman, J.R., Heath, W.F., Bursell, S. & King, G.L. 1993. Correlation of diacylglycerol level and protein kinase C activity in rat retina to retinal circulation. *Am J Physiol Endocrinol Metabol,* 265(5): E783-E793.

[134] Derubertis, F.R. & Craven, P.A. 1994. Activation of protein kinase C in glomerular cells in diabetes: mechanisms and potential links to the pathogenesis of diabetic glomerulopathy. *Diabetes,* 43(1): 1-8.

[135] Thallas-Bonke, V., Thorpe, S.R., Coughlan, M.T., Fukami, K., Yap, F.Y., Sourris, K.C., Penfold, S.A., Bach, L.A., Cooper, M.E. & Forbes, J.M. 2008. Inhibition of NADPH oxidase prevents advanced glycation end product–mediated damage in diabetic nephropathy through a protein kinase C-α–dependent pathway. *Diabetes,* 57(2): 460-469.

[136] Klann, E., Roberson, E.D., Knapp, L.T. et al., 1998. A role for superoxide in protein kinase C activation and induction of long-term potentiation. *J Biol Chem*. 273: 4516–4522.

[137] Noh, H. & King, G. 2007. The role of protein kinase C activation in diabetic nephropathy. *Kidney Int,* 72(: S49-S53.

[138] Jones, S., O'donnell, V., Wood, J., Broughton, J., Hughes, E. & Jones, O. 1996. Expression of phagocyte NADPH oxidase components in human endothelial cells. *Am J Physiol Heart Circ Physiol,* 271(4): H1626-H1634.

[139] Pagano, P.J., Clark, J.K., Cifuentes-Pagano, M.E., Clark, S.M., Callis, G.M. & Quinn, M.T. 1997. Localization of a constitutively active, phagocyte-like NADPH oxidase in rabbit aortic adventitia: enhancement by angiotensin II. *Proc Natl Acad Sci,* 94(26): 14483-14488.

[140] Greiber, S., Münzel, T., Kästner, S., Müller, B., Schollmeyer, P. & Pavenstädt, H. 1998. NAD (P) H oxidase activity in cultured human podocytes: effects of adenosine triphosphate. *Kidney Int,* 53(3): 654-663.

[141] Patterson C, Ruef J, Madamanchi NR, Barry-Lane P, Hu Z, Horaist C, Ballinger CA, Brasier AR, Bode C, Runge MS, 1999: Stimulation of a vascular smooth muscle cell NAD(P)H oxidase by thrombin: evidence that p47phox may participate in forming this oxidase in vitro and in vivo. *J Biol Chem*. 274:19814–19822.

[142] Hink, U., Li, H., Mollnau, H., Oelze, M., Matheis, E., Hartmann, M., Skatchkov, M., Thaiss, F., Stahl, R.A. & Warnholtz, A. 2001. Mechanisms underlying endothelial dysfunction in diabetes mellitus. *Circ Res,* 88(2): e14-e22.

[143] Guzik, T.J., Mussa, S., Gastaldi, D., Sadowski, J., Ratnatunga, C., Pillai, R. & Channon, K.M. 2002. Mechanisms of increased vascular superoxide production in human diabetes mellitus Role of NAD (P) H oxidase and endothelial nitric oxide synthase. *Circulation,* 105(14): 1656-1662.

[144] Kim, Y.K., Lee, M., Son, S.M., Kim, I.J., Lee, W.S., Rhim, B.Y., Hong, K.W. & Kim, C.D. 2002. Vascular NADH oxidase is involved in impaired endothelium-dependent vasodilation in OLETF rats, a model of type 2 diabetes. *Diabetes,* 51(2): 522-527.

[145] Etoh, T., Kakimoto, M., Sonoda, N., Kobayashi, K., Kuroda, J., Sumimoto, H. & Nawata, H. 2003. Increased expression of NAD (P) H oxidase subunits, NOX4 and p22phox, in the kidney of streptozotocin-induced diabetic rats and its reversibity by interventive insulin treatment. *Diabetologia,* 46(10): 1428-1437.

[146] Ellis, E., Grant, M.B., Murray, F.T., Wachowski, M.B., Guberski, D.L., Kubilis, P.S. & Lutty, G.A. 1998. Increased NADH oxidase activity in the retina of the BBZ/Wor diabetic rat. *Free Radic Biol Med,* 24(1): 111-120.

[147] Ceriello, A., Ihnat, M.A. & Thorpe, J.E. 2009. The "metabolic memory": is more than just tight glucose control necessary to prevent diabetic complications? *J Clin Endocrinol Metabol,* 94(2): 410-415.

[148] Liu S, Lee I.M., Song Y, Van Denburgh M, Cook N.R., Manson J.E., Buring J.E., 2006. Vitamin E and risk of type 2 diabetes in the women's health study randomized controlled trial. *Diabetes*, 55:2856–62.

[149] Rhee, S., Jeong, Y. & Choi, J. 2005. Effects of vitamin E on phospholipase A2 activity and oxidative damage to the liver in streptozotocin-induced diabetic rats. *Ann Nutr Metabol,* 49(6): 392-396.

[150] Devaraj, S., Leonard, S., Traber, M.G., Jialal, I., 2008. Gamma-tocopherol supplementation alone and in combination with alpha-tocopherol alters biomarkers of oxidative stress and inflammation in subjects with metabolic syndrome. *Free Radic Biol Med.* 44:1203–1208

[151] Minamiyama, Y., Takemura, S., Bito, Y., Shinkawa, H., Tsukioka, T., Nakahira, A., Suehiro, S. & Okada, S. 2008. Supplementation of α-tocopherol improves cardiovascular risk factors via the insulin signalling pathway and reduction of mitochondrial reactive oxygen species in type II diabetic rats. *Free Radic Res,* 42(3): 261-271.

[152] Davi, G., Ciabattoni, G., Consoli, A., Mezzetti, A., Falco, A., Santarone, S., Pennese, E., Vitacolonna, E., Bucciarelli, T., Costantini, F., Capani, F., Patrono, C., 1999. In vivo formation of 8-iso-prostaglandin f2alpha and platelet activation in diabetes mellitus: effects of improved metabolic control and vitamin E supplementation. *Circulation.* 99, 224–229

[153] Wu, J.H., Ward, N.C., Indrawan, A.P., Almeida, C., Hodgson, J.M., Proudfoot, J.M., Puddey, I.B. & Croft, K.D. 2007. Effects of α-tocopherol and mixed tocopherol supplementation on markers of oxidative stress and inflammation in type 2 diabetes. *Clin Chem,* 53(3): 511-519.

[154] Montero, A., Munger, K.A., Khan, R.Z., Valdivielso, J.M., Morrow, J.D., Guasch, A., Ziyadeh, F.N. & Badr, K.F. 2000. F2-isoprostanes mediate high glucose-induced TGF-&bgr; synthesis and glomerular proteinuria in experimental type I diabetes. *Kidney Int,* 58(5): 1963-1972.

[155] Je, H., Shin, C., Park, H., Huh, I. & Sohn, U. 2001. The comparison of vitamin C and vitamin E on the protein oxidation of diabetic rats. *J Auton Pharmacol,* 21(5): 231-236.

[156] Schleicher, E.D., Wagner, E. & Nerlich, A.G. 1997. Increased accumulation of the glycoxidation product N (epsilon)-(carboxymethyl) lysine in human tissues in diabetes and aging. *J Clin Investig,* 99(3): 457.

[157] Jialal, I., Devaraj, S. & Venugopal, S. 2002. Oxidative stress, inflammation, and diabetic vasculopathies: the role of alpha tocopherol therapy. *Free Rad Res,* 36(12): 1331-1336.

[158] Sakamoto, W., Fujie, K., Handa, H., Ogihara, T. & Mino, M. 1989. In vivo inhibition of superoxide production and protein kinase C activity in macrophages from vitamin E-treated rats. *Int J Vitam Nutr Res,* 60(4): 338-342.

[159] Kunisaki, M., Bursell, S., Clermont, A.C., Ishii, H., Ballas, L.M., Jirousek, M.R., Umeda, F., Nawata, H. & King, G.L. 1995. Vitamin E prevents diabetes-induced abnormal

retinal blood flow via the diacylglycerol-protein kinase C pathway. *Am J Physiol Endocrinol Metabol,* 269(2): E239-E246.

[160] Koya, D., Lee, I., Ishii, H., Kanoh, H. & King, G.L. 1997. Prevention of glomerular dysfunction in diabetic rats by treatment with d-alpha-tocopherol. *Clin J Am Soc Nephrol,* 8(3): 426-435.

[161] Yülek, F., Or, M., Özoğul, C., Isik, A.C., Ari, N., Stefek, M., Bauer, V. & Karasu, C. 2007. Effects of stobadine and vitamin E in diabetes-induced retinal abnormalities: involvement of oxidative stress. *Arch Med Sc,* 38(5): 503-511.

[162] Hamblin M, Smith HM, Hill MF., 2007. Dietary supplementation with vitamin E ameliorates cardiac failure in type I diabetic cardiomyopathy by suppressing myocardial generation of 8-iso-prostaglandin F2-alpha and oxidized glutathione. *J Card Fail,* 13(10): 884-892.

[163] Boaz, M., Smetana, S., Weinstein, T., Matas, Z., Gafter, U., Iaina, A., Knecht, A., Weissgarten, Y., Brunner, D. & Fainaru, M. 2000. Secondary prevention with antioxidants of cardiovascular disease in endstage renal disease (SPACE): randomised placebo-controlled trial. *The Lancet,* 356(9237): 1213-1218.

[164] Skyrme-Jones, R.A.P., O'Brien, R.C., Berry, K.L. & Meredith, I.T. 2000. Vitamin E supplementation improves endothelial function in type I diabetes mellitus: a randomized, placebo-controlled study. *J Am Coll Cardiol,* 36(1): 94-102.

[165] Heart Outcomes Prevention Evaluation (HOPE) Study Investigators, 2000. Effects of ramipril on cardiovascular and microvascular outcomes in people with diabetes mellitus: results of the HOPE study and MICRO-HOPE substudy. *Lancet.* 355: 253-259.

[166] Lonn E, Yusuf S, Hoogwerf B, Pogue J, Yi Q, Zinman B, Bosch J, Dagenais G, Mann JFE, Gerstein HC, 2002. Effects of vitamin E on cardiovascular and microvascular outcomes in high-risk patients with diabetes: Results of the HOPE study and MICRO-HOPE substudy. *Diabetes Care.* 25:1919-1927.

[167] Lee, E.Y., Lee, M.Y., Hong, S.W., Chung, C.H. & Hong, S.Y. 2007. Blockade of oxidative stress by vitamin C ameliorates albuminuria and renal sclerosis in experimental diabetic rats. *Yonsei Med J,* 48(5): 847-855.

[168] Sridulyakul, P., Wongeak-in, N. & Patumraj, S. 2010. Increased nitric oxide level in diabetic rats from vitamin C supplementation: an in vivo detection using diaminofluorescein. *Asian Biomed,* 2(5): 371-379.

[169] Eriksson, J. & Kohvakka, A. 1995. Magnesium and ascorbic acid supplementation in diabetes mellitus. *Ann Nutr Metabol,* 39(4): 217-223.

[170] Paolisso, G., Balbi, V., Volpe, C., Varricchio, G., Gambardella, A., Saccomanno, F., Ammendola, S., Varricchio, M. & D'Onofrio, F. 1995. Metabolic benefits deriving from chronic vitamin C supplementation in aged non-insulin dependent diabetics. *J Am Coll Nutr,* 14(4): 387-392.

[171] Mullan, B.A., Young, I.S., Fee, H. & McCance, D.R. 2002. Ascorbic acid reduces blood pressure and arterial stiffness in type 2 diabetes. *Hypertension,* 40(6): 804-809.

[172] Regensteiner, J.G., Popylisen, S., Bauer, T.A., Lindenfeld, J., Gill, E., Smith, S., Oliver-Pickett, C.K., Reusch, J.E. & Weil, J.V. 2003. Oral L-arginine and vitamins E and C improve endothelial function in women with type 2 diabetes. *Vasc Med,* 8(3): 169-175.

[173] Mazloom, Z., Hejazi, N., Dabbaghmanesh, M.H., Tabatabaei, H.R., Ahmadi, A. & Ansar, H. 2011. Effect of vitamin C supplementation on postprandial oxidative stress and lipid profile in type 2 diabetic patients. *Pakistan J Biol Sci: PJBS,* 14(19): 900-904.

[174] Ting, H.H., Timimi, F.K., Boles, K.S., Creager, S.J., Ganz, P. & Creager, M.A. 1996. Vitamin C improves endothelium-dependent vasodilation in patients with non-insulin-dependent diabetes mellitus. *J Clin Investig,* 97(1): 22.

[175] Timimi, F.K., Ting, H.H., Haley, E.A., Roddy, M., Ganz, P. & Creager, M.A. 1998. Vitamin C improves endothelium-dependent vasodilation in patients with insulin-dependent diabetes mellitus. *J Am Coll Cardiol,* 31(3): 552-557.

[176] Chen, H., Karne, R.J., Hall, G., Campia, U., Panza, J.A., Cannon, R.O., Wang, Y., Katz, A., Levine, M. & Quon, M.J. 2006. High-dose oral vitamin C partially replenishes vitamin C levels in patients with type 2 diabetes and low vitamin C levels but does not improve endothelial dysfunction or insulin resistance. *Am J Physiol Heart Circ Physiol,* 290(1): H137-H145.

[177] Jackson, T.S., Xu, A., Vita, J.A. & Keaney, J.F. 1998. Ascorbate prevents the interaction of superoxide and nitric oxide only at very high physiological concentrations. *Circ Res,* 83(9): 916-922.

[178] Sherman, D.L., Keaney, J.F., Biegelsen, E.S., Duffy, S.J., Coffman, J.D. & Vita, J.A. 2000. Pharmacological concentrations of ascorbic acid are required for the beneficial effect on endothelial vasomotor function in hypertension. *Hypertension,* 35(4): 936-941.

[179] Darko, D., Dornhorst, A., Kelly, F., Ritter, J. & Chowienczyk, P. 2002. Lack of effect of oral vitamin C on blood pressure, oxidative stress and endothelial function in Type II diabetes. *Clin Sci,* 103(4): 339-344.

[180] Corradini, E., Foglia, P., Giansanti, P., Gubbiotti, R., Samperi, R. & Lagana, A. 2011. Flavonoids: chemical properties and analytical methodologies of identification and quantitation in foods and plants. *Nat Prod Res,* 25(5): 469-495.

[181] Middleton, E., Kandaswami, C. & Theoharides, T.C. 2000. The effects of plant flavonoids on mammalian cells: implications for inflammation, heart disease, and cancer. *Pharmacol Rev,* 52(4): 673-751.

[182] Batra P and Sharma AK, 2013 Anti-cancer potential of flavonoids: recent trends and future perspectives 3 *Biotechnology* DOI 10.1007/s13205-013-0117-5

[183] Selway, J.W. 1986. Antiviral activity of flavones and flavans. *Progr Clin Biol Res,* 213: 521-536.

[184] Rice-Evans, C.A., Miller, N.J. & Paganga, G. 1996. Structure-antioxidant activity relationships of flavonoids and phenolic acids. *Free Radic Biol Med,* 20(7): 933-956.

[185] Heim, K. E.; Tagliaferro, A. R.; Bobilya D. J. Flavonoid antioxidants: chemistry, metabolism and sructure-activity relationships. *J Nutr Biochem*. 2002, 13, 572-584

[186] Groot, H.d. & Rauen, U. 1998. Tissue injury by reactive oxygen species and the protective effects of flavonoids. *Fund Clin Pharmacol,* 12(3): 249-255.

[187] Narayana K.R., Reddy M.S., Chaluvadi M.R., Krishna D.R., 2001. Bioflavonoids classification, pharmacological, biochemical effects and therapeutic potential. *Indian J Physiol Pharmacol*; 33: 2-16.

[188] Wu, C. & Yen, G. 2005. Inhibitory effect of naturally occurring flavonoids on the formation of advanced glycation endproducts. *J Agr Food Chem,* 53(8): 3167-3173.

[189] Yamabe N, Yokozawa T, Oya T and Kim M, 2006. Therapeutic potential of (-) epigallocatechin 3-Ogallate on renal damage in diabetic nephropathy model rats. *J Pharmacol Exp Therapeut,* 319: 228-236.

[190] Urios, P., Grigorova-Borsos, A. & Sternberg, M. 2007. Flavonoids inhibit the formation of the cross-linking AGE pentosidine in collagen incubated with glucose, according to their structure. *Eur J Nutr,* 46(3): 139-146.

[191] Kim, H.Y., Lee, J.M., Yokozawa, T., Sakata, K. & Lee, S. 2011. Protective activity of flavonoid and flavonoid glycosides against glucose-mediated protein damage. *Food Chem,* 126(3): 892-895.

[192] Goodarzi, M., Zal, F., Malakooti, M. & Sadeghian, M.S.S. 2006. Inhibitory activity of flavonoids on the lens aldose reductase of healthy and diabetic rats. *Acta Medica Iranica,* 44(1).

[193] Jung, S.H., Lee, Y.S., Lee, S., Lim, S.S., Kim, Y.S. & Shin, K.H. 2002. Isoflavonoids from the rhizomes of Belamcanda chinensis and their effects on aldose reductase and sorbitol accumulation in streptozotocin induced diabetic rat tissues. *Arch Pharm Res,* 25(3): 306-312.

[194] Kim, J., Kim, J.H., Jun, H., Yu, Y.S. & Kim, K. 2010. Inhibition of protein kinase C δ attenuates blood-retinal barrier breakdown in diabetic retinopathy. *Am J Clin Pathol,* 176(3): 1517-1524.

[195] Frank, R.N., 2004. Diabetic retinopathy. *New Engl J Med.* 350: 48–58

[196] Kumar, B., Gupta, S.K., Srinivasan, B., Nag, T.C., Srivastava, S. & Saxena, R. 2012. Hesperetin ameliorates hyperglycemia induced retinal vasculopathy via anti-angiogenic effects in experimental diabetic rats. *Vasc Pharmacol,* 57(5): 201-207.

[197] Kandhare, A.D., Raygude, K.S., Ghosh, P., Ghule, A.E. & Bodhankar, S.L. 2012. Neuroprotective effect of naringin by modulation of endogenous biomarkers in streptozotocin induced painful diabetic neuropathy. *Fitoterapia,* 83(4): 650-659.

[198] Valsecchi, A.E., Franchi, S., Panerai, A.E., Rossi, A., Sacerdote, P. & Colleoni, M. 2011. The soy isoflavone genistein reverses oxidative and inflammatory state, neuropathic pain, neurotrophic and vasculature deficits in diabetes mouse model. Eur J Clin Pharmacol, 650(2): 694-702.

[199] Wang, G., Li, W., Lu, X., Bao, P. & Zhao, X. 2012. Luteolin ameliorates cardiac failure in type I diabetic cardiomyopathy. *J Diabetes Complications,* 26(4): 259-265.

[200] Manuel y Keenoy, B., Vertommen, J. & De Leeuw, I. 1999. The effect of flavonoid treatment on the glycation and antioxidant status in Type 1 diabetic patients. *Diabetes, Nutr Metabol,* 12(4): 256-263.

[201] Pandey, K.B., Mishra, N. & Rizvi, S.I. 2009. Myricetin may provide protection against oxidative stress in type 2 diabetic erythrocytes. *Int J Biosci,* 64(9): 626.

[202] Kamalakkannan, N. & Prince, P.S.M. 2006. Antihyperglycaemic and Antioxidant Effect of Rutin, a Polyphenolic Flavonoid, in Streptozotocin-Induced Diabetic Wistar Rats. *Basic Clin Pharmacol Toxicol,* 98(1): 97-103.

[203] Sattanathan, K., Dhanapal, C., Umarani, R. & Manavalan, R. 2011. Beneficial health effects of rutin supplementation in patients with diabetes mellitus. *JAPS,* 1(08): 227-231.

[204] Hao, H., Shao, Z., Tang, D., Lu, Q., Chen, X., Yin, X., Wu, J. & Chen, H. 2012. Preventive effects of rutin on the development of experimental diabetic nephropathy in rats. *Life Sci.*

[205] Cervantes-Laurean, D.D. Schramm, E.L. Jacobson, I. Halaweish, G.G. Bruckner, G.A., 2006. Boissonneault. Inhibition of advanced glycation end product formation on collagen by rutin and its metabolites. *J Nutr Biochem*. 17: 531–540

[206] Campanero, M.A., Escolar, M., Perez, G., Garcia-Quetglas, E., Sadaba, B. & Azanza, J.R. 2010. Simultaneous determination of diosmin and diosmetin in human plasma by ion trap liquid chromatography–atmospheric pressure chemical ionization tandem mass spectrometry: Application to a clinical pharmacokinetic study. *J Pharmaceut Biomed Anal,* 51(4): 875-881.

[207] Srinivasan S, Pari L, 2012. Ameliorative effect of diosmin, a citrus flavonoid against streptozotocin-nicotinamide generated oxidative stress induced diabetic rats. *Chem Biol Interact*. 195: 43–51

[208] Tang, D., Wei, Y., Gao, Y., Yin, X., Yang, D., Mou, J. & Jiang, X. 2011. Protective effects of rutin on rat glomerular mesangial cells cultured in high glucose conditions. *Phytother Res,* 25(11): 1640-1647.

[209] Machha, A., Achike, F.I., Mustafa, A.M. & Mustafa, M.R. 2007. Quercetin, a flavonoid antioxidant, modulates endothelium-derived nitric oxide bioavailability in diabetic rat aortas. *Nitric Oxide,* 16(4): 442-447.

[210] Alkhamees, O.A. 2013. Morin a Flavonoid Exerts Antioxidant Potential in Streptozotocin-induced Hepatotoxicity. *Br J Pharmacol Toxicol* 4(1): 10-17, 2013

[211] Kapoor, R. & Kakkar, P. 2012. Protective role of morin, a flavonoid, against high glucose induced oxidative stress mediated apoptosis in primary Rat hepatocytes. *PloS one,* 7(8): e41663.

[212] Coskun, O., Kanter, M., Korkmaz, A. & Oter, S. 2005. Quercetin, a flavonoid antioxidant, prevents and protects streptozotocin-induced oxidative stress and β-cell damage in rat pancreas. *Pharmacol Res,* 51(2): 117-123.

[213] Anjaneyulu, M. & Chopra, K. 2004. Quercetin, an anti-oxidant bioflavonoid, attenuates diabetic nephropathy in rats. *Clin Exp Pharmacol Physiol,* 31(4): 244-248.

[214] Mahmoud AM, Ashour MB, Abdel-Moneim A, Ahmed OM, 2012. Hesperidin and naringin attenuate hyperglycemia-mediated oxidative stress and proinflammatory cytokine production in high fat fed/streptozotocin-induced type 2 diabetic rats. *J Diabetes Complications*. 26: 483-490.

[215] Shi, X., Liao, S., Mi, H., Guo, C., Qi, D., Li, F., Zhang, C. & Yang, Z. 2012. Hesperidin Prevents Retinal and Plasma Abnormalities in Streptozotocin-Induced Diabetic Rats. *Molecules,* 17(11): 12868-12881.

[216] Annadurai, T., Muralidharan, A.R., Joseph, T., Hsu, M., Thomas, P. & Geraldine, P. 2012. Antihyperglycemic and antioxidant effects of a flavanone, naringenin, in streptozotocin–nicotinamide-induced experimental diabetic rats. *J Physiol Biochem,* 68(3): 307-318.

[217] Tsai, S., Huang, C., Mong, M., Kam, W., Huang, H. & Yin, M. 2011. Anti-inflammatory and antifibrotic effects of naringenin in diabetic mice. *J Agr Food Chem,* 60(1): 514-521.

[218] Soto, C., Pérez, J., García, V., Uría, E., Vadillo, M. & Raya, L. 2010. Effect of silymarin on kidneys of rats suffering from alloxan-induced diabetes mellitus. *Phytomedicine,* 17(14): 1090-1094.

[219] Wang, G.G., Lu, X.H., Li, W., Zhao, X. & Zhang, C. 2011. Protective effects of luteolin on diabetic nephropathy in STZ-induced diabetic rats. *Evid Base Compl Alternative Med,* article ID 323171, 7 pages.

[220] Qian, L., Wang, H., Chen, Y., Chen, F., Ma, Y., Bruce, I.C. & Xia, Q. 2010. Luteolin reduces high glucose-mediated impairment of endothelium-dependent relaxation in rat aorta by reducing oxidative stress. *Pharmacol Res,* 61(4): 281-287.

[221] El-Bassossy, H.M., Abo-Warda, S.M. & Fahmy, A. 2013. Chrysin and Luteolin Attenuate Diabetes-Induced Impairment in Endothelial-Dependent Relaxation: Effect on Lipid Profile, AGEs and NO Generation. *Phytother Res*. doi: 10.1002/ptr.4917.

[222] Panda, S. & Kar, A. 2007. Apigenin (4 ', 5, 7-trihydroxyflavone) regulates hyperglycaemia, thyroid dysfunction and lipid peroxidation in alloxan-induced diabetic mice. *J Pharm Pharmacol*, 59(11): 1543-1548.

[223] Ihm, S., Lee, J., Kim, S., Seung, K., Schini-Kerth, V.B., Chang, K. & Oak, M. 2009. Catechin prevents endothelial dysfunction in the prediabetic stage of OLETF rats by reducing vascular NADPH oxidase activity and expression. *Atherosclerosis*, 206(1): 47-53.

[224] Fu, Z., Yuskavage, J. & Liu, D. 2013. Dietary Flavonol Epicatechin Prevents the Onset of Type 1 Diabetes in Nonobese Diabetic Mice. *J Agr Food Chem*, 61(18): 4303-4309.

[225] Kim, M.J. & Lim, Y. 2013. Protective Effect of Short-Term Genistein Supplementation on the Early Stage in Diabetes-Induced Renal Damage. *Mediat Inflamm*, 2013: 1-14

[226] Roghani, M., Vaez Mahdavi, M., Jalali-Nadoushan, M., Baluchnejadmojarad, T., Naderi, G., Roghani-Dehkordi, F., Taghi Joghataei, M. & Kord, M. 2013. Chronic Administration of Daidzein, a Soybean Isoflavone, Improves Endothelial Dysfunction and Attenuates Oxidative Stress in Streptozotocin-induced Diabetic Rats. *Phytother Res*, 27(1): 112-117.

[227] Fukui, T., Noma, T., Mizushige, K., Aki, Y., Kimura, S. & Abe, Y. 2000. Dietary troglitazone decreases oxidative stress in early stage type II diabetic rats. *Life Sci*, 66(21): 2043-2049.

[228] Dobsak P, Courderot-Masuyer C, Siegelova J, Svacinova H, Jancik J, Vergely-Vanriessen C, Rochette, 2001. Antioxidant properties of aminoguanidine: a paramagnetic resonance test. *Scripta Med* (BRNO) 74: 45–50.

[229] Elmalí, E., Altan, N. & Bukan, N. 2004. Effect of the sulphonylurea glibenclamide on liver and kidney antioxidant enzymes in streptozocin-induced diabetic rats. *Drugs in R & D*, 5(4): 203-208

[230] Haendeler, J., Hoffmann, J., Zeiher, A.M. & Dimmeler, S. 2004. Antioxidant effects of statins via s-nitrosylation and activation of thioredoxin in endothelial cells a novel vasculoprotective function of statins. *Circulation*, 110(7): 856-861.

[231] Gumieniczek, A., Hopkała, H., Roliński, J. & Bojarska-Junak, A. 2005. Antioxidative and anti-inflammatory effects of repaglinide in plasma of diabetic animals. *Pharmacol Res*, 52(2): 162-166.

Chapter 3

Anti-Diabetic Effects of Nigerian Indigenous Plant Foods/Diets

Elizabeth A. Udenta, Ikemefuna C. Obizoba and Oluwafemi O. Oguntibeju

Additional information is available at the end of the chapter

http://dx.doi.org/10.5772/57240

1. Introduction

Plants play important role in the cycle of nature. This is because life on earth basically depends on them. Plants provide man with all his needs as regards food, shelter, clothing, flavours and fragrance as well as medicine. They are naturally occurring substances that produce almost all the foods that animals as well as humans eat. They have unique potential to make their own food through photosynthesis. All foods that people eat naturally come directly or indirectly from plants. Food is fundamental to human survival. It is basic for averting hunger, satisfying one's palate and maintaining health of every human being. It is used as a status symbol, making people happy, emotionally and socially content, and constitutes a form of cultural expression. It is also used in the performance of various rituals and rites as well as for therapeutic purposes. Culture has a lot of influence on the kind of foods people eat and how they eat them. Traditional foods, was adopted to describe all foods from a particular culture, available from local sources and culturally acceptable as appropriate and desirable foods [1]. The direct and indirect food sources as regards nutrition are simply described as and categorized into two major sources - plant and animal foods, respectively.

Despite the unique role of plant foods as irreplaceable food sources for humans, not all plant foods are available or edible worldwide. Traditional plant foods are those plants grown for food in varying proportions within the farming system operating in any particular locality; or gathered in wild or semi-wild conditions; and are accepted by the community, through custom, habit and tradition as appropriate and desirable foods [1, 2]. They are categorized as those that are consumed as traditional dietary staples and those consumed as components of accompanying relishes and sauces. These traditional foods are often used in sciences as basis for ensuring and optimizing utilization of indigenous foods and their health benefits by individuals, households and communities. The use of plant foods for therapeutic purposes represents one of the biggest human uses of the natural flora of the world [3]. This is because of their health-enhancing bioactive constituents [4]. In the last four decades, there has been considerable interest in resurrecting health-promoting potentials of indigenous plant foods in developing countries and integrating their use into modern medical system. The reasons for this interest are varied and include, i) the negative impact of nutrition transition that increase epidemic of diet-related non-communicable chronic diseases (NCDs) in such regions; ii) high cost of medicare, which put modern health care out of reach of the poor; iii) low adherence to drug prescriptions; and iv) side effects of medicinal plant and herbal medicine extracts and/or preparations, because out of ignorance the consumers consume them as food supplements that are safe at any dose. This is not true for any of the high biologically active medicinal plants. Most of them cannot be consumed habitually as local foods without adverse effects. There was need to challenge reduced interest in and demand for drugs amidst poor health management in these poor regions. Pharmaceutical preparations from medicinal plants created a new expanding market as herbal components of health foods and preventive medicine under "nutraceuticals" or "nutriceuticals". Culhane [5] defined them as products produced from food and sold in pills, powders and other medicinal forms not generally associated with food and are shown to have a physiological benefit or provide protection against chronic diseases. Chronic diseases are largely preventable diseases. Diet-related NCDs are diseases of long duration and generally slow in progression [6]. They are relatively difficult to manage. The high cost and side effects of these supplements still limit their use and have made this approach an unsustainable alternative strategy for chronic disease management and prevention.

Carbohydrate food sources form the greatest percentage [50-60%) of the daily diet for different segments of the population [7]. In Nigeria, starchy staples (cereals, roots/tubers) and legumes constitute the major part of the traditional diets, up to 70% and 25%, respectively [8, 9, 10]. Physiologically, chronic restriction of carbohydrate–rich sources, mainly supplied by plant foods, may pose a serious threat to Nigeria's survival. Diabetics are particularly adversely affected due to misinformation and inability to seek dietetic intervention. Such dietary misinformation has led to starvation and the development of psychosocial problems in diabetics. This is because they feel denied and full of anxiety in anticipation of lifestyle changes [11].

Type 2 diabetes is more common in Nigeria. There was increase in the average prevalence rate from 2.7% [12] to 3.9% [13] and annual increase of 0.3%. Over the years, diet was implicated both as one of the aetiological factors to the development of diabetes [14] as well as a key component in diabetes management [7, 15]. Plant foods are the most important dietary sources to meet the nutritional needs of majority of the population in sub-Saharan Africa and Asian subcontinent [16]. Dietary fibre is a component of carbohydrate in plant foods shown to modulate post-prandial blood glucose after discovery of the "dietary fibre hypothesis" by Cleave [17] and Burkitt et al. [18]. Roles of phytochemicals and antioxidant constituents of plant foods were reported [4]. On this basis, plant foods hold good promise for diabetes

http://dx.doi.org/10.5772/57240

management. There are mounting scientific evidence to date on their various health-promoting properties.

The global concern for the diversification of the uses of plant foods to improve normal and therapeutic nutrition for diabetes control has shifted scientists' interest to enhancing the potential sources of beneficial constituents in plant foods. Plant foods have generated increasing research interest because of their anti-diabetic potentials. There is need to integrate traditional plant foods within local research and innovative systems, in accordance with local needs, food habits and priorities. Currently, documentations on Nigerian indigenous plant foods with anti-diabetic properties are either scattered or lacking. Most reviews on anti-diabetic potentials of plants both locally [19, 20, 21] and internationally [22, 23, 24] were done on medicinal plants. Evidently, not all medicinal plants and herbs used locally are edible. Similarly, not all identified food crops have anti-diabetic potentials. Most of the plants assayed pharmacologically present some difficulties in their dietetic application in humans. They create a gap in optimizing their health-promoting potentials. This paper focuses on some Nigerian indigenous plant foods with anti-diabetic potentials, parts used, their individual effects as reported *in vitro*/*in vivo* and the extent to which the elucidated parts of the plants were incorporated into the traditional diets for good glycaemic control. The scientific evidence for health benefits of the identified plant foods are summarized in tabular format, and the strength of the evidence is discussed in general terms. Optimization of the utilization of some commonly consumed indigenous anti-diabetic plant foods and their diversification would enhance good diabetes management, improve health of people with diabetes in Nigeria and offer more sustainable health benefits for the indigenous inhabitants.

2. Plant foods in human nutrition and health

Plant foods have remained the ultimate source of nutrients for larger population of the world. They are simply described as irreplaceable food resources for humans, which exclude animal sources. Besides, they are available, affordable and acceptable. They are used for socio-cultural, diabolic, nutritional and therapeutic purposes. These foods contain many chemical compounds needed for metabolic functions in varying proportions. Some of these chemical compounds are non-nutrients that are beneficial to man and others provoke some adverse reactions depending on the levels of intake, interrelationships of nutrients and food habits. Plant foods are classified as cereals, roots and tubers, legumes (pulses, oil seeds and nuts), vegetables and fruits [25]. In order to accommodate these various constituents in foods provided by plants foods, three main categories were established according to the major nutrients they provide. They include the macronutrients (carbohydrate, protein, fat and water), micronutrients (minerals and vitamins) and non-nutrient components (dietary fibre, phytochemicals, anti-nutrients, food toxicants and additives). Metabolic functions of these nutrients and non-nutrients were reviewed by several authors. Bennett [16] observed that plant foods provide the bulk of daily calories for humans [85%) and about 65% of the protein, an assortment of minerals and vitamins, unsaturated fats and phytochemicals in a characteristic manner that reflects current dietary recommendations aimed at promoting health and reducing diet-related chronic diseases. Thomas [26] concluded that the contribution a food makes to nutrient intake of a person depends on the quantity consumed per 100g, the amount consumed per meal and the frequency of consumption.

Obviously, plant foods have other values related to human nutrition and health apart from their nutritional importance. Plant foods are one of the elements in virtually all cultures, with symbolic and ritualistic values that link language and religion. In many cultures, especially the Asian countries, distinction between food and medicine as therapeutic agents is obscure as the traditional vegetable diets provide the people with disease fighting arsenals that serve both protective/preventive and curative functions. For this reason, foods are widely recognized as the primary health provider.

The bioactive compounds or secondary metabolites are the non-nutrient components in plant foods. They have some nutritional effects and health benefits. They are those substances contained in foods which supply no nutrients. They could contain some compounds that are beneficial to health or toxic to humans and/or act as antagonists to nutrients in foods [27]. They include tannins and other phenolic compounds (phenols, flavonoids, isoflavonoids), saponins, glucosinolates, alkaloids [28, 29], phytate and dietary fibre [30]. These chemical compounds are found in different classes and parts of plant foods in varying amounts. They are more concentrated in plant storage organs (leaves and seeds) than other parts of the plants [22]. These constituents have their individual health-promoting qualities that compel people to combine the different food sources to achieve healthy eating and maintain good health. Several authors [27, 31-35] studied therapeutic potentials and metabolic effects of foods rich in dietary fibre and phytochemical constituents. These include lower risk of colon cancer, promotion of early satiety and normal laxation, moderation of post-prandial blood glucose responses and improved insulin sensitivity, reduction in total and low density lipoprotein (LDL)-cholesterol, regulation of appetite and enhancement of sodium and fluid balance. They are also used to treat constipation and prevent development of diverticulosis and diverticulitis. These are features of a dietary pattern to treat and prevent obesity and its co-morbidities (especially type 2 diabetes mellitus). These two conditions are closely linked because hyperglycaemia and hypercholesterolaemia are well-known cardiovascular risk factors in type 2 diabetes mellitus. Invariably, diets adequate in dietary fibre are usually rich in micronutrients and phytochemicals, and frequently less calorically dense and lower in fat and added sugars. However, environmental factors, cultural food habits and insufficient nutritional information about health benefits of traditional plant foods still pose a problem to healthy food choices. Drewnowski and Gomez-Carneros [29] reported that most of the bioactive compounds are bitter, acrid or astringent and aversive to the consumer and may be wholly incompatible with consumer acceptance. These caused increasing epidemic of diet-related diseases across the regions. They suggest the need to take sensory properties and food preferences into account when advocating for increased consumption and diversification of rich sources of these secondary metabolites in plant foods. The challenge of achieving adequate supply of energy and nutrient intake as well as the health-promoting compounds from plant-based foods/diets without compromising the health of an individual, forms the basis for current dietary recommendations aimed at promoting consumption of plant foods to reduce diet-related NCDs.

3. Plant foods utilization in Nigeria

Nigeria's diverse ethnic groups (over 250] are accommodated under three main ethnic regions - Igbo (in the East), Yoruba (in the West) and Hausa-Fulani (in the North). The country has a beautiful climate, which endows it with very rich biodiversity. A variety of plant foods (maize, rice, sorghum, millet, yam, cassava, cocoayam and legumes) are mainly produced as subsistence food crops in Africa. They are more commonly and widely consumed in Nigeria and other developing countries than in the developed world. They are relatively available, affordable and acceptable. They contribute appreciably to the nutrient intake (energy, protein, fat, vitamins and minerals) of the less developed world. In Nigeria, starchy staples (cereals, roots/tubers) and legumes constitute the major part of the traditional diets (up to 70% and 25%, respectively) [8]. However, cereals are the major staples in the north with much higher intake of animal protein sources (mutton, beef and milk), while starchy roots and tubers are the main staples in the south with relatively more consumption of legumes [10]. These foods contribute appreciably to nutrient intake of southerners [36]. The plant foods are cultivated, gathered wild or are semi-wild.

Roots and tubers are the thickened underground starch storage organs of some plants, propagated vegetatively from the underground stems and their stem cuttings. These edible roots and tubers belong to several families and are formed by both monocotyledons (yams and cocoyams) and dicotyledons (cassava and sweet potatoes) [37]. Cereals are seeds of grass family (Gramineae). Cereals are important crops which serve as industrial raw materials and staple foods for the world over [38]. Cereals are the most widely cultivated and consumed crops globally. World cultivated cereals include wheat, maize, rice, barley, oats, rye, sorghum, millet, wild rice and hungry rice (acha). In Nigeria, the starchy staples (maize, rice, sorghum, millet, yam, cassava, cocoayam and plantain) are utilized in many different forms for preparation of various dishes. Their nutritional importance is that they provide most of the energy, contain high carbohydrate, low protein and appreciable amount of minerals and vitamins, especially the B-complex vitamins. They form the base and usually constitute the major ingredients in the traditional dishes. Some dishes are light and serve as breakfast. Others are solid and frequently made palatable in combination with a variety of legumes and by the addition of palm oil, vegetables and fruits, a range of spices, various sauces and fish/meats. They serve as main meals and eaten later in the day. Processing and preparation methods of these starchy staples and their recipes vary with ethic groups and geographical locations. Each of these staples irrespective of the preparation methods produces a thick paste known as "foofoo" eaten with soups/sauces. These dishes are highly cherished and consumed daily in all parts of Nigeria [39]. These starchy staples are also used to produce complementary foods and local snacks as roasted/fried/baked products or drinks. Some like yam, cocoyam, 'okoho' (*Cissus pulponea* root) are also used to thicken traditional soups.

Legumes are flowering plants in the family Fabaceae (or Leguminosae) that have pods, which contain beans or peas. According to Okafor [40], a list of edible woody leguminous plants, consisting of 150 species covering 103 genera in 48 families was recorded in Nigeria. Legumes rank second to the grasses as source of fodder (for animal) and food for man. The plants are most commonly known as pulses, peas or beans [38]. They contain more protein and less carbohydrate than cereals. There are two main types of legumes: those containing high protein

[25-35%) and oil content [15-45%) and those containing moderate protein [18-24%) and less than 5% oil content. They are oil seeds and pulses, respectively. The most common forms in which legumes are used – they may be cooked alone as pottage, or eaten in combination with any starchy staple of choice. The more widely consumed legumes include cowpea, pigeon pea, soyabean, bambara-groundnut, african yam bean, groundbean and lima bean. It is due to their high protein content that legumes are widely used in combination with cereals for production of nutritious complementary foods for infants and young children both in Nigeria and other developing countries, in both industrial and household levels. This is because legumes are deficient in sulphur-containing amino acids (methionine and cystine) and contain high amount of lysine. Cereals are deficient in lysine and rich in the sulphur-containing amino acids. Legumes play very important culinary roles as soup thickeners. Many of the leguminous seeds are used for thickening soups, sauces and stews in Nigeria [41]. These soup thickeners are condiments/ingredients used in preparation of local soups to alter their consistency and give them special flavour [42]. Traditionally, roots/tubers (yam and cocoayam, 'okoho'), vegetables (okro, 'ogbamu' leaves), legumes (grain legumes/oil seeds and nuts) and fungi are used for thickening soups. Soups made from them are basically prepared with meat and/or fish (when available), oil, vegetables, crayfish, pepper and other condiments and water to obtain watery or thick consistencies depending on their composition. These soups are traditionally consumed in combination with cereals and starchy roots/tubers, processed into a form of paste known as "foofoo". Soups are very important accompaniment to main dishes in Nigeria. Ene-Obong et al. [39] recorded 110 soup recipes out of 322 recipes in all the 6 geo-political zones in Nigeria. The total number of recipes documented reflects the biodiversity of the Nigerian food system. The high viscous property possessed by these leguminous soup thickeners is associated with their dietary fibre content, implicated in attenuation of post-prandial blood glucose and control of lipid metabolism [32].

Vegetables are succulent herbaceous plants that are harvested and eaten whole or in part, raw or cooked as part of a main dish or salad [43]. They can be classified into leaves (green, fluted pumpkin), stems/whole shoot (asparagus, elephant grass, 'achara'), roots (carrot), flowers, immature fruit (fresh corn, okra), mature green fruits (peppers), ripe fruit (tomato), fresh pod (vegetable cowpea), bulbs (onions), tubers (irish potatoes, yams) and fungi (mushrooms, puffballs). There are over 500 known edible vegetables in Africa. Some of these are valued for their bulking effect/thickening power and others may be used as garnishes or spices. Vegetables are generally low in calories and protein. They are valued most for high vitamins and minerals contents. They are low in sodium and rich in potassium, which helps to lower blood pressure [44, 45]. They also contain dietary fibre and phytochemicals (pigments and other compounds that impart flavour to foods), which have heart-disease fighting properties. However, fruits and vegetables consumption is generally low in Nigeria despite their recognition as very important food items to reduce nutrient deficiencies from inadequate intake of minerals and vitamins [46].

Composition of vegetables depends on their species, part of plant and stage of maturity. Spices are vegetables used as ingredients, which contribute to the taste and flavour of foods. The flavour of vegetables is due to sugars, organic acids, minerals salts, volatile sulphur compounds and tannins. The strong flavour of some vegetables (onions and cabbage) is due to their sulphur-containing compounds. Non-volatile acids such as malic, citric, oxalic and

http://dx.doi.org/10.5772/57240

succinic may also contribute to flavour in vegetables. The colour of vegetables depends on the pigments they contain. Spices are known to exert several physiological effects including antidiabetic influence [47]. Anthocyanins impart the blue, purple and red colours to vegetables such as tomatoes, garden eggs and red peppers. Chlorophyll imparts green colour to green leafy vegetables and carotenoids are responsible for the yellow colour in carrots, sweet potatoes and maize. Green leafy vegetables also contain carotenoids but this is masked by the more intense green of chlorophyll. The indigestible dietary fibres – cellulose, hemicelluloses and lignin give the vegetables their characteristics structure. However, some vegetables also contain pectin as storage carbohydrate, which has been linked to reduction of post-prandial hyperglycaemia. Data collection and assessment of commonly consumed foods in all the 6 geo-political zones in Nigeria published by Ene-Obong et al. [39] showed that fruit consumption was conspicuously absent in all the areas. Fruits are the fleshy or dry ripened ovary of a plant, enclosing the seeds. They are commonly eaten raw and used for desserts. Green and yellow vegetables are rich sources of beta-carotene and essential minerals. Most fruits, particularly the citrus species are abundant in vitamin C. These vitamins play antioxidant roles in the body and needs to be supplied in the diet.

4. Diabetes and its public health importance

The term "Diabetes" has been defined by many authors from different perspectives. However, the similarity in these definitions is that diabetes is a chronic metabolic disorder, characterized by high blood glucose (hyperglycemia), associated with impaired carbohydrate, fat and protein metabolism, resulting from either insufficient or no release of insulin by pancreas in the body [48, 49]. Diabetes mellitus is a chronic life-long disease, which has been known to mankind for over 2000 years. It requires careful monitoring and control. Currently, diabetes ranks fourth worldwide among the NCDs (cardiovascular diseases, cancers, chronic respiratory diseases and diabetes) with prevalence rates of 30%, 13%, 7% and 2%, respectively WHO [50]. It has been projected that by 2020 -2025, the number of people in the developing world with diabetes will increase by more than 2.5 fold; from 84 million in 1995 to 228 million in 2025 [7] and that 70% of deaths due to type 2 diabetes will occur in developing countries. Diabetes mellitus is increasingly being recognized as a major public health problem in developing countries.

Aetiological classification of diabetes mellitus includes type I diabetes (immune-mediated and idiopathic), type 2 diabetes, gestational diabetes and other specific types [48, 49]. However, types 1 and 2 diabetes mellitus appeared to have gained much more popularity among researchers and have generally been considered as the two major categories. In Africa, type 2 diabetes is the predominant form of diabetes in sub-Saharan Africa, accounting for over 90% of cases. The IDF Atlas [51] estimated that 10.8 million people have type 2 diabetes in sub-Saharan Africa in 2006 and this would rise to 18.7 million by 2025, an increase of 80%, as such exceeding the predicted worldwide increase of 55% [52]. In the past, the estimates on mortality of diabetes as the leading cause of death for sub-Saharan Africa were amongst the lowest for all regions globally [53]. This was attributed to Africa's rich biodiversity and high consumption of natural foods, which are rich in complex carbohydrates, proteins and dietary fibre.

There is enormous and escalating economic and social cost of treating type 2 diabetes. Sifelani [54] observed that the number of people seeking medical assistance for diabetes is rising in Africa at a time when health experts reported the continent's overburdened health systems are ill equipped to diagnose the disease. Majority of the poor cannot afford the cost of treatment. Cost of treating diabetes accounts for about 10% of the national income of most countries in Sub-Saahara Africa. National surveys in most parts of Africa indicate that diabetes cases are on the rise due to rapid urbanization as well as fast changing diets which are displacing the traditional ones in favour of the western diets [55]. This makes a compelling case for attempts to reduce the risk of developing diabetes.

Nigeria is among the top 5 countries that have the highest number of people affected by type 2-diabetes in sub-Saharan Africa. Nigeria has about 1.2 million people; South Africa, 841,000; the Democratic Republic of Congo, 552,000; Ethiopia, 550,000 and Tanzania, 380,000 living with diabetes. A national survey had an average prevalence rate of 2.7% with similar pattern in both sexes. There are slightly varying prevalence rates in different geographical locations [12]. Some sporadic figures on prevalence rates of diabetes in Nigeria were published. Cooper *et al.* [56] studied rural areas in Nigeria and found the prevalence of diabetics to be 2.8%. Wokoma [57] reported that the prevalence of diabetes in Nigeria ranges from 1% to 6%. International Diabetes Federation (IDF) [13] and [51] reported 2.2% and 3.9%, respectively, for type 2 diabetes in Nigeria. The annual increase was 0.3% in prevalence rate. A good number of people still live with it undiagnosed. The prevailing trend to replace the consumption of more complex forms of traditional diets with high intake of refined carbohydrates (Western) diets, in Nigeria, calls for great concern and urgent action. This is because carbohydrate (CHO) foods form over 70% of the local diets. The bleak account of national prevalence poses great challenges to individuals and the nation. Diabetes mellitus is a significant contribution to medical morbidity and mortality risk worldwide. Many factors are involved in its aetiology. The general risk factors include age, obesity, physical inactivity and family history/ previous history of gestational diabetes and poor eating habits. This is because intakes of good sources of dietary fibre such as fruits, vegetables, whole and high fibre grain products and legumes are low due to changes in dietary habit (nutrition transition) across the globe [58]. The main diabetes related risk factors include hyperglycaemia, hyperinsulinaemia/insulin resistance and microalbuminuria/proteinuria [59].

5. An overview of pathogenesis of type 2 diabetes mellitus

Several pathogenic processes are involved in the development of diabetes. Type 2 diabetes is characterized by excessive hepatic glucose production, reduced insulin action and insulin resistance. These alter the utilization of endogenously produced insulin at the target cells. These precipitate hyperglycaemia [60]. The pathogenesis of type 2 diabetes rests on the relationship between carbohydrate metabolism and insulin action. Consumed complex carbohydrates are metabolized to their monosaccharide constituents (glucose, galactose and fructose) in the gut. These monosaccharides have roles in nutrition. Glucose metabolism and absorption receive more attention in relation to diabetes. Glucose, absorbed into the blood stream, elevates blood glucose level. This rise in blood glucose stimulates the secretion of insulin from the beta-cells of the pancreas to regulate blood sugar levels by increasing active transport of glucose into fat and muscle cells. Post-prandially, blood glucose is absorbed and transported via the portal vein to the liver. The liver maintains blood glucose levels by converting glucose into glucose-6-phosphate and glycogen (glucogenesis). The increased insulin secretion from the pancreas and subsequent cellular utilization of glucose lowers blood glucose levels. Lower blood glucose level decreases insulin secretion. In diseased condition, insulin production is decreased to inhibit glucose uptake into the cells, which precipitates hyperglycaemia. The insulin secreted by the pancreas at this time is not used by the target cells. Hyperglycaemia is a common effect of uncontrolled diabetes and overtime, it causes serious damage to many body systems, particularly, the blood vessels and nerves. Common symptoms include glucosuria, frequent urination (polyuria), excessive thirst (polydypsia), excessive hunger (polyphagia), sudden weight loss, extreme tiredness and blurred vision.

Decreased amount of insulin in circulation decreases lipogenesis and increases lipolysis. Increased lipolysis releases fatty acids from adipose tissues. Fatty acids are also absorbed from the intestinal tract. The rapid release of fatty acids in the blood leads to hyperlipidaemia. The blood level of cholesterol increases, causing the development of atherosclerosis to occur at an earlier age than in non-diabetics and is more pronounced [61]. Elevated circulating levels of free fatty acids derived from adipocytes are the most likely link between insulin resistance and type 2 diabetes [60]. They contribute to insulin resistance by inhibiting glucose uptake, glycogen synthesis and glycolysis, and increasing hepatic glucose production. This leads to a decrease in intracellular concentration of glucose by a reduction in glucose-6-phosphate levels, implicating the glucose transport system as the rate-controlling step for free fatty acid-induced insulin resistance [62].

Free radicals and enhanced oxidative stress with reduced blood levels of anti-oxidants were implicated in the pathogenesis of diabetes and more importantly, in the development of diabetic complications [60, 63]. Free radicals are highly reactive molecules (charged superoxide, hydroxyl radical and nitric oxide). The uncharged hydrogen peroxide species is capable of damaging cellular molecules, DNA, proteins and lipids. These produce altered cellular functions. Oxidative stress is a serious imbalance between the production of free radicals and antioxidant defences. This causes potential tissue damage [64]. Antioxidants play protective role against the effects of hyperglycaemia and free fatty acids *in vitro*. They neutralize free radicals effects in experimentally-induced diabetes in animal models [60] and reduce the severity of diabetic complications [63].

6. Dietary approaches to the management of type 2 diabetes mellitus

A diet is a combination of foods individuals or community habitually eat to exist or live, or use for therapeutic purposes. Diet is known for many years to play a key role as a risk factor for chronic diseases [7]. Conventionally, type 2 diabetes is controlled with diet alone or diet and hypoglycaemic drugs (in combination with insulin in few cases where pancreas produces no insulin because of age). Objectives of dietary management of diabetes are to: achieve optimal blood glucose and blood lipid concentrations; provide appropriate energy for reasonable weight, prevent, delay and treat diabetes-related complications and improve health through optimal nutrition [65]. The general practice is to counsel people with diabetes on moderation of their food intake through proper food selection with incorporation of low GI foods that contain slowly digestible carbohydrates and increased consumption of dietary fibre-rich foods in combination with increased physical activity. Most often, diabetics are misinformed and advised to consume only those foods with low GI values. The restriction has two adverse effects: either the diabetics become too rigid with their food selection which might cause starvation and frequent hypoglycaemic attacks [66] or consume more carbohydrate per meal from the low GI diets. These precipitate poor diabetic control (hyperglycaemia). This has resulted in reduced intake or total avoidance of starchy staples and overall poor diabetes management in Nigeria with its attendant high cost of medical treatment. The types of foods/diets eaten in Nigeria vary tremendously and depend on several factors. Climate, environment, cost and availability of foods, and religious beliefs are among the factors. There are also significant differences in eating habits between the rural and urban populations. The latter increasingly adapt to western food habits [67]. The promotion of indigenous mixed diets still remains a powerful weapon in the fight against diabetes.

7. Dietary recommendations for type 2 diabetes mellitus

Nutrients are needed in certain amounts for good health. The type of food/diet people eat, in all their cultural variety, is a key universal factor that defines and affects people's health, growth and development. However, due to some environmental, genetic, physiological and metabolic factors, humans become susceptible to conditions that influence the body's homeostasis, nutrient intake and metabolism. To meet the challenges of optimizing nutrient utilization for specific conditions, dietary recommendations are made for various diet-related diseases. These are based on the causal factors and aim of dietary intervention in a particular disease condition. These involve consideration for the key nutrients in metabolic functions, their daily required amounts with reference to age and sex, their food sources and individual quantities of selected foods. These foods must offer desirable short or long-term health benefits without adverse effects. Dietary recommendations for prevention of diet-related chronic diseases and for people with diabetes were published by WHO [7] and American Diabetes Association [15], respectively. One major emphasis in these recommendations is that these diets should be close to normal (family) diet. In diabetes mellitus, the three energy-giving nutrients are involved. Based on this, adequate supply and intake of carbohydrate, protein and fat as well as micronutrients (vitamins and minerals) becomes an important factor to consider in diet and glycaemic control. The diet should contain 50-60% carbohydrate, 30-35% and 10-15% protein relative to the individual's total daily caloric allowance. Fruits, vegetables and spices are rich in bioactive constituents [68, 69]. Bioactive constituents (dietary fibre, phytochemicals and anti-oxidants) of plant foods are receiving attention with regard to their roles in diabetes management. Most studies used different fibre sources (legumes, cereals and leaves) at different levels of incorporation [5-15%) into single meals of subjects [70, 71, 72, 73]. These studies tend to support the American Diabetes Association (ADA) position [15] that the public should consume adequate amounts of dietary fibre from a variety of plant foods. Unfortunately, recommended dietary fibre intakes 20-35g per day for healthy adults and the aged [7], and 5g per day for children [74], respectively, are not being met. Recent studies have shown that high carbohydrate, high fibre diets have low glycaemic index and reduce blood cholesterol and triglyceride levels. This more flexible glycaemic index concept replaces the therapeutic distinction between simple versus complex carbohydrates. Quantification of bioactive compounds *in vivo* is costly and time consuming. Liu [75] reported that synergistic effects of phytochemicals in fruits and vegetables are best acquired through whole-food consumption, not from expensive dietary supplements. It is recommended that consumers should eat 400g or 5 servings of fruits and vegetables from a wide variety of fruits and vegetables/day.

One limitation of dietary recommendations is the problem of translating them into practical terms. This appears to be a major gap in knowledge, which should be explored to translate the accumulated scientific evidence of plant foods benefits into practical terms. FAO/WHO/UNU [76] recommended the food-based dietary guideline (FBDG) to address problem of dietary inadequacies and poor nutrient intake. This ensures supply of nutrients per 1000kcal (nutrient density) of the traditional diet as consumed relative to standard values. The concept is used to express required, desirable nutrient intake and population goals relative to energy intake. It strongly emphasizes that food-based approaches are the only sustainable strategy to improve the nutritional status of all. Its major advantages are - it is easy to adopt and implement; emphasizes changes that promote adequate vitamins and minerals, and reduce risks of food-borne illness, obesity, diabetes, cancers and CVD. It also portrays long term effects of diets as consumed [76]. For instance, a total of 15-20g dietary fibre/1000kcal and sodium 1000mg/1000kcal are recommended. McCarty [33] proposed a dietary 'phytochemical index' as a means of improving phytochemical nutrition of clients/patients. This index is the percentage of dietary calories derived from foods rich in phytochemicals. Calories derived from fruits, vegetables, legumes, whole grains, nuts, seeds, fruit/vegetable juices, soy products, wine, beer and cider- and foods compounded therefrom, would be counted in this index.

Harden et al. [77] advocated direct evaluation of GI of many meal combinations based on indigenous, more widely and frequently consumed foods. Two principal approaches were used to study the effects of increasing carbohydrate and fibre in diabetes management:

i. supplementation of the low fibre foods with fibre-rich sources (for instance, guar gum, flours from tallow tree, counter wood tree seeds and locust bean); and

ii. selective use of dietary fibre–rich foods.

Selective and holistic use of dietary fibre content of a mixed meal than the soluble non-starch polysaccharides (NSP) supplements has currently become of research interest. It is because the supplementation approach compromises sensory properties of indigenous food products with anti-diabetic potentials at clinically effective and acceptable levels [78]. Translation of the nutrient recommendations for specific conditions into foods for easy culinary application and appropriate nutrient intake is an integral part towards achieving the goals of dietary recommendations.

8. Problems associated with use of medicinal plants/traditional medicine and diabetes control

WHO reported that in several countries and areas, about 80% of the third world countries and 40-60% of total world population use traditional medicine instead of orthodox medicine for health-care. The process of extraction and purification of plant extracts affect the unit cost [3]. These expensive products are unaffordable for the low income countries. The low demand for drugs led to the use of medicinal plants as herbal components of health foods and for preventive medicine. This new expanding market gave rise to nutraceuticals (nutriceuticals). Culhane [5] reported nutraceuticals as "foods derived from a naturally occurring substance (in pills or powder or other medicinal forms), which can and should be consumed as part of the daily diet, and serves to regulate or otherwise affect a particular body process when ingested". These foods are known as medicinal foods, phytofoods, phytonutrients and functional foods. All of these terms meant substances that may or may not be considered as foods or parts of food but provide health benefits when eaten. However, more people prefer traditional medicine. This is because it provides holistic treatment (treatment that caters for the spirit, body and soul). The need for traditional medicine arose from the indigenous knowledge. This showed that aetiology of diseases does not only come from physiological imbalance and psychological causes as in orthodox medicine, but can come from spiritual causes, astral influence, esoteric causes and imbalance in cosmic natural forces. This could be associated with the belief by some diabetic patients that their condition is diabolical (personal communication). Every region has had, at one time or the other in its history, a form of traditional medicine. However, distinction exists between the use of traditional medicine and traditional plant foods as regards therapeutic agents used in diabetes management and health promotion. The misconception in the use of these indigenous medicinal plants precipitated self-medication when such plants are used. This poses serious problem in diabetes control in Nigeria. Consumers take medicinal plants, herbal products and nutraceuticals as food and think they are safe at any dose. Concerns raised about the interaction between herbal preparation and drugs are that herbal remedies might – i) increase the effect of an antidiabetic drug and plunge blood sugar to dangerously low level; ii) decrease the effect of blood pressure medication and cause high blood pressure and stroke; iii) decrease the effect of an anti-infection agent, letting the infection get out of control; iv) increase or decrease the effect of a blood thinner such as warfarin and cause either bleeding episode or formation of a dangerous clot. The combination of orthodox and traditional medicines has negative impact on people with diabetes in Nigeria. This may explain high incidence of cases of uncontrolled diabetes and associated complications in patients admitted in hospitals in Nigeria. The major link between the use of traditional medicine and traditional plant foods is that their uses are community-based and indigenous. Each community has its own peculiar approach to health and diseases even at the level of ethno-pathological perception of diseases and therapeutic behaviours. This gives indigenous knowledge in agriculture, medicine and health its diverse and pluralistic nature. The implication is that success for use of any indigenous plant foods that possess antidiabetic potential when incorporated into the family diets, could offer sustainable health benefits to the community/consumers of such plant foods.

9. Bioactive constituents and their effects on diabetes

Several terms have been used to describe the therapeutic potentials of plants. Health-promoting activities, bioactive constituents, medicinal properties (often used in orthodox and traditional medicine), natural plant products and biological response modifiers are examples of such terms. All plants, especially the wild ones, are potential sources of biological active molecules. These compounds protect plants against predators and other damage but are not directly essential for growth. They are known as secondary chemical compounds or metabolites. The plant constituents useful extractable substances in their storage organs (leaves and seeds/roots) in quantities sufficient to be economically useful as raw materials for various scientific technological and commercial applications [3].

Some plant constituents appear to be disease specific. The plants for consideration when a hypoglycaemic property of a plant is elucidated were reported. Ivorra et al. [28] studied different compounds isolated from plants with attributable hypoglycaemic activity. They gave a broad classification as follows: polysaccharides and proteins; steroids and terpenoids; alkaloids; flavonoids and related compounds. Drewnowski and Gomez-Carneros [29] and Noor et al [23] reported phenols and polyphenols, flavonoids, isoflavones, terpenes and glucosinolates in vegetables and fruits; Thompson et al. [79] included phytate in bean flour, which reduced GI. Iwu et al. [80] found alkaloids in yam. Several studies have published similar effects with dietary fibre (non-starch polysaccharides, NSPs) [31, 73]. A new classification of dietary fibre (water-soluble and insoluble dietary fibre) was based on their solubility characteristics [81]. The soluble dietary fibre is highly viscous and has added viscosity as functional property in the evaluation food/diets. These NSPs lower blood glucose level by impeding glucose absorption from the gastrointestinal tract and reduce post-prandial hyperglycaemia. The water-insoluble NSP are mainly obtained from structural carbohydrates (cellulose and lignin of cell walls) of starchy roots/tubers and cereals. The water-soluble NSP are obtained from storage carbohydrates (gum and hemicellulose) of legumes and as pectin from fruits and vegetables. The phytochemicals are basically sourced from fruits and vegetables.

Widely used parameters for clinical studies in diabetes are post-prandial blood glucose, glycaemic index (GI) and glycaemic load (GL). Jenkins et al. [82] introduced the concept of GI to classify both single foods and mixed meals on the basis of their potential for increasing the blood glucose concentration. The starchy foods have high GI (>70%) compared to the low values (<50%) for vegetables, fruits, legumes. The GL is defined as the product of the amount of available carbohydrate in a certain amount of food and its GI divided by 100 [83]. Low GI-based diets tend to maintain glucose and insulin at a moderate level avoiding the hyperglycaemic state [84]. This is based on advantages of the GI concept: i) GI and GL are determined both on single and mixed meals; ii) they permit proper selection and combination of low and high GI foods to achieve good glycaemic control and prevent hyperglycaemia; iii) they prevent fear of excessive intake of low or high GI foods and resultant hypoglycaemia/hyperglycaemia; and iv) hyperinsulinaemia is abated when both GI and GL are considered in dietary counselling. The link between GI and GL simply means that although both GI and GL elicit information on carbohydrate content of foods in relation to their blood glucose response. GI is associated with the quality of carbohydrate in a food/meal while GL relates to the overall quantity of carbohydrate in the same food/meal [85]. However, when these low GI (low GL) foods are habitually consumed in large amounts, high glycaemic effect may manifest over time. Based on this, attention is drawn to researchers on the limitation of the use of glycaemic index values alone in diabetes management. The practical application of the Gl, used in combination with other information on food composition, is promising in guiding good food choices, especially for people with diabetes. Englyst et al. [87] proposed the inclusion of rapidly digested starch (RDS) and slowly digested starch (SDS) to account for limitations of GI. More recently, resistant starch (RS) has received attention as one of the components of carbohydrate foods that are closely linked to glycaemic control [86]. Salijata *et al.* [34] observed that the justification of similarity of RS with NSP is that RS assays as insoluble fibre and has the physiological benefits of soluble fibre. They reviewed the importance of high amylose content and high amylose:amylopectin ratio in foods/diets in the post-pandrial glycaemic and insulinaemic responses. A higher amylose lowers digestibility of starch due to positive correlation between amylose level and formation of RS [88]. Plants with these hypoglycaemic activities collectively exert their effects in two major ways. They either improve insulin sensitivity to glucose at the peripheral cells to increase glucose uptake and reduce hyperglycaemia. Or, they act on insulin production-related actions to improve insulin production and control of blood sugar homeostasis.

Evans et al. [60] has reported that pathogenesis of diabetes is better appreciated and should be discussed in line with hyperglycaemia and elevated free fatty acid in the blood in relation to oxidative stress and production of free radicals. Some plants with hypolipidaemic activities were included by several authors as those that may assist in diabetes control. This is because diabetes and cardiovascular disease are closely related. The active ingredients identified *in vivo* for this purpose are antioxidants (vitamin A, beta-carotene, vitamin E and tannins) [89, 90]. The degree of these constituents in foods and their relative importance varies with the chemical compound, specie, part and age of the plant as well as environment. From the above perspective, the following operational definition will be used for documenting the antidiabetic potential/effects of identified plant foods. *Anti-diabetic plant foods/diets* are those plant foods/diets that contain any of the chemical compounds, shown to reduce hyperglycaemia or induce hypoglycaemia through their effect on the improvement of insulin resistance or insulin supply to the peripheral cells.

http://dx.doi.org/10.5772/57240

10. Documentation of anti-diabetic potentials of selected Nigerian indigenous plant foods

The 1978 Alma Ata declared that traditional medicine is the surest means to achieve total health care coverage of the world's population. This has encouraged the use of medicinal plants. Currently, the active ingredients in most plants with anti-diabetic potentials are elucidated pharmacologically. Consequently, it was a bit difficult to identify edible Nigerian indigenous plants from huge database on medicinal plants. Information on their constituents of nutritional importance was lacking. Invariably, not all traditional medicinal plants qualify as plant foods. Bosch et al. [91] as cited in Ogbu et al. [92] reported that the total number of species of edible plants in primary use in Africa is 1004. However, a little above 50% of the number of medicinal plants was reported as 1975. In Nigeria, Federal Environmental Protection Agency (FEPA) shows that 20 species of the plants were in extinction since 1950. Another 431 species are endangered, 45 species are classified as rare, 20 species are vulnerable and 305 species are endemic [93]. Not all plants with antidiabetic potentials published online may be available or edible in Nigeria. The local herbalists keep secret the information on health benefits of indigenous crops to enhance their patronage. Preliminary identification of the anti-diabetic potentials of these plant foods becomes necessary to improve their food diversification and consumption.

11. Sequence for literature review

Surveys on traditional food systems are commonly used to document information on indigenous foods with health-benefits [94]. Google search was used to review literature on published works on ethnobotanical surveys in northern and southern regions of Nigeria. These were used to identify commonly consumed indigenous plants. Some related unpublished works were also used to supplement published data. Information obtained include botanical names of the plant foods where available, habitat (cultivated (C), wild (W) or semi-wild (S)), part used, culinary uses, anti-diabetic potentials/effects of single foods and diets and corresponding references. From the profile of edible indigenous plant foods, those that have antdiabetic potentials were selected based on their bioactive constituents, proven to be active ingredients in attenuating post-prandial blood glucose. Additional information on anti-diabetic effects of some of the plant foods/diets evidenced by *in vivo* or *in vitro* studies were also elucidated.

12. Results

The concept of food groups of plant origin was used to present the results on documentation of Nigerian indigenous plant foods and those with anti-diabetic potentials. This was to encourage increased diversification and culinary uses. These food groups include fruits, vegetables, spices and condiments, grain legumes, nuts and oil seeds as well as starchy roots/

tubers/fruits and cereals. Forty-eight families of plant foods were identified. Out of 241 plant species (spp) identified, 80 fruits, 77 vegetables, 68 spices and condiments, 22 grain legumes/nuts/oil seeds and 19 starchy roots/tubers/fruits and cereals were documented. Twelve out of 22 grain legumes/nuts/oil seeds and 11 out of 19 roots/tubers/cereals were soup thickeners. Only 3 spp of fruits, 16 spp of vegetables, 27 spp of spices/condiments/grain legumes and 10 spp of starchy staples have anti-diabetic potentials *in vivo or in vitro* (Table 1]. Twenty-five indigenous diets as consumed had anti-diabetic effects (Tables 2]. Three of the *Candida tropicalis* fermented low GI starchy staple (cassava/maize/sorghum) flours were used to formulate high dietary fibre diets using food-based approach of 10% protein and 20g total dietary fibre/1000kcal in a 1:2 ratio of soluble: insoluble dietary fibre. The diets were composed of fermented cassava/maize/sorghum flours (commonly used to prepare thick paste traditionally known as "foofoo". They are eaten with traditional soup blended with *Cola gigantea* flour (a soup thickener) and other standard ingredients for rat bioassay to mimick traditional diets as consumed. These diets reduced post-prandial blood glucose concentrations of the diabetes-induced adult rats. More of the most commonly consumed vegetables than fruits were cultivated. The indigenous diets that had anti-diabetic effects did not contain any fruit group in their various recipes. They contained vegetables as part of the ingredients. This observation supports the report by Ene-Obong et al. [39]. It showed that fruit consumption was conspicuously absent in a survey of commonly consumed foods in all the 6 geo-political zones in Nigeria. The implication is that fruit intake as source of anti-oxidants and phytochemicals in Nigeria is disturbingly low and needs urgent intervention strategies. The low percentage of plants with proven anti-diabetic potentials underscores the need to explore anti-diabetic potentials of Nigerian rich biodiversity towards diversification of their utilization to optimize their health benefits. One significant observation (Table 2] is that apart from the *Afzelia*-cowpea pudding, all the diets investigated by various authors were based on starchy staples. These foods have high nutrient density and are consumed frequently and appreciably. They serve as desirable vehicles to improve utilization and consumption of phytochemical – and anti-oxidant–rich indigenous foods for improved diabetes control and prevention. However, the limitation of the work is that the identified diets were mostly reports from diets consumed in Southern Nigeria. There are wide variations in recipes used for the same traditional diets in many ethnic groups in Nigeria. The diets in this study may serve more or less as preliminary and/or available research work rather than representive of all Nigerian traditional diets. Another limitation is the differences in their concept and determination of "50g of digestible carbohydrate" of reference and experimental foods/diets. Some studies correctly determined the digestible carbohydrate contents of the food samples used, and some simply obtained the carbohydrate content by difference (proximate analysis). These discrepancies in the analytical methods pose some problems in the use of such available data. It calls for further clinical evidence-based studies to authenticate these claims for proper application in culinary practices and optimization of their health benefits.

Family name	Botanical name	C/W/S	Part studied and form in which the food was prepared for assay	Type of assay (AM = animal model)	Potential active ingredients	Anti-diabetic property	References
FRUITS							
Oleaceae	*Carica papaya*	W	Fruit	*In vivo*	Dietary fibre	Not determined	[95]
Myrtaceae	*Psidium guajava Linn.*	C	Fruit and fruit juice	*In vivo* (humans)			[96, 97]
Chrysobalanaceae	*Parinari curatollifolia*	W	Fresh fruit, paste		High viscosity	Not determined	[98]
VEGETABLES							
Bombacaceae	*Adansonia digitata*	W	Leaves extract	*In vivo*	Mucilage	Anti-hyperglycaemic	[99]
Cucurbitaceae	*Citrulus lanatus*	C	Seeds flour	*In vitro*	Dietary fibre	Not determined	[100]
Cucurbitaceae	*Telfairia occidentalis*	C	Ground leaves pulp	*In vitro; In vivo* (AM)	High phytochemical constituents (alkaloids, tannins, flavonoids, steroids, anthacyanin, carotenoides)	Antioxidant; anti-hyperglycaemic	[101, 102]
Cucurbitaceae	*Momordica charantia*	S	Fruit extract	*In vivo*	Phytochemicals	Anti-oxidant, anti-hyperglycaemic	[45, 24]
	Vernonia amygdalina	C	Ground leaf pulp	In vitro	High phytochemical constituents (alkaloids, tannins, flavonoids, steroids, anthacyanin, carotenoides)	Hypoglycaemic	[102, 103]
Labiatae	*Occimum gratissimum*	S	Ground leaf pulp	*In vitro*	The same constituents	Not determined	[102]
	Gnetum africana	S	Ground leaf pulp	*In vitro*	The same constituents	Not determined	[102]
Tiliaceae	*Corchorus olitorus*	W	Ground leaf pulp	*In vitro*	The same constituents	Not determined	[102]

Family name	Botanical name	C/W/S	Part studied and form in which the food was prepared for assay	Type of assay (AM = animal model)	Potential active ingredients	Anti-diabetic property	References
Fabaceae	*Pterocarpus santalinoides*	W	Ground leaf pulp	*In vitro*	The same constituents	Not determined	[102]
	Pterocarpus mildbreadii	S	Ground leaf pulp	*In vitro*	The same constituents	Not determined	[102]
	Abelmoschus esculentus	W	Pod	*In vivo* (animal model)	Mucilage, dietary fibre	Antioxidant anti-hyperglycaemic	[99, 104, 105, 106]
	Solanium melongena	C	fruit	*In vitro*	Phytochemical (anthocyanin)	Anti-oxidant	[45]
	Solanum tuberosum	C	Stem	*In vitro*	Resistant starch	Anti-hyperglycaemic	[45]
	Moringa olifera	S	Leaves and seeds extracts	*In vivo* in human & AM	Phytochemicals	Anti-hyperglycaemia; anti-lipidaemia	[107]
SPICES AND CONDIMENTS/ GRAIN LEGUMES, NUTS, OIL SEEDS							
Alliaceae	*Allium cepa var. aggregatum*	W	Dried bulb powder	*In vivo* (human & AM)	Anthocyanins	Anti-hyperglycaemia	[24, 47]
Alliaceae	*Allium sativa*	C	Bulb extract	*In vivo* (human/AM)	Anthocyanins (allicin)	Anti-hyperglycaemia	[47]
Euphorbiaceae	*Ricinus communis*	C	Seeds extract	*In vivo* (AM)	Not determined	Anti-hyperglycaemia	[108]
	Gongronema latifolium	C	Ground leaves pulp		High phytochemical constituents (alkaloids, tannins, flavonoids, steroids, anthacyanin, carotenoides)	Not determined	[102]
	Murraya koenigii	W	Leaves extract	*In vivo* (AM)	Not determined	Hypoglycaemic	[24, 47]

http://dx.doi.org/10.5772/57240

Family name	Botanical name	C/W/S	Part studied and form in which the food was prepared for assay	Type of assay (AM = animal model)	Potential active ingredients	Anti-diabetic property	References
	Zingiber officinale	W	Fresh or dried rhizome powder	*In vivo*	Not determined	Antihyperglycaemia	[24, 47]
	Piper nigrum	C	Fruit extract	*In vitro*	Flavonoids	Anti-oxidant	[45]
Piperaceae	*Piper guineense*	W	Fruit extract	*In vitro*	Flavonoids	Anti-oxidant	[45]
Vitaceae	*Cissus pulponea syn. rotundofolia*	W	Stem flour	*In vivo* (AM)	High viscosity, dietary fibre	Hypoglycaemic	[70]
Basidiomycetes	*Pleurotus tuberegium*	C	Sclerotium flour	*In vitro*	Dietary fibre	Not determined	[42]
Caesalpiniaceae	*Afzelia Africana*	W	Seeds flour	*In vitro*	Dietary fibre	Hypoglycaemic	[42, 73]
Caesalpiniaceae	*Brachystegia nigerica* Hoyle ex A. P. D. Jones	W	Seeds flour	*In vitro*	Dietary fibre	Not determined	[42]
Caesalpiniaceae	*Detarium microcarpum*	W	Seeds flour	*In vitro*	Dietary fibre	Hypoglycaemic	[42, 73]
Fabaceae	*Mucuna pruriens* (L.) D. C. var. utilis	C	Seeds flour	*In vitro*	Dietary fibre	Not determined	[42]
Fabaceae	*Mucuna sloanei* Fawcett	C	Seeds flour	*In vitro*	Dietary fibre	Not determined	[42]
Fabaceae	*Vigna unguiculata* (L.) Walp var. *unguiculata*	C	Seeds flour	*In vivo*	Dietary fibre	Antihyperglycaemic, anti-hyperlipidaemic	[106, 109]
Fabaceae	*Vigna unguiculata*	C	Seeds flour	*In vivo*	Not determined	Antihyperglycaemia, anti-hyperlipidaemia	[109]

Family name	Botanical name	C/W/S	Part studied and form in which the food was prepared for assay	Type of assay (AM = animal model)	Potential active ingredients	Anti-diabetic property	References
	(L.) Walp var. *dekindtiana*						
Fabaceae	*Arachis hypogea* (L.)	C	Seeds flour	*In vitro*	Mucilage	Not determined	[38]
Fabaceae	*Glycine max.* (L.)	C	Seeds flour	*In vitro*	Dietary fibre	Not determined	[110]
Irvingiaceae	*Irvingia gabonensis*	C	Seeds flour	*In vitro*	Soluble dietary fibre	Anti hypoglycaemic	[106, 111]
Irvingiaceae	*Irvingia wombulu*	S	Seeds flour	*In vitro*	Soluble dietary fibre	Anti-hypoglycaemic	[106, 111]
Lauraceae	*Bielschmedia gabonensis* (Meisn) Benth. ex Hook. f.	W	Seeds flour	*In vitro*	High viscosity, dietary fibre, low GI	Not determined	[112]
Papilionaceae	*Sphenostylis sternocarpa* (a. Rich.) Harms	C	Seeds flour	*In vitro*	Dietary fibre	Antihyperglycaemia, anti-hyperlipidaemic	[109]
Papilionaceae	*Vigna subterranean* (L.) Verdc.	C	Seeds flour	*In vitro*	Dietary fibre	Antihyperglycaemia, anti-hyperlipidaemic	[106, 109]
Papilionaceae	*Cajanus cajan* (L.) Millip.	C	Seeds flour	*In vivo*	Dietary fibre	Anti-hyperglycaemic	[42]
Sterculiaceae	*Cola gigantea*	W	Seeds flour	*In vitro*	High viscosity, dietary fibre, low GI	Not determined	[112]
Sterculiaceae	*Garcina cola*	C	Nuts		Not determined	Anti-oxidant, hypoglycaemic	[113, 114, 24]
STARCHY/ROOTS/TUBERS/FINGERS & CEREALS							
Dioscoreaceae	*Dioscorea documentum*	C	Tubers extract	*In vivo* (AM)	Alkaloids	Hypoglycaemic	[24]
Dioscoreaceae	*Dioscorea alata*	C	Tuber flour	*In vitro*	Dietary fibre	Not determined	[115]

Family name	Botanical name	C/W/S	Part studied and form in which the food was prepared for assay	Type of assay (AM = animal model)	Potential active ingredients	Anti-diabetic property	References
			Seeds flour	*In vitro*	Dietary fibre	Anti-hyperglycaemia	[116, 117, 118]
Poaceae	*Oryza sativa*	C	Seeds flour	*In vivo*	Dietary fibre, polyphenols and phytic acid	Anti-hyperglycaemic	[119]
Poaceae	*Zea mays*	C	Seeds, *Candida tropicalis* fermented flour	*In vitro*	Dietary fibre, low GI	Not determined	[120]
Poaceae	*Sorghum bicolor*	C	Seeds, *Candida tropicalis* fermented flour	*In vitro*	Dietary fibre, low GI	Not determined	[120]
Euphorbiaceae	*Manihot esculenta*	C	Roots, *Candida tropicalis* fermented flour	*In vitro*	Dietary fibre, low GI	Not determined	[120]
	Ipomea batatas	C	Leaf and stem extracts; stem	*In vivo* (AM)	Flavones ; dietary fibre	Anti-oxidant, hypoglycaemia;	[24, 121]
Musaceae	*Musa paradisica*	C	Unripe fruit flour	*In vivo* (animal model)	Saponins, flavonoids, tannins & alkaloids	Anti-oxidant, hypoglycaemia	[89]
	Abrus precatorius		Seeds flour	*In vivo* (AM)	Not determined	Hypoglycaemic	[24, 114]

C = Cultivated; W = Wild; Semi-wild = S

Table 1. List of identified Nigerian indigenous plant foods (single foods) with anti-diabetic potentials/effects by food groups

Name of local diet as consumed/ snacks/drinks	**Description of diet**	**Type of assay AM= animal model**	**Potential active ingredients**	**Anti-diabetic property**	**Ref.**
Detarium macrocarpum soup meal	Traditional soup prepared with *Detarium* seed flour, meat, fish, red palm oil, salt, spinach, fresh tomatoes, waterand consumed with boiled *Oryza sativa* seeds	*In vivo* (humans)	Dietary fibre	Hypoglycaemic	[122]
Detarium bread meal	Breadrolls prepared with *Detarium* seed flour and other basic bread ingredients (hydrogenated fat, improver, fresh yeast, water)	*In vivo* (humans)	Dietary fibre	Anti-hyperglycaemic	[123]
Sphenostylis sternocarpa gruel	Gruelprepared with *Sphenostylis* seed flour and water to produce a gruel	*In vivo* (humans)	Dietary fibre	Anti-Hyperglycaemic	[124]
Afzelia-cowpea moi-moi	Moi-moi (*V. unguiculata* seed pudding) prepared with *Afzelia* seed flour	*In vivo* (humans)	Dietary fibre	Anti-Hyperglycaemic	[72]
Gari with *afang* soup	Gari *with Gnetum africanum* leaf-based traditional soup prepared with modified recipe by Ana (125)	*In vivo* (AM)	Not determined	Anti-Hyperglycaemic	[126]
Pounded yam with *edikang ikong* soup	*Talinum triangulare* and *Telfairia occidentalis* leaves-based traditional soup prepared with modified recipe by Ana (125) and consumed with boiled yam (*Dioscorea rotundata)* tuber pounded into a thick dough	*In vivo* (AM)	Not determined	Anti-Hyperglycaemic	[126]
Ekpang nkukwo	Cocoayam *(Colocasia esculentum) corm/* wateryam (*Dioscorea alata) tuber* pudding prepared with modified recipe by Ana (125)	*In vivo* (AM)	Not determined	Anti-Hyperglycaemic	[126]
Plantain porridge with beans	*Musa paradisiaca* fruit cooked with *V. unguiculata* to produce a savoury dish with modified recipe Ana (125)	*In vivo* (AM)	Not determined	Anti-Hyperglycaemic	[126]
Afzelia-plantain based biscuits	*Afzelia* seed and plantain (*Musa paradisiaca*) finger flours prepared with other basic biscuit ingredients (baking fat, salt and water without sugar)	*In vivo* (humans)	Dietary fibre	Anti-Hyperglycaemic	[71]
Yam flour with *'ewedu'*	Cooked, thick paste made from *Dioscorea rotundata* tuber flour (*amala*) consumed with traditional soup	*In vivo* (humans)	Low GI	Hypoglycaemic	[127]

Name of local diet as consumed/ snacks/drinks	Description of diet	Type of assay AM= animal model	Potential active ingredients	Anti-diabetic property	Ref.
(Corchorus olitorius) soup	prepared with *Corchorus olitorius* leaves, tomato sauce, beef, salt, local spices				
Fermented cassava flour with *'ewedu' (Corchorus olitorius)* soup	Cooked, thick paste made from *Manihot esculenta* tuber flour (*lafun)*consumed with traditional soup prepared with *Corchorus olitorius* leaves	*In vivo* (humans)	Low GI	Hypoglycaemic	[127]
Maize flour with *'ewedu' (Corchorus olitorius)* soup	Cooked, thick paste made from *Zea mays* flour consumed with raditional soup prepared with *Corchorus olitorius* leaves	*In vivo* (humans)	Low GI	Hypoglycaemic	[127]
Fermented cassava flour with "ogbono soup	Cooked, thick paste made from *Manihot esculenta* flour (*lafun)* consumed with traditional soup prepared with Irvingia spp seeds	*In vivo* (humans)	High viscosity; reduced digestibility	Hypoglycaemic	[128]
Plantain flour with 'ogbono'soup	Cooked, thick paste made from *Musa parasidiaca* flourconsumed with traditional soup prepared with *Irvingia* spp seeds	*In vivo* (humans)	High viscosity; reduced digestibility	Hypoglycaemic	[128]
Fermented cassava flour with "egusi soup'	Cooked, thick paste made from *Manihot esculenta* root flourconsumed with traditional soup prepared with *Colocynthis citrillus* seeds	*In vivo* (humans)	High viscosity; reduced digestibility	Hypoglycaemic	[128]
Plantain flour with 'egusi soup'	Cooked, thick paste made from *Musa parasidiaca* flourconsumed with traditional soup prepared with *Colocynthis citrillus* seeds other ingredients	*In vivo* (humans)	High viscosity; reduced digestibility	Hypoglycaemic	[128]
Fermented cassava flour with pepper soup	Cooked, thick paste made from *Manihot esculenta* root flourconsumed with traditional soup prepared with *piper spp* and other ingredients	*In vivo* (humans)	High viscosity; reduced digestibility	Hypoglycaemic	[128]
Plantain flour with pepper soup	Cooked, thick paste made from *Musa parasidiaca* flourconsumed with traditional soup prepared with *piper spp* and other ingredients	*In vivo* (humans)	High viscosity; reduced digestibility	Hypoglycaemic	[128]

Name of local diet as consumed/ snacks/drinks	Description of diet	Type of assay AM= animal model	Potential active ingredients	Anti-diabetic property	Ref.
Boiled yam with fish stew	Boiled yam (*D. rotundata*) consumed with stew prepared fish, vegetable oil, fresh tomatoes, red pepper and vegetables	*In vivo* (human)	Dietary fibre	Anti-hyperglycaemic; anti-hyperlipidaemic	[129]
Cassava flour with vegetable soup	Cooked, thick paste made from *Manihot esculenta* root flourconsumed with traditional soup prepared with 'soup thickener' fresh vegetables, beef/fish, vegetable oil, fresh tomatoes and red pepper	*In vivo* (human)	Dietary fibre	Anti-hyperglycaemic; anti-hyperlipidaemic	[129]
Yam flour with vegetables stew	Cooked, thick paste made from *D. rotundata tuber* flour consumed with traditional soup prepared with 'soup thickener' fresh vegetables, beef/fish, vegetable oil, fresh tomatoes and red pepper	*In vivo* (human)	Dietary fibre	Anti-hyperglycaemic; anti-hyperlipidaemic	[129]
Boiled beans and boiled plantain with beef/fish stew	Boiled cowpea (*V. unguiculata*) and boiled *Musa parasidiaca* consumed with traditional soup prepared with 'soup thickener' fresh vegetables, beef/fish, vegetable oil, fresh tomatoes and red pepper	*In vivo* (human)	Dietary fibre	Anti-hyperglycaemic; anti-hyperlipidaemic	[129]
Fermented cassava/*C. gigantea* blend	*Candida tropicalis* fermented *Manihot esculenta* root flour blended with *Cola gigantea* seed flour and other basic ingredients for rat study to provide 10% protein and 20g total dietary fibre/ 1000kcal	*In vivo* (AM)	Dietary fibre, protein	Anti-hyperglycaemia	[130]
Fermented maize/ *C. gigantea*	*Candida tropicalis* fermented *Zea mays* seed flour blended with *Cola gigantea* seed flour and other basic ingredients for rat study to provide 10% protein and 20g total dietary fibre/1000kcal	*In vivo* (AM)	Dietary fibre, protein	Anti-hyperglycaemia	[130]
Fermented sorghum/C. gigantea	*Candida tropicalis* fermented *Sorghum bicolor* seed flour blended with *Cola gigantea* seed flour and other basic ingredients for rat study to provide 10%	*In vivo* (AM)	Dietary fibre, protein	Anti-hyperglycaemia	[130]

http://dx.doi.org/10.5772/57240

Name of local diet as consumed/ snacks/drinks	Description of diet	Type of assay AM= animal model	Potential active ingredients	Anti-diabetic property	Ref.
	protein and 20g total dietary fibre/ 1000kcal				
C = Cultivated; W = Wild; Semi-wild = S					

Table 2. List of identified Nigerian indigenous plant-based diets with anti-diabetic effects

13. Conclusions and recommendations

Diet therapy, undisputedly, has long been recognized as key tool in the clinical management of diabetes. The challenge centres on how to translate the existing scientific evidence into practical terms for individual and household application in the management of diabetes mellitus. Relatively, a few clinical studies were published in Nigeria. Widely used parameters for diabetes-related clinical studies in Nigeria are post-prandial blood glucose response, anti-oxidant activity, lipid profiles and GI of diets. Most of the studies conducted on single foods were on dietary fibre. Much more indepth research is needed on phytochemical constituents of the rich national flora as regards phytochemical index and diabetes control. This is because health benefits of these indigenous plants are of public health importance. Based on recent documentation, Nigeria is rich in varieties of plant foods. Only a few varieties or cultivars were captured relative to diverse nature of Nigeria. It has generated a database for future investigations. Relevant research outputs on the plant foods would encourage diversification and increase consumption to maintain dietary adequacy and optimize their health benefits/ therapeutic potentials.

Much of the *in vivo* studies on antidiabetic effects of indigenous diets were conducted on human subjects. Levels of incorporation of fruits and vegetables into the traditional recipes are inadequate. The recipes used for traditional diets vary from one region/ethnic group to another in Nigeria. The variations in recipes for these diets might influence their nutrient concentrations and effects on blood glucose level. It is imperative to fill this gap using FBDG. This guideline proposed by FAO/WHO/UNU [76] has not been embraced and applied widely to enhance their health benefits in communities despite its advantages over the traditional and orthodox medicine. Rat study model to simulate this approach using high dietary fibre plant-based diet showed that traditional mixed diet as consumed can attenuate post-prandial blood glucose concentration in diabetic adult rats. There is research need to focus on wider varieties of traditional diets as consumed in Nigeria.

The goal for optimizing the use of indigenous plants with anti-diabetic potentials to control and prevention type 2-diabetes rests on conducting controlled clinical trials using food-based approach as the last step to establish their efficacy in humans. Evidently, these diets adequate in macronutrients, micronutrients and phytochemicals can retard and prevent diabetic complications. Optimum utilization of these indigenous anti-diabetic plant foods in Nigeria and their diversification would enhance management of diabetes and improve health of people in the communities.

Author details

Elizabeth A. Udenta[1*], Ikemefuna C. Obizoba[1] and Oluwafemi O. Oguntibeju[2]

*Address all correspondence to: elizabeth.udenta@unn.edu.ng

1 Department of Home Science, Nutrition and Dietetics, Faculty of Agriculture, University of Nigeria, Nsukka, Nigeria

2 Oxidative Stress Research Centre, Department of Biomedical Sciences, Cape Peninsula University of Technology, Bellville, South Africa

References

[1] Kuhnlein, H. V. and Receveur, O. Dietary change and traditional food systems of indigenous peoples. *Annual Review of Nutrition* 1996; 16: 117-142

[2] Food and Agriculture Organization (FAO). *Promoting under-exploited food plants in Africa- A brief for policy makers.* FAO/UN, Rome; 1987.

[3] Balandrin, M.F., Klocke, J. A., Wurtele, E. S & Bollinger, W. H. Natural plant chemicals: Sources of industrial and materials. *Science* 1985; 228: 1154-1160.

[4] Nyam News. *Phytochemicals*. Caribbean Food and Nutrition Institute, Jamaica, W.I. 2005; (1) & (2): 1-4.

[5] Culhane, C. *Nutraceuticals /funtional foods - an exploratory survey on Canada's potential (for Agriculture and Agro-food Canada).* Summary report, International Food Focus Limited Toronto ON.Ca; 1995 p9.

[6] World Health Organization (WHO). *The world health report* WHO 2009, Geneva, Switzerland.

[7] WHO *Diet, nutrition and the prevention of chronic diseases.* Report of a joint WHO/FAO Expert Consultation. Geneva, Switzerland; 2003.

[8] Okeke, E. C., Mbah., B. N. & Nwosu, M. O. Field survey of indigenous African food crops and useful plants, food preparations from them and home gardens. UNU/

INRA Programme on Natural Resources Survey, Nairobi Kenya Series No. B5 (c); 1993.

[9] Europa. Nigeria In: *Africa South of the Sahara*, 27th Edition; 1998. p780 – 806.

[10] Maziya-Dixon, B., Akinyele, I. O., Oguntona, E. B., Sanusi, R. A. and Harris, E. Nigeria food consumption survey 2001 – 2003. Ibadan, Nigeria. IITA; 2004

[11] Nicholas, K. Diabetes education and psychological care. *Practical Diabetes International* 1996; 13: 383- 355.

[12] Federal Ministry of Health. National Expert Committee on Non-Communicable Diseases in Nigeria: Report of a national survey. Federal Ministry of Health, Lagos, Nigeria;1992

[13] International Diabetes Federation (IDF) *Diabetes Atlas*, 2nd ed.. Brussels, IDF; 2003.

[14] Hoet, J. J. The role of foetal and infant growth and nutrition in the causality of diabetes and cardiovascular disease in later life. Sub-Committee on Nutrition News 1992; 14: 10 - 13.

[15] American Diabetes Association. Nutrition recommendations and principles for people with diabetes. (Position statement). *Diabetes Care* 1999; 22 Supplement 1.

[16] Bennet, B. C. Plant as foods. Economy Botany. UNESCO-Encyclopedia of Life Support Systems (EOLSS); 2009.

[17] Cleave, T. L. The neglect of natural principles in current medical practice. *Journal of the Royal Naval Medical Service* 1956; 42: 55-82

[18] Burkitt, D. P., Walter, A. R. P & Painter, N. S. Dietary fibre and disease. *Journal of American Medical Association* 1974; 299: 1068-1074.

[19] Olowokudejo, J. D., Kadiri, A. B. & Travih, V. A. An ethnobotanical survey of herbal markets, and medical plants in Lagos state of Nigeria. *Ethnobotanical leaflets* 2008; 12: 851-865.

[20] Odugbemi, T. & Ayoola, A. Medicinal plants from Nigeria: an overview. In: Odugbemi, T. (ed.). *A text book of medicinal plants from Nigeria*. Lagos, Nigeria: University of Lagos press; 2008. p 9-17.

[21] Fred-Jaiyesimi, A. A. & Ajibesin, K. K. Ethnobotanical survey of toxic plants and plants parts in Ogun state, Nigeria. *International Journal of Green Pharmacy* 2012; 6 (3): 174-179.

[22] Chan, C., Ngoh, G. & Yusoff, R. A brief review of antidiabetic plants: Global distribution, active ingredients, extraction techniques and mechanisms. *Pharmacognosy Reviews* 2012; 6 (11): 22-28

[23] Noor, A., Bansal, V.S. & Vijayalakshmi, M. A. Current update on anti-diabetic biomolecules from key traditional Indian medicinal plants. *Current Science* 2013; 104 (6): 721-727.

[24] Mukesh, R. and Namita, P. Medicinal plants with anti-diabetic potential- A review. *American – Euroasian Journal of Agriculture and Environmental Sciences* 2013; 13 (1): 81-94

[25] Osagie, A. U. and Eka, O. U. *Nutritional quality of plant foods.* Ugbowo, Benin City: Ambik Press; 1998.

[26] Thomas, B., editor. *Manual of Dietetic Practice*. Second edition. Oxford, London. Blackwell Scientific Publication; 1994.

[27] Soetan, K.O. Pharmacological and other beneficial effects of anti-nutritional factors in plants – a review. *African Journal Biotechnology* 2008; 7 (25): 4713-4721.

[28] Ivorra, M. D., Paya, M. & Villa, A. A review of natural products and plants as potential anti-diabetic drugs, *Journal of Ethnopharmacology* 1989; 27: 243-275.

[29] Drewnowski, A & Gomez-Carneros, C. Bitter taste, phytonutrients and the consumer: A review. *American Journal of Clinical Nutrition* 2000; 72, 1424-1435.

[30] Gibson, R. S. The role of diet-and host-related factors in nutrient bioavailability and thus in nutrient-based dietary requirement estimates. *Food and Nutrition Bulletin* 2007; 28 (1) (supplement): S77-S100

[31] Jenkins, D. J. A., Kendall, C. W. C., Marchie, A., Jenkins, L. A., Livia, S. A. A., Ludwig, D. S., Neal, D. B. & Anderson, J. W. Type II diabetes and the vegetarian diet. *American Journal of Clinical Nutrition* 2003; 78 (3): 610S – 616S.

[32] Champ, M., Langkilde, A., Brouns, F., Kettlitz, B & Collet, Y. Advances in dietary fibre characterization. 1. Definition of dietary fibre, physiological relevance, health benefits and analytical aspects. *Nutrition Research Reviews* 2003; 16: 71-82.

[33] McCarty, M. F. Proposal for a dietary "phytochemical index". *Medical Hypothesis* 2004; 63 (5): 813-817.

[34] Salijata, M.G., Singhal, R. S & Kulkarni, P. R. Rsistant starch: A review. *Comprehensive Review in Food Science and Food Safety* 2000; 5: 54-93.

[35] Vikas, K., Amit, K. S. Harinder, P. S. M. & Klaus, B. Dietary roles of phytate and phytase in human nutrition: A review. *Food Chemistry* 2010; 120: 945-959.

[36] Okeke, E. C. (1988). Dietary habits, nutrients intake and energy expenditure of low income rural farm households in the derived Savana area of Anambra State, Nigeria. Ph.D. Thesis, Department of Home Science and Nutrition, University of Nigeria, Nsukka.

[37] FAO. FAO production year book. Food and Agriculture handbook. Rome. FAO/UN 495; 1985.

[38] Enwere, N. J. *Foods of plant origin*. 1st ed. Nsukka, Nigeria: Agro–Orbis Publications; 1998.

[39] Ene-Obong, H. N., Sanusi, R. A., Udenta, E. A., William, I. O., Anigo, K. M., Chibuzo, E. C., Aliyu, H. M., Ekpe, O. O. & Davidson, G. I. Data collection and assessment of commonly consumed foods and recipes in six geo-political zones in Nigeria: Important for the development of a National Food Composition Database and dietary assessment, *Food chemistry* 2013 (in press) http://dx.doc.org/10./016/j.fdchem. 2013.01.102.

[40] Okafor, J. C. Edible indigenous edible plants in the rural economy of the Nigerian forest zone. In: Okali, D. U. U. (ed). *The Nigerian rain forest ecosystem*. 1979. p262.

[41] Udenta, E.A., Thomas, J. and Ellis P. R. Documentation and botanical characterization of leguminous seed crops and polysaccharide plant materials used as thickening agents in Southern Nigeria. A final project report (FAO Project PR. 18496) presented to FAO at King's College, London in June, 2004.

[42] Ene-Obong, H.N. and Carnovale, E. Nigerian soup condiments: Traditional processing and potential as dietary fibre sources. *Food Chemistry* 1992; 43: 29-34.

[43] Uzo, J. O. Vegetable crops in Nigeria's agriculture. In: Mbah, B. N. and Nnanyelugo, D. O. (ed.) *Food crop production, utilization and nutrition.* Ibadan, Nigeria: Dotan publications limited; 1989. p39-44.

[44] Smith, I. F. Use of Nigerian leafy vegetables for diets modified in sodium and potassium. Nigerian Journal of Nutritional Sciences 1983; 4, 21-27.

[45] Dias, J. S. Nutritional quality and health benefits of vegetables: A Review. *Food and Nutrition Sciences* 2012; 3: 1354-1374.

[46] Garrow, J. S. and James, W. P. T. (eds.) *Human nutrition and dietetics.* 9th ed. Edinghburgh, United Kingdom: Churchill Livingston, 1998.

[47] Scrinivasan, K. Plant foods in the management of diabetes mellitus: Species as beneficial anti-diabetic food adjuncts. *International Journal of Food Sciences and Nutrition* 2005; 56 (6): 399-414.

[48] WHO. *Diagnosis and classification of diabetes mellitus and its complications*. Report of a *WHO consultation.* Part 1. World Health Organisation, Geneva (document WHO/NCD/NCS/99.2) (1999).

[49] American Diabetes Association (ADA). Diagnosis and classification of diabetes mellitus. *Diabetes Care* 2012; 35 (Supplement 1) S64-S71

[50] WHO. *The global burden of disease*: 2004 Update. Geneva, Switzerland: WHO; 2008.

[51] International Diabetes Federation (IDF). Diabetes Atlas (3rd ed.). *Diabetes Voice* 2007; 52 (1), 46-48.

[52] Levitt, N. S. Diabetes in Africa: Epidemiology, management and healthcare challenges. In: Global burden of cardiovascular diseases. *Heart* 2008; 94: 1376-1382.

[53] Roglic, G., Unwin, N. & Bennett, P. The burden of mortality attributable to diabetes. *Diabetes Care* 2005; 28: 2130-2135.

[54] Sifelani, T. *Diabetes in Africa; A day in black history.* Harare, Zimbabwe; 2006.

[55] Mbanya, J. N., Motala, A. A., Sobngwi, E., Assah, F. K. & Enoru, S. T. Diabetes in sub-Saharan Africa. Lancet 2010; 375: 22254-2266

[56] Cooper, R., Rotimi, C., Kaufman, J., Owoaje, E., Fraser, H., Forester, T., Wilks, R., Riste, L. K. and Cruikshank, J. K.. Prevalence of NIDDM among populations of the African Diaspora. *Diabetes Care* 1997; 20.

[57] Wokoma, F. S. Hypertension in non-isulin dependent diabetes mellitus patients in Nigeria. *Diabetes International* 2002; 9 (3): 58.

[58] Popkin, B. M. The shift in the stage of Nutritional Transition in the Developing World Differs from past experiences. *The Journal of Public Health* 2002; 5:205-214.

[59] Geissler, B. & Powers, A. R. *Human nutrition.* Amsterdam ; Elsevier Applied Science Publisher; 2005.

[60] Evans, J.L., Goldfine, I. D., Maddux, B. A. & Grodsky, G. M. Oxidative stress and stress-activated signaling pathways: A unifying hypothesis of type diabetes mellitus. *Endocine reviews* 2002; 23: 299-622.

[61] Khan, A & Ahmed, I. Biochemical nature of diabetes mellitus. *Diabetes Journal* 1993; 5: 9-15.

[62] Shulman, G.I. Cellular mechanism of insulin resistance. *Journal of Chemical Investigation* 2000; 106, 171-176.

[63] Lipinski, B. Pathophysiology of oxidative stress in diabetes mellitus. *Journal of Diabetes Complications,* 15, 203-210.

[64] Halliwell, B. Anti-oxidant characterization, methodology and mechanism. Biochemical Pharmacology 1995; 49:1341-1348.

[65] Association for Dietetics in Southern Africa (ADSA) *Dietary management of patients with diabetes mellitus.* Position paper: 1996.

[66] Macdonald, I. Diabetes and hypoglycaemia: An update. *Carbohydrate* 1998; 9 (1): 1-3.

[67] Naidu, R. Dietary management of diabetes in Africa. (Review). *Diabetes International* 2000; 10 (1).

[68] Asif, M. The role of fruit, vegetables and spices in diabetes. *Journal of Nutrition, Pharmacology and Neurological Diseases* 2013; 1 (1): 27-35.

[69] Khan, A. & Safdav, M. Role of diet, nutrients, species and natural products in diabetes mellitus. *Pakistan Journal of Nutrition* 2003; 2 (1): 1-12.

[70] Onyechi, A. U., Judd, P. A. & Ellis P. R. African plant foods rich in non - sugar polysaccharides reduce post-prandial blood glucose and insulin concentrations in healthy human subjects. *British. Journal of Nutrition,* 1998; 80: 419 – 428.

[71] Odo, I. F. The post-prandial blood glucose response of diabetes to snacks (biscuits) developed from *Afzelia Africana* and plantain (Musa paradisiaca) flours. B. Sc. Thesis, Department of Home Science, Nutrition and Dietetics, University of Nigeria, Nsukka; 1998.

[72] Odenigbo, U. M. Incorporation of *Afzelia africana* (Akpalata) in Dietary management of Type 2 Diabetes mellitus in Nnewi, Anambra State, Nigeria. Ph. D. Thesis. Department of Home scienece and Nutrition, University of Nigeria, Nsukka; (2001).

[73] Onyechi, U. A. A comparative study of the effect of three plant foods high in soluble non starch polysaccharide on rat metabolism. *Nigerian Journal of Nutritional Sciences* 2009b; 30 (1): 122- 129.

[74] Kritchevsky, D. Dietary fibre. *Annual Review of Nutrition* 1988; 8: 301 - 328.

[75] Liu, R. H. Potential synergy of phytochemicals in cancer prevention: Mechanism of action. *The Journal of Nutrition* 2004; 134: 3479S-3485S.

[76] FAO/WHO/UNU. *Preparation and use of food-based dietary guidelines*. Report of a joint FAO/WHO Consultation, Nicosia, Cyprus. 1996. p.15-29

[77] Harden, K. E., Judd, P. A. & Hockaday, T. D. R. Glycaemic responses in type 2 diabetic patients to various mixed meals taken at home. *Diabetes Medicine* 1993; 10: 654-659.

[78] Ellis, P. R. The effect of fibre on diabetes. In: Hill M. (ed.). *The right fibre for the right disease*. International congress and symposium series, 236. London; The Royal Society of Medicine Press Ltd; 1999.

[79] Thompson, L. U., Button, C. L. & Jenkins, D. J. A. Phytic acid and calcium affect the *in vitro* rate of navy bean starch digestion and blood glucose response in humans. *American Journal of Clinical Nutrition* 1987; 46: 467-473.

[80] Iwu, M. M., Okunji, C. O. Aka, P. Diodcoretine: the hypoglycaemic principle of Dioscorea documentum tubers. Planta Medica1990; 56; 119-120.

[81] Gray, J. *Carbohydrates: nutritional and health aspects*. Europe: International Life Science Institute; 2003. p1-30.

[82] Jenkins, D. J. A., Wolever, T. M. S. & Taylor, R. H. Glycaemic index of foods: a physiological basis for carbohydrate exchange. *American Journal of Clinical Nutrition* 1981; 134: 362-366.

[83] Brennam, C. S. Dietary fibre, glycaemic response and diabetes. *Molecular Nutrition and Food Research* 2005; 49: 560-570.

[84] Augustin, L. S., Franceschi, S., Jenkins, DJA., Kendall, C. W. C., & La Vecehia, C. Glycaemic index in chronic disease: A Review. *European Journal of Clinical Nutrition* 2002; 56: 1049-1071.

[85] Mendosa, D. The glycaemic index. Mendosa.com living with diabetes (no date).

[86] Nugent, A. P. Health properties of resistant starch. *British Nutrition Foundation Nutrition Bulletin* 2005: 30, 27-54.

[87] Englyst, K. N., Vinoy, S., Englyst, H. N. & Lang, V. Glycaemic index of cereal products explained by their content of rapidly and slowly available glucose. *British Journal of Nutrition* 2003; 89: 329-339.

[88] Berry, C. S. Resistant starch, formation and measurement of starch that survives exhaustive digestion with amylolytic enzymes during the determination f dietary fibre. *Journal of Cereal Science* 1986 ; 4: 301-314.

[89] Atawodi, S. E. Anti-oxidant potential of African medical plants. *African Journal of biotechnology* 2005; 4 (2): 128- 133

[90] Eleazu, C. O & Okafor, P.N. Anti-oxidant effect of unripe plantain (*Musa paradisica*) on oxidative stress in alloxan-induced diabetic rabbits. *International Journal of Medicine and Biomedical Research* 2012; 1 (3): 232-241.

[91] Bosch, C. H., Siemonsma, J. S. Lemmens, R. H. M. J. & Oyen, L.P.A. Plant resources of tropical Africa basic list of species and commodity grouping. PROTA Programme. Wageningen, The Netherlands: 2002. p7-12.

[92] Ogbu, J. U., Essien, B. A. Essien, J. B. & Anaele, M. U. Conservation and management of genetic resources of horticultural crops in Nigeria: Issues and biotechnological strategies. *Journal of Horticulture and Forestry*, 2010; 2 (9): 214-222.

[93] Adejuwon, J. O. Biotic resources. In: Ajaegbu, H. I. St. Mathew-Daniel, B. J. & Uya, O. E (eds). Nigeria: *A people united, a future assured*. Calaber; Gabumo publishers: 2000. p91-96.

[94] Kuhnlein, H., Erasmus, B., Cree-Kanashiro, H., Englberger, L. Okeke, C., Turner, N., Allen, L. & Bhattacharjee, L on behalf of the whole group. Indigenous peoples' food systems for health: finding interventions that work. *Public Health Nutrition 2006*; 9 (8): 1013-1019.

[95] Boogmans, B. Ethnobotanical survey of West African vegetable food in the Netherlands. NHN, Leiden University. (no date).

[96] Cheng, J. T. & Yang R.S. Hypoglycaemic effect of guava juice in mice and human subjects. *American Journal of Clinical medicine* 1983; 11 (1-4): 74-76.

[97] Jimenze-Escrig, A., Rincon, M., Pulido, R., & Saura-Calixto, F. Guava fruit (*Psidium guajawa* Linn.) as a new source of anti-oxidant and dietary fibre. *Journal of Agricultural and Food Chemistry* 2001; 49: 5489-5493

[98] Alyegba, S. S., Roy, M. & Ioryem, D. B. Ethnobotamical survey of edible wild plants in TIV communication of Benue state, Nigeria. *Journal of Natural Science Research* 2013; 3 (7): 17

[99] Woolfe, M. L., Chaplin, M. F., & Otchere, G. Studies on mucilages extracted from okra fruits (*Hibiscus esculentus* L.) and baobab leaves (*Adansonia digitata* L.). *Journal of the Science of Food and Agriculture* 1977; 28 (6): 519-529.

[100] Ibeanu, V. N., Onyechi, U. A., & Ugwuanyi, G. U. Nutrient and dietary profile of dehulled and undehulled seeds of sweet princess water melon (Citrullus lanatus) consumed in Nigeria. *International Journal of Basic and Applied Sciences* 2012; 12 (6): 249-252.

[101] Eseyin, O. A., Oforah, E., Dooka, B. D. Preliminary study of hypoglycaemi action of the extract of leaf of *Telfairia occidentalis* in normoglycaemic guinea pigs. *Global Journal of Pure and Applied Science* 2000; 6: 639-641.

[102] Onyeka, E. U. & Nwambekwe, I. O. phytochemical profile of some leafy vegetables in South-east, Nigeria. *Nigerian Food Journal* 2007; 25 (1): 67-76

[103] Nwanjo, H. U. Efficacy of aqueous leaf extract of *Vernonia amygdalina* on plasma lipoprotein and oxidative status in diabetic rat models. *Nigerian Journal of Physiological Sciences* 2005; 20 (1-2): 39-42.

[104] Adetunji, F. O. Anti-oxidant degradation in six indigenous okra *Abelmoschus esculentus* (L) Moench varieties during storage in Nigeria. *Journal of Food Technology* 2008; 6(5): 227-230.

[105] Zhenzhong, X., & Hongium, S. Effects of okra capsule combined with valsartan in treatment of early diabetic nephropathy with microalbuminuria. *Modern Journal of Integrated Traditional Chinese and Western Medicine* 2010; 3.

[106] Tanya, A.K. N., Mbofung, C. M. F. & Keshinro, O.O. Soluble and insoluble fibre content of some Cameroonian foodstuffs. *Plant Foods for Human Nutrition* 1997; 51: 199-207.

[107] Fahey, J. W. Moringa oleifera: A review of the medical evidence for its nutritional therapeutic and prophylactic properties. Part I. *Trees for Life Journal* 2005; 1(5).

[108] Rao, M. U., Screenivasulu, M., Chengalah, B., Reddy, K. J. &Chetty, C. M. Herbal medicines for diabetes mellitus: A review. *International Journal of PharmTech Research* 2010;. 2 (3): 1883-1892.

[109] Rotimi, S.O., Olayiwola, I. Ademuyiwa, O & Adamson, I. Improvement of diabetic dyslipidemia by legumes. *African Journal of Food, Agriculture, Nutrition and Development* 2013; 13 (2): 7606-7623

[110] FAO. *Legumes in human nutrition*. No. 20, Rome; 1982.

[111] Adamson, I., Okafor, C. & Abu, B. A. A supplement of dikanut (*I. gabonensis*) improves treatment of type 2 diabetes. *West African Journal of Medicine* 1990; 9: 108-115.

[112] Udenta, E. A. and Obizoba, I. C. Physico-chemical profile and *in vitro* glycaemic index of two under-utilized leguminous seeds used as soup thickeners in Nigeria. A paper presented at the Nutrition Society of Nigeria 42nd Annual General Meeting and Sientific Conference on "Nutrition, Food Security, MDGs and National Development" held at Nelrose Hotel, Asaba, Delta State, Nigeria from 18th-22nd September, 2012. Book of Abstract 2012pT47: p67.

[113] Adebayo, S. A., & Oladele, O. I. Medicinal values of kolanuts in Nigeria: Implications for extension service delivery. *Life Science Journal* 2012; 9(2): 887-891.

[114] Monago, C. C., & Alumunah, E. O. Anti-diabetic effect of chloroform-methand extract of *Abrus precatorius* Linn seed in alloxan diabetic rabbits. Journal of Applied Science, Environment and Management 2005; 9 (1): 85-88

[115] Wireko-Manu, F., Maxiya-Dixon, B., Asiedu, R., Oduro, I. & Ellis, W. O. Exploiting the health benefits of water yam; its total dietary fibre composition.. A paper presented at the Nutrition Congress Africa 2012, held at University of the Free State, Bloemfontein, South Africa, from 30th September – 4th October, 2012. Book of Abstract 2012: p118.

[116] Onwurah, I. N. E. Crystallinity and polysaccharide chains of β-glucan in white sorghum, SK_{5912}. *International Journal of Biological Macromolecules* 2001; 29: 281-286.

[117] Saleh, A. S. M., Zhang, Q, Chen J. & Shen, Q Millet grains: Nutritional quality processing and potential health benefits. *Comprehensive Reviews in Food Science and Food Safety* 2013; 12: 281-295.

[118] Dyles, L., & Rooney, L. W. Sorghum and millet phenols and anti-oxidants. *Journal of Cereal Science* 2006; 44: 236-251.

[119] Babu, P. D., Subhasree, R. S., Bhkyraj, R. &Vidhhylaksmi, R. Brown rice- beyond the colour reviving a lost health food- A review. American-Eurasian Journal of Agronomy 2009; 2 (2): 67-72.

[120] Udenta, E. A. and Obizoba, I. C. Physico-chemical profile and *in vitro* glycaemic index of *Candida tropicalis* fermented Nigerian starchy staple flours. A paper presented at the Nutrition Congress Africa 2012, held at University of the Free State, Bloemfontein, South Africa, from 30th September – 4th October, 2012. Book of Abstract 2012: p112.

[121] Olowu A.O., Adeneye, A. A. & Adeyemi, O. O. Hypoglycaemic effect of *Ipomea batatas* acqueous leaf and stem extract in normal and streptozotocin-induced hyperglycaemic rats. *Journal of Natural Pharmaceutics,* 2 (2), 56-61.

[122] Onyechi, U. A. The effect of *Detarium macrocarpium* soup meal on the plasma glucose and insulin levels of healthy non-diabetic adults. *Nigerian Journal of Nutritional Sciences* 2009a; 30 (1): 10 – 18.

[123] Onyechi, U. A. The physiological effect of *Detarium* bread meal on the post-prandial profile of non-insulin dependent diabetes mellitus (NIDDM) subjects. *Nigerian Journal of Nutritional Sciences* 2010; 31 (1): 47-52.

[124] Ngwu, E. K., Ndiokwelu, I.C, Ibaro, U. & Nwachi, I.C. Effect of African yambean gruel consumption on the health characteristics of diabetics in a rural community. *Journal of Dietitians Association of Nigeria* 2011: 3.

[125] Ana, A. '*A taste of Calabar' selected Efik recipes to warm your stomach*. Gazeen, Lagos. 2000.

[126] Ani, A. I., Atangwho, I. J., Agiang, M.A. & Alozie, Y.E. Biochemical effects of some traditional Nigerian diets in experimental diabetic rat models. *International Journal of Biochemistry Research* 2012; 2 (2): 70-77.

[127] Fasanmade, A. A. & Anyakudo, M. M. C. Glycaemic indices of selected Nigerian flour meal products in male type 2 diabetic subjects. *Diabetologia Croatica* 2007; 36 (2): 33-38.

[128] Ikewuchi, C. C. & Ikewuchi, J. C. Rate of *in vitro* digestion of some Nigerian foods by salivary α-amylase: implications for the management of post-prandial glucose levels. *The Pacific Journal of Science and Technology* 2009; 10 (2): 835-841.

[129] Ikem, R. T. Kolawole, B. A., Ojofeitimi, E. O. Salawu, A. Ajose, O. A. Abiose, S. & Odewale, F. A. Controlled comparison of a high fibre diet on the glycaemic and lipid profile of Nigerian clinic patients with type 2 diabetes. *Pakistan Journal of Nutrition* 2007; 6 (2): 111-116.

[130] Udenta, E. A., Ohagwa, H.O., Mbah, U. C., Odo, A.U. & Obizoba, I.C. Effects of antidiabetic diets based on fermented cassava, maize and sorghum and unfermented *Cola gigantea* on biochemical composition of diabetic adult rats. A paper presented at the 2nd Federation of African Nutrition Societies on "Accelerating Nutrition Actions for Africa's Development" held at International Conference Centre, Abuja, Nigeria from 11th-15th September, 2011

Chapter 4

Some Selected Medicinal Plants with Antidiabetic Potentials

A.A. Oyagbemi, M. Salihu, O.O. Oguntibeju,
A.J. Esterhuyse and E.O. Farombi

Additional information is available at the end of the chapter

http://dx.doi.org/10.5772/57230

1. Introduction

1.1. General overview of diabetic mellitus

Diabetes mellitus is a metabolic disorder that is characterized by hyperglycemia associated with impairment in insulin secretion and/or insulin action as well as aberrations in intermediary metabolism of carbohydrates, proteins and lipids. Several reports indicate that annual incidence rate of diabetes mellitus will increase in the future worldwide, especially in the developing countries [1]. The effects of diabetes mellitus include long-term damage, dysfunction and failure of various organs. Diabetes mellitus may present with classical characteristic features such as blurring of vision, excessive thirst (polydypsia), excessive feeding (polyphagia) excessive urination (polyuria), and weight loss. In its most severe forms, ketoacidosis may develop leading to stupor, coma and, in absence of effective treatment death ensues [2].

Often symptoms are not severe, or may be absent, and consequently hyperglycaemia sufficient to cause pathological and functional changes may be present for a long time before the diagnosis is made. On the other hand, other chronic features of diabetes mellitus include progressive development of the specific complications of retinopathy with potential blindness. Nephropathy that may lead to renal failure with risk of foot ulcers, amputation, including reproductive dysfunction [3-6]. People with diabetes are at increased risk of developing cardiovascular, peripheral vascular and cerebrovascular disease [7-8]. These include processes which destroy the beta cells of the pancreas with consequent insulin deficiency and ultimately resulting in insulin resistance. The abnormalities of carbohydrate, fat and protein metabolism have also been shown to result in deficient action of insulin on target tissues resulting from insensitivity or lack of insulin [9-10].

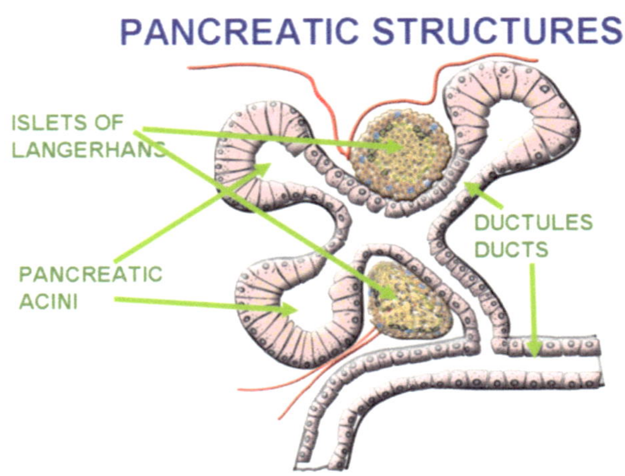

Figure 1. The structure of the pancreas which houses islets of Langerhans

Insulin resistance was recently reported to be associated with obesity and type 2 diabetes[11]. Recent studies suggest that a complex interaction between inflammation, endoplasmic reticulum stress, oxidative stress, mitochondrial dysfunction and autophagy dysregulation play an important role in insulin resistance. The stress-activated c-Jun N-terminal kinase (JNK) has been increasingly recognized as a central mediator of insulin resistance [11] and suppression of the JNK pathway has been shown to improve insulin resistance and glucose tolerance. Also, hyperhomocysteinemia (HHcy) was found to induce insulin resistance in adipose tissue via activation of JNK pathway [12].

2. Classifications of diabetic mellitus

The terms type 1 and type 2 are used for classification based on aetiological factors. The terms insulin-dependent and non-insulin-dependent are used for classifying pathophysiological conditions of diabetes mellitus regardless of the aetiological factors. However, it has been noticed that failure to administer insulin in an insulin-dependent condition can lead to ketosis and with resultant life threatening condition. In the same vein patients whose conditions do not require insulin treatment for prevention of ketosis or for survival are known to require insulin for glycaemic control and such patients are considered to be in a non-insulin-dependent state [13].

http://dx.doi.org/10.5772/57230

2.1. Type 1 diabetes mellitus

Type 1 diabetes mellitus is caused by insulin deficiency due to destruction of pancreatic β-cells principally via an autoimmune reaction that can be triggered by different factors [14]. It can also develop in association with certain hereditary factors, such as Human Leukocyte Antigen (HLA) alleles. Typically, destruction of pancreatic β-cells progresses to absolute deficiency in insulin. This condition develops rapidly in young people and has been found to occur in any age group [14]. Similarly, autoantibodies against islet antigens (islet-associated antibodies) have been shown to increase in the early phase of the disease. Hence, pancreatic β-cell destruction involves autoimmune mechanisms. Therefore, type 1 diabetes mellitus is also known as 'autoimmune' type 1 diabetes mellitus [14, 15-16].

2.2. Type 2 diabetes mellitus

Type 2 diabetes mellitus is one of the most common diseases of the western world and is associated with cardiovascular disease [17]. Type 2 diabetes mellitus (formerly called NIDDM, type II or adult-onset) is characterized by insulin resistance in peripheral tissue and an insulin secretory defect of the beta cell. This is the most common form of diabetes mellitus and is highly associated with a family history of diabetes, old age, obesity and lack of exercise. It is more common in women, especially women with a history of gestational diabetes. Type 2 diabetes mellitus is characterized by derangement of carbohydrate, protein and fat metabolism [18]. Insulin resistance and hyperinsulinemia eventually lead to impaired glucose tolerance [19].

Defective beta cells become exhausted, further fuelling the cycle of glucose intolerance and hyperglycaemia. The aetiology of type 2 diabetes mellitus is multifactorial with evidence of genetic involvement [20-21]. Types of diabetes mellitus of various known aetiologies are grouped together to form the classification called "other specific types." This group includes persons with genetic defects of beta-cell function (this type of diabetes was formerly called MODY or maturity-onset diabetes in youth) or with defects of insulin action; persons with diseases of the exocrine pancreas, such as pancreatitis or cystic fibrosis; persons with dysfunction associated with other endocrinopathies (e.g., acromegaly); and persons with pancreatic dysfunction caused by drugs, chemicals or infections. Diabetic cardiomyopathy (DCM) has also been extensively reported in type 2 diabetes mellitus [22-25]. DCM is recognized as asymptomatic progressing structural and functional remodelling in the heart of diabetics, in the absence of coronary atherosclerosis and hypertension. Diabetic cardiomyopathy is a fairly common cause of heart failure in the native population with type-2 diabetes mellitus and results in high morbidity and mortality [22]. Few of the classical symptoms of DCM include marked left ventricular (LV) systolic dysfunction, dysfunction of coronary microcirculation, in relation with glycaemic levels, insulin resistance, sympathetic overdrive, endothelial dysfunction, abnormalities of the angiotensin-renin system, and remodelling/hypertrophy, diastolic dysfunction and impairment of coronary flow reserve (CFR) may be associated in DM [22-24].

3. Global impact of diabetic mellitus

Diabetes mellitus is a disease common to all parts of the world [26]. It is a common and very prevalent disease affecting the citizens of both developed and developing countries. It has been estimated that 25% of the world population is affected by this disease [27]. Currently, India has got the largest number of diabetics and is being called as diabetic capital of the world. Diabetes has significant health consequences for individuals and communities. In fact, many countries face large increases in the number of people suffering from diabetes. The World Health Organization estimated that about 30 million people suffered from diabetes in 1985 and the number increased to more than 171 million in 2000. Additionally, it has been estimated that the number will increase to over 366 million by 2030 and that large increases will occur in developing countries, especially in people aged between 45 and 64 years [28].

A large disparity in total health spending for diabetes among the top 80 most populous countries exists, varying from USD 1.3 million to USD 198.0 billion. The country with the highest total expenditure, the United States of America, will spend 52.7% of the global expenditure. India, the country with the largest population of people living with diabetes, will spend an estimated USD 2.8 billion or less than 1% of the world total. The total diabetes spending in the 18 countries in IDF's African Region will be only USD 1.2 billion, 0.3% of the global total [29]. The absolute level of health expenditure in developing countries appears to be quite low. The lowest 20 spending countries in the top 80 most populated countries will spend less than USD 50 per person per year for managing diabetes and diabetes-related complications. Expenditure at this level cannot even cover the annual wholesale cost of a generic oral agent capable of preventing acute, life-threatening hyperglycaemia [29]. Considering the health services and therapeutic treatments needed to manage diabetes and diabetes-related complications, more health care resources are required to provide adequate diabetes care in the poor countries.

4. Diabetic mellitus and oxidative stress

Diabetes mellitus is associated with an increased risk of cardiovascular diseases mediated via oxidative stress. ROS can directly damage lipids, proteins or DNA and modulate intracellular signaling pathways, such as mitogen activated protein kinases and redox sensitive transcription factors causing changes in protein expression with irreversible oxidative modifications [30-31]. Hyperglycaemia-induced mitochondrial dysfunction and endoplasmic reticulum stress has been shown to promote reactive oxygen species (ROS) accumulation, accelerates cellular damage and significantly contributes to the diabetic complications development and progression [30, 32-33]. PA *et al.* [34] described the mechanism of cardiovascular dysfunction in diabetes mellitus (Figure 2).

http://dx.doi.org/10.5772/57230

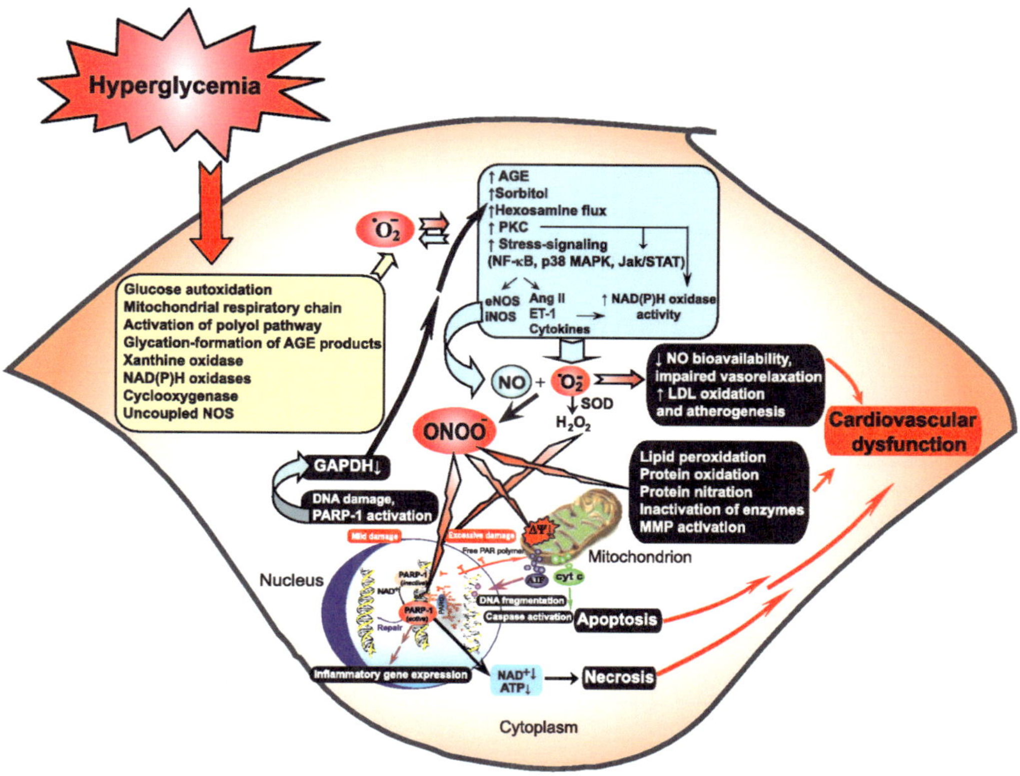

Figure 2. Mechanisms of cardiovascular dysfunction in diabetes: role of superoxide and peroxynitrite. Hyperglycaemia induces increased superoxide anion (O2•–) production via activation of multiple pathways including xanthine and NAD(P)H oxidases, cyclooxygenase, uncoupled nitric oxide synthase (NOS), glucose autoxidation, mitochondrial respiratory chain, polyol pathway, and formation of advanced glycation end products (AGE). Hyperglycaemia-induced increased superoxide generation may also favour an increased expression of nitric oxide synthases (NOS) through the activation of NFκB, which may increase the generation of nitric oxide (NO). Superoxide anion may quench NO, thereby reducing the efficacy of a potent endothelium-derived vasodilator system. Superoxide can also be converted to hydrogen peroxide (H_2O_2) by superoxide dismutase (SOD) and interact with NO to form a reactive oxidant peroxynitrite (ONOO–), which induces cell damage via lipid peroxidation, inactivation of enzymes and other proteins by oxidation and nitration, and activation of matrix metalloproteinases (MMPs) among others. This figure was adapted from [34].

Hyperglycaemia-induced oxidative stress also mediates endothelial dysfunction which plays a central role in the pathogenesis of micro- and macro-vascular diseases with resultant increase in pro-inflammatory cytokines and induction of apoptosis and impairment of nitric oxide release. Hyperglycaemia induces vascular damage probably through a single common pathway - increased intracellular oxidative stress- linking four major mechanisms, namely the polyol pathway, advanced glycation end-products (AGEs) formation, the protein kinase C (PKC)-diacylglycerol (DAG) and the hexosamine pathways [35]. However, synthetic drugs against diabetes mellitus have been reported with avalanche of side effects (Table 1) as reported by Kavishankar *et al*. [36].

Agent	Mechanism	Site of action	Advantages	Side effects
Sulphonylureas	Stimulating insulin production by inhibiting the K-ATP channel	Pancreatic beta cells	Effective and inexpensive	Hypoglycaemia and weight gain.
Metformin	Decreases insulin resistance	Liver	Weight loss Does not cause hypoglycaemia	Nausea and diarrhoea. Hypoglycaemia occurs when combined with sulfonylurea or insulin
Thiazolidinediones	Reduce insulin resistance by activating PPAR-γ	GI tract	Low risk	Increased liver enzymes, weight gain, oedema, mild anaemia
α-glucosidase inhibitors	Reduces intestinal glucose absorption	Fat, muscle	Decreases postprandial plasma triglyceride levels	Diarrhoea, abdominal pain, flatulence; Serum levels of transaminases increases at doses

Adapted from Kavishankar *et al.* [36].

Table 1. Synthetic drugs and their side effects

5. Drug-induced diabetic mellitus and their mechanisms of action

The most common drugs that are currently being used for the experimental induction of diabetes are alloxan and streptozotocin (STZ). Streptozotocin (STZ) is a synthetic antineoplastic agent that is classified as an anti-tumour antibiotic and is chemically related to other nitrosureas used in cancer chemotherapy [37]. Intra-venous injection of 60mg/kg dose of streptozotocin in adult Wistar rats, makes pancreas swell and at last causes degeneration in Langerhans islet beta cells and induces experimental diabetes mellitus in 2-4 days [37]. Both alloxan and STZ have been extensively documented for the induction of diabetes via free radical generation and depletion of antioxidant defense system [38-40]. STZ has been reported to significantly decrease the activity of erythrocytes antioxidative enzymes catalase (CAT), superoxide dismutase (SOD) and glutathione peroxidase (GPx) [38-39]. Several drugs, with pharmacological properties including theophylline, aspirin, isoniazid and nalidixic acid can cause transient hyperglycaemia in over dosage, but only streptozotocin, alloxan and the rodenticide vacor are likely to cause permanent diabetes. Alloxan and the product of its reduction, dialuric acid, establish a redox cycle with the formation of superoxide radicals that undergo dismutation to produce hydrogen peroxide via Fenton reaction [41]. Similarly, the reactive oxygen species results in simultaneous massive increase in cytosolic calcium concentration causes rapid destruction of B cells. In the same vein, streptozotocin enters the B cell via a glucose transporter (GLUT2) and causes alkylation of DNA. DNA damage induces activation of poly ADP-ribosylation, a process that is more important for the diabetogenicity of streptozotocin than DNA damage itself. More so, Poly ADP-ribosylation leads to depletion of cellular NAD+ and ATP [41]. Enhanced ATP dephosphorylation after streptozotocin treatment supplies a substrate for xanthine oxidase resulting in the formation of superoxide radicals. Also, streptozotocin liberates toxic amounts of nitric oxide that inhibits aconitase activity and participates in DNA damage [41].

6. Some scientifically validated antidiabetic plants

Recently, Etuk *et al.* [42] reported that the following medicinal plants have been validated scientifically as potent antidiabetic plants: *Acacia arabica* (Lam.) Muhl. ex Willd. (Family:

Mimosaceae), *Aegle marmelos* (L.) Correa ex Roxb. (Family: Rutaceae), *Allium cepa* L. (Family: Liliaceae), *Allium sativum* L. (Family: Alliaceae), *Aloe vera* (L.) Burm.f. (Family: Aloaceae), *Anthemis mobilis* Linn. (Family: Compositae), *Areca catechu* L. (Family: Arecaceae), *Artemisia pallens* Wall. ex DC. (Family: Compositae), *Annona squamosa* L. (Family: Annonaceae), *Andrographis paniculata* Nees (Family: Acanthaceae), *Aerva lanata* (L.) Juss. ex Schult. (Family: Amaranthaceae), *Asteracantha longifolia* Nees (Family: Acanthaceae), *Azadirachta indica* A. Juss. (Family: Meliaceae), *Biophytum sensitivum* (L.) DC. (Family: Oxalidaceae), *Bombax ceiba* L. (Family: Bombacaceae), *Beta vulgaris*

L. (Family: Chenopodiaceae), *Brassica juncea* (L.) Czern. (Family: Brassicaceae), *Barleria lupulina* Lindl. (Family: Acanthaceae), *Boerhavia diffusa* L. (Family: Nyctaginaceae), *Brickellia veronicaefolia* A. Gray (Family: Asteraceae), *Cassia auriculata* L. (Family: Leguminosae), *Caesalpinia bonducella* (L.) Roxb. (Family: Cesalpinaceae), *Capparis decidua* (Forsk.) Edgew. (Family: Capparidaceae) *Cajanus cajan* (L.) Millsp. (Family: Fabaceae), *Citrullus colocynthis* (L.) Schrad. (Family: Cucurbitaceae), *Coccinia indica* Wight & Arn. (Family: Cucurbitaceae), *Casearia esculenta* Roxb. (Family: Flacourtiaceae), *Catharanthus roseus* (L) G. Don. (Family: Apocynaceae), *Camellia sinensis* Kuntze (Family: Theaceae), *Coriandrum sativum* L. (Family: Apiaceae).

7. Antidiabetic plants in clinical trials

The following antidiabetic plants are currently under clinical trials viz:

Allium cepa L., Clerodendron phlomoides Linn., Cinnamomum tamala (Buch.-Ham.) T. Nees & Eberm., Coccinia indica Wight & Arn., Enicostemma littorale Blume, Ficus bengalensis L., Momordica charantia L., Pterocarpus marsupium Roxb., Cyamopsis tetragonolobus (L.) Taub., Cephalandra indica Naud., Casearia esculenta Roxb., Cannabis indica (Lam.) E. Small & Cronq., and Syzygium cumini L. when subjected to clinical trials, showed promising hypoglycaemic effects [43]. *Other potent antidiabetic plants in this category include Cecropia obtusifolia, Marrubium vulgare, Asteracantha longifolia Nees L., Panax quinquefolius L, Gymnema Sylvestre, Phyllanthus amarus, Opuntia streptacantha Lem.* They were found to produce beneficial effects on carbohydrate and lipid metabolisms when administered as an adjunct on patients with type 2 diabetes [44]. These plants have been reported to improve glucose tolerance in healthy human subjects and diabetic patients, caused significant reduction in blood glucose, glycosylated haemoglobin and glycosylated plasma proteins comparable to an oral hypoglycaemic drug [45].

8. General mechanism (s) of action of medicinal plants with antidiabetic property

Different mechanisms of action of medicinal plants with anti-diabetic have been extensively described. These include inhibition of renal glucose reabsorption [46], stimulation of insulin secretion from beta cells of islets or/and inhibition of insulin degradative processes, reduction in insulin resistance [47] regenerating and/or repairing pancreatic beta cells with increasing the size and number of cells in the islets of Langerhans [45]. Stimulation of insulin secretion [48] and stimulation of glycogenesis and hepaticglycolysis [49] with antidiabetic plants is well established. Also, protective effect on the destruction of the beta cells and improvement in digestion along with reduction in blood sugar urea has been documented [50]. Prevention of pathological conversion of starch to glucose, and inhibition of β-galactocidase, α-glucocidase and alpha-amylase with concomitant capacity to lower cortisol has also been reported [51-52]. Antioxidant activity of antidiabetic plant against oxidative stress which is involved in pancreatic ß-cell dysfunction has been reported as one of the mechanisms of action of anti-diabetic plants [53]. Similarly, some plant families reported for antidiabetic activity are shown below (Table 2).

9. Antioxidant activity of medicinal plants with antidiabetic activity

One of the major pathogenic mechanisms of diabetes mellitus include generation of oxidative stress, increase generation of free radicals and an impaired antioxidant defence system with concomitant imbalance of the oxidant/antioxidant status [54]. Inhibition of this cascade of oxidative processes has been reported to prevent the onset and development of diabetic complications [55]. Antidiabetic plants have been documented to scavenge free radicals, quench electronically excited compounds, reduce hydroperoxide formation, and attenuate production of reactive oxygen species (ROS) through modulation of several enzymes including xanthine oxidase, cyclooxygenase, lipoxygenase, microsomal monooxygenase, NADH oxidase and mitochondrial succinoxidase [56]. More so, plant phytonutrients such as polyphenols are known to enhance the endogenous antioxidative system, improve oxidant antioxidant balance, prevent oxidative damage, decrease lipid peroxidation, increase plasma total antioxidant capacity and induce antioxidant enzymes including superoxide dismutase, catalase and glutathione peroxidase [57].

http://dx.doi.org/10.5772/57230

Botanical	Family
Mangifera indica	Anacardiaceae
Senna occidentalis	Fabaceae
Euphorbia convuludiodes	Euphobiaceae
Khaya senegalensis	Meliaceae
Acacia nilotica	Mimosaceae
Vernonia amygdalina	Asreraceae
Fiscus thonnigii	Moraceae
Angeissus leiocarpus	Combretaceae
Gossypium hirsutum	Malvaceae
Vitillarta paradoxa	Sapotaceae
Anacardium occidentalis	Anacardiaceae
Anana senegalensis	Anonaceae
Psidium guajava	Myrtaceae
Moringa oleifera	Mringaceae
Azadirachata indica	Meliaceae
Alluvium cepa	Liliaceae
Ctrus medica	Rutaceae
Parkta filicoidea	Mimosaceae
Allium sativum	Liliaceae
Balanites aegyptiaca	Zygophyliaceae
Bauhinia reticulate Casalpiniaceae	Casalpiniaceae
Adapted from Etuk et al., 2010	

Table 2. Some plant families reported for antidiabetic activity

10. Plant phytochemicals associated with antidiabetic activity

Photochemicals or phytonutrients are chemical compounds that occur naturally in plants that have protective or disease preventive properties [58]. Each type of fruit or vegetable may contain hundreds of phytochemicals. They have been reported to show multiple beneficial effects in combating diabetes and diabetes related complications [58]. The widest known groups of phytochemicals are the alkaloids, terpenes, and phenolics. Plant constituents such as polysaccharides, peptides, alkaloids, glycopeptides, triterpenoids, amino acids, steroids, xanthone, flavonoids, lipids, phenolics, coumarins, iridoids, alkyl disulphides, inorganic ions and guanidines are reported to have antidiabetic activities [49, 59]. More interestingly, the following phytochemicals are reported to have antidiabetic activity, aminoacids like hypoglycin A and hypoglycin B, alkaloids like catharanthine, leurosine, lochnerine, arecoline and vindoline, pinitol, epicatechin, S-methyl cysteine sulphoxide, S-allyl cysteine sulphoxide, andrographolide, allicin (thio-2-propene-1- sulfinic acid S-allyl ester), shamimin, beta vulgarosides I–IV, glycoside of leucopelargonidin and leucodelphinidin, mangiferin, marsupsin, pterosupin, pterostilbene, salacinol, swerchirin, trigonelline, berberine, harmane, norharmane, pinoline, quercetin, chlorogenic acid, hesperidin, naringin, epigallocatechin gallate, charantin, galactonmannan, lactucain C, kaempferol glucosides, caffeoyl glucoside, bakuchiol, swerchirin, thysanolactone, bellidifolin and kolaviron have been documented for potential phytonutrients [60].

11. Plant phytochemicals associated with insulinomimetic activity

They stimulate Beta cell rejuvenation, regeneration and stimulation increase insulin level, Irneccerepatoser insulin secretion and reduction of insulin binding on the insulin [34]. Some of the plant phytochemicals associated with insulinomimetic activity include the following: Abies pindrow Pinaceae, Acacia arabica (Leguminosae), Agrimony eupatoria (Rosaceae), Aloe barbadensis (Liliaceae), Annona squamosa (Annonaceae), Averrhoa bilimbi (Oxalidaceae), Bixa orellana (Bixaceae), Boerhaavia diffusa (Nyctaginaceae), Camellia sinensis (Theaceae), Capsicum frutescens (Solanaceae), Cinnamomum zeylanicum (Lauraceae), Clausena anisata (Rutaceae), Eucalyptus globulus (Myrtaceae), Ficus religiosa (Moraceae), Hibiscus rosa (Malvaceae), Helicteres isora (Sterculiaceae), Ipomoea batata (Convolvulaceae) Juniperus communis (Pinaceae), Olea europia (Oleaceae), Swertia chirayata (Gentianaeae), Scoparia dulcis (Scrophulariaceae),Tinospora crispa (Menispermaceae) Urtifca dioica (Urticaceae), Vinca rosea (Apocynaceae), Zingiber officinale (Zingiberaceae).

12. Some selected medicinal plants with antidiabetic potentials in Nigeria

In Nigeria, two plants, *Mangifera indica and Vernonia amygdalina* have been ranked highest for their antidiabetic property. Diabetes mellitus is known to affect 3% on average of adult Nigerians [61] and the prevalence in northern Nigerian is put at 1.6% [62]. Some of the selected medicinal plants with antidiabetic potentials in Nigeria are listed below.

Mangifera indica, Angeissus leiocarpus, Fiscus thonnigii, Khaya senegalensis,. Euphorbia convuludiodes, Acacia nilotica, Vernonia amygdalina,Cassia goratensis,Cassia arereh, Calotropis procera, Senna occidentalis, Alluvium cepa, Ipomoea batatas, Vitex gekowskii,Ctrus medica, Parkta filicoidea, Allium sativum, Anacardium occidentalis, Azadirachata indica,Vitillarta paradoxa, Gossypium hirsutum,

Lawsonia inermis, Moringa oleifera, Psidium guajava, Bauhinia reticulate, Balanites aegyptiaca, Lannea kerstingii, Daucus carota, Zizyphus spina, Anana senegalensis, Eugenia caryophyllata, Blighia sapida.

The leaves of *Mangifera indica* are used as an antidiabetic agent in Nigerian folk medicine. The hypoglycemic activity of *Mangifera indica* has been reported in both rats and mice [63-64]. Aqueous extract of the leaves of *Mangifera indica* were found to possess hypoglycaemic activity against glucose-induced hyperglycaemia but not with normoglycaemic or STZ-induced diabetic rats and mice respectively [63-64]. The hypoglyceamic effect of this plant was thought to be by reduction of intestinal absorption of glucose. Antihyperglycaemic activity of aqueous stem bark extract of *Mangifera indica* was also reported by Ojewole [65]. The extract from the stem bark of *Mangifera indica* administered intraperitoneally in streptozotocin induced diabetics rats produced a significant reduction in blood glucose level in rats Ojewole [65].

In Nigeria, the leaves of *Vernonia amygdalina* Del. (VA) and *Azadirachta indica* A. Juss (AI) have been used traditionally as a remedy against diabetes mellitus [66]. Atangwho et al. [66] reported that significant antidiabetic effect of the combination therapy was achieved when VA and AI were combined. The mechanism of action of the combination therapy was proposed as attenuation of oxidative stress, insulin mimetic action and β-cell regeneration. The presence of flavonoids such as luteolin, luteolin 7-*O*-*β*-glucuronoside, and luteolin 7-*O*-*β*-glucoside has been shown to be responsible for the antioxidant activity of *Vernonia amygdalina* [67]. The presence of these flavonoids could therefore contribute significantly to the antidiabetic property of *Vernonia amygdalina*.

Etuk and Mohammed [68] reported that 200 mg/kg of *V. amygdalina, C. procera, C. goratensis* and *M. indica* aqueous extracts produced a significant ($p < 0.05$) reduction in the blood glucose levels of the rats in alloxan-induced diabetic mellitus. In the same vein, *A. leicarpus, C. arereh* and *G. hirsutum* extracts produced a non-significant reduction ($p > 0.05$) in blood glucose levels in rats after treatment. Similarly, aqueous extracts of *M. Oleifera, S. occidentalis* and *K. senegalensis* were found to produce a minimal effect (about 4% reduction) on the alloxan-induced hyperglycemia in rats (Etuk and Mohammed, 2009). In summary, Etuk and Mohammed (2009) reported that 200mg/kg body weight of *Vernonia amygdalina* (67%), *Calotropis procera* (59%), *Cassia gorotensis* (53%) and *Magnifera indica* (35%) extracts produced a significant (p < 0.0.5%) reduction in blood glucose levels in diabetic rats while *Angeissus leiocarpus* (30%), Cassia arereh (19%), *Gossypium hirsutum* (17%), *Khaya senegalensis* (4%), *Senna occidentalis* (4%) and *Moringa oleifera* (4%) produced a nonsignificant ($p < 0.05\%$) effect.

Previous study showed that aqueous leaves extract of *Psidium guajava* (PG) at 250 mg/kg showed statistically significant hypoglycaemic activity on alloxan-induced diabetic rats [69]. A 4-week supplementation of PG (125 and 250 mg/kg) in streptozotocin (STZ)-induced diabetic rats was shown to protect pancreatic tissues, including islet β-cells, against lipid peroxidation and DNA strand breaks induced by STZ, thereby reducing the loss of insulin-positive β-cells and insulin secretion [70]. More so, PG was found to markedly inhibited pancreatic nuclear factor-kappa B protein expression induced by STZ and restored the activities of antioxidant enzymes, including superoxide dismutase, catalase, and glutathione peroxidase [70].

1 ml *Allum cepa* solution (0.4 g A. cepa/rat) has been shown to increase the fasting serum high-density lipoprotein levels and caused reduction of hyperglycaemia in streptozotocin (STZ) diabetic rats [71]. The hypoglycaemic and hypolipidaemic activities of A. cepa were associated with antioxidant activity via decrease superoxide dismutase (SOD) activity while no increased lipid hydroperoxide and lipoperoxide concentrations in diabetic rats treated with A. cepa [71]. In another experiment, onion juices exerted antioxidant and antihyperglycemic effects on alloxan-induced diabetes and consequently ameliorated liver and renal damage associated with alloxan toxicity [72].

Flavonoids from *Ipomoea batatas* leaf (FIBL) was reported to have anti-diabetic activity on alloxan-induced diabetic mice [73]. FIBL treatment (50, 100, and 150 mg/ kg body weight) for 28 days resulted in a significant decrease in the concentration of fasting blood glucose (FBG), total cholesterol (TC) and triglyceride (TG) in diabetes mellitus mice [73]. Also, FIBL significantly increased body weight (bw) and serum high-density lipoprotein cholesterol (HDL-c) level [73]. Stress and inflammation-related p38 mitogen-activated protein kinase activity and tumour necrosis factor-α production of diabetic rats were significantly depressed by *Ipomoea batatas* administration [74]. Similarly, histological examination also revealed improvement of pancreatic β-cells mass after treatments with *Ipomoea batatas* [74]. *Blighia sapida* has also been reported to have several ethnomedicinal uses of which various preparations and extracts have been made for the treatment of diseases such as dysentery, epilepsy, yellow fever and diabetes [75]. Saidu *et al.* [76] recently reported that *Anacardium occidentale* leaves at 300mg/kg body weight showed significant hypoglycaemic activity in alloxan-induced diabetic rats comparable to the standard drug-metformin.

13. Conclusion

Diabetes mellitus is a metabolic disorder in the endocrine system. It is known to be a dreadful disease that is found in all parts of the world with a serious threat to the health of mankind. Diabetes mellitus affect most of the people of both developed and developing countries. There are lots of synthetic drugs that have been used to control and to treat diabetic patients with partial recovery from this dreaded disease. Alternative to these synthetic agents, plants provide a potential source of hypoglycemic drugs and are widely used in several traditional systems of medicine to prevent diabetes. Several medicinal plants have been investigated for their beneficial use in different types of diabetes. Several phytonutrients have been identified from medicinal plants and this presents an exciting opportunity for the development of new types of therapeutics for diabetes mellitus. Most abundant phytonutrients present in medicinal plants are the alkaloids, terpenes, and phenolics. Phytomedicine has been used since ancient time in many parts of the world where access to modern medicine is limited. Despite considerable progress in the treatment of diabetes by oral hypoglycemic agents, search for newer drugs continues because the existing synthetic drugs have several limitations as shown in table 1. The treatment of diabetes with synthetic drugs in the developing countries is expensive due to poverty and lack of access to Medicare. Hence, phytotherapy has significant role to play in

http://dx.doi.org/10.5772/57230

the developing countries compared to synthetic drugs because it is safe, less expensive and available as a gift of nature.

Author details

A.A. Oyagbemi[1,2], M. Salihu[3], O.O. Oguntibeju[4], A.J. Esterhuyse[4] and E.O. Farombi[1*]

*Address all correspondence to: olatunde_farombi@yahoo.com

1 Drug Metabolism and Toxicology Unit, Department of Biochemistry, College of Medicine, Nigeria

2 Department of Veterinary Physiology, Biochemistry & Pharmacology, University of Ibadan, Nigeria

3 Biochemistry Unit, Department of Biological Sciences, College of Natural Sciences, Al-Hikmah University, Ilorin, Nigeria

4 Oxidative Stress Research Centre, Department of Biomedical Sciences, Faculty of Health & Wellness Sciences, Cape Peninsula University of Technology, Bellville Campus, South Africa

References

[1] Kameswara Rao B, Rajasekhar MD, Sreelatha A, and Apparao C. Treatment of diabetes mellitus: Plant drugs vs oral hypoglycemic agents and insulin. In Recent Progress in Medicinal Plants, 14, pp. 279-296, Biopharmaceuticals Studium Press, Houson, TX, USA; 2006.

[2] Shin HJ, Kim JH, Yi JH, Han SW, Kim HJ. Polyuria with the Concurrent manifestation of Central Diabetes Insipidus (CDI) & Type 2 Diabetes Mellitus (DM). Electrolyte & Blood Pressure 2012; 10(1):26-30.

[3] Smolek MK, Notaroberto NF, Jaramillo AG, Pradillo LR. Intervention with vitamins in patients with nonproliferative diabetic retinopathy: a pilot study. Clinical Ophthalmology 2013; 7:1451-1458.

[4] Lidén MK. Prevention and protection in diabetic nephropathy. Lakartidningen 2013; 110(21):1025-1027.

[5] Westerberg DP (2013). Diabetic ketoacidosis: evaluation and treatment. American Family Physician. 87(5):337-346

[6] Liu J, Wang S, Feng L, Ma D, Fu Q, Song Y, Jia X, Ma S. Hypoglycemic and antioxidant activities of paeonol and its beneficial effect on diabetic encephalopathy in streptozotocin-induced diabetic rats. Journal of Medical Foods 2013; 16(7):577-586.

[7] Bell DS. Diabetes: a cardiac condition manifesting as hyperglycemia. Endocrine Practice 2008; 14(7):924-932.

[8] Yoshimura M, Anzawa R, Mochizuki S. Cardiac metabolism in diabetes mellitus. Current Pharmaceutical Design 2008; 14(25):2521-2526.

[9] Andreozzi F, Gastaldelli A, Mannino GC, Sciacqua A, Succurro E, Arturi F, Folli F, Perticone F. Increased carotid intima-media thickness in the physiologic range is associated with impaired postprandial glucose metabolism, insulin resistance and beta cell dysfunction. Atherosclerosis 2013; 229(2):277-281.

[10] Simopoulos AP. Dietary omega-3 Fatty Acid deficiency and high fructose intake in the development of metabolic syndrome, brain metabolic abnormalities, and non-alcoholic Fatty liver disease. Nutrients 2013; 5(8):2901-2923.

[11] Li H, Yu X. Emerging Role of JNK in Insulin Resistance. Current Diabetes Reviews 2013; Sep;9(5):422-428.

[12] Li Y, Zhang H, Jiang C, Xu M, Pang Y, Feng J, Xiang X, Kong W, Xu G, Li Y, Wang X. Hyperhomocysteinemia promotes insulin resistance by inducing endoplasmic reticulum stress in adipose tissue. J Biological Chemimstry 2013; 288(14):9583-92.

[13] Sutradhar SR, Ali L, Khan AK, Siddiqui NI, Sarker CB, Rahman S, Huq MH, Debnath CR. Ketosis resistance in under thirty diabetic subjects. Mymensingh Medical Journal 2004; 13(2):134-137.

[14] Chhabra P, Brayman KL. Stem cell therapy to cure type 1 diabetes: from hype to hope. Stem Cells Translational Medicine 2013; 2(5):328-336.

[15] Ting C, Bansal V, Batal I, Mounayar M, Chabtini L, El Akiki G, Azzi J. Impairment of immune systems in diabetes. Advances in Experimental Medicine & Biology 2012; 771:62-75.

[16] Thompson JA, Perry D, Brusko TM. Autologous regulatory T cells for the treatment of type 1 diabetes. Current Diabetes Reports 2012; 12(5):623-32.

[17] Psallas M, Manes C. Incretins in type 2 diabetes mellitus: cardiovascular and anti-atherogenic effects beyond glucose lowering. Hippokratia Medical Journal 2012; 16(2):100-105.

[18] Pathak R, Pathak A (2012). Study of life style habits on risk of type 2 diabetes. International Journal of Applied & Basic Medical Research 2012; 2(2):92-96.

[19] Santaguida L, Balion C, Hunt D. Diagnosis, prognosis, and treatment of impaired Satyavati GV, Tandon N, Sharma M (1989). Indigenous Plant Drugs For Diabetes Melli-

tus 2008. [updated 1989 October; Available from: http://www.rssdi.org/1989_october/article1.pdf

[20] Ramirez-Garcia SA, Cabrera-Pivaral CE, Huacuja-Ruiz L, Flores-Alvarado LJ, Pérez-García G, González-Rico JL, López-Velázquez A, Topete-González, LR,Rosales-Góme RC, Candelario-Mejía G, Villa-Ruano N. [Implications in primary health care of medical genetics and genomic in type 2 diabetes mellitus]. Review in Medical Institute & Sociology 2013; 51(3):e6-e26.

[21] Morgan AR. Determining genetic risk factors for pediatric type 2 diabetes. Current Diabetes Reports 2012; 12(1):88-92.

[22] Muhammad Z, Hashmi A. Frequency of diabetic cardiomyopathy among type-2 diabetics presenting as heart failure. Journal of College of Physicians & Surgeons- Pakistan 2013; 23(8):538-542.

[23] Patil MB, Burji NP. Echocardiographic evaluation of diastolic dysfunction in asymptomatic type 2 diabetes mellitus. Journal of Association of Physicians- India 2012; 60:23-26.

[24] Shrestha NR, Sharma SK, Karki P, Shrestha NK, Acharya P. Echocardiographic evaluation of diastolic function in asymptomatic type 2 diabetes. Journal of Nepal Medical Association 2009;Jan-Mar;48(173):20-23.

[25] Galderisi M. Diastolic dysfunction and diabetic cardiomyopathy: evaluation by Doppler echocardiography. Jornal of American College of Cardiology 2006; Oct 17;48(8): 1548-1551.

[26] Adebola PO, Grierson DS and Afolayan AJ. An ethnobotanical study of plants used for the treatment of diabetes in the Eastern Cape Province, South Africa. African Journal of Biotechnology 20055; 4(12): 1458-1460.

[27] Erasto P, Adebola PO, Grierson DS and Afolayan AJ. An ethnobotanical study of plants used for the treatment of diabetes in the Eastern Cape Province, South Africa. African Journal of Biotechnology 2005; 4(12): 1458-1460.

[28] Wild SH, Roglic G, Sicree R, Green A, King H. Global Burden of Diabetes Mellitus in the Year 2000. Available from http://www3.who.int/whosis/menu.cfm?

[29] Ping Zhang, Xinzhi Zhang, Jonathan Brown, Dorte Vistisen, Richard Sicree, Jonathan Shaw, Gregory Nichols. Global healthcare expenditure on diabetes for 2010 and 2030. Diabetes research and clinical practice 2010; 78: 293-301.

[30] Diogo CV, Suski JM, Lebiedzinska M, Karkucinska-Wieckowska A, Wojtala A, Pronicki M, Duszynski J, Pinton P, Portincasa P, Oliveira PJ, Wieckowski MR. Cardiac mitochondrial dysfunction during hyperglycemia--the role of oxidative stress and p66Shc signaling. International Journal of Biochemistry & Cell Biology 2013; Jan; 45(1):114-122.

[31] Yang H, Jin X, Kei Lam CW, Yan SK. Oxidative stress and diabetes mellitus. Clinical Chemistry & Laboratory Medicine 2011; 49(11):1773-1782.

[32] Folli F, Corradi D, Fanti P, Davalli A, Paez A, Giaccari A, Perego C, Muscogiuri G. The role of oxidative stress in the pathogenesis of type 2 diabetes mellitus micro- and macrovascular complications: avenues for a mechanistic-based therapeutic approach. Current Diabetes Reviews 2011; 7(5):313-324.

[33] Madonna R, De Caterina R. Cellular and molecular mechanisms of vascular injury in diabetes-part I: pathways of vascular disease in diabetes. Vascular Pharmacology 2011; 54(3-6):68-74.

[34] Patel DK, Prasad SK, Kumar R, Hemalatha S. Asian Pacific Journal of Tropical. An overview on antidiabetic medicinal plants having insulin mimetic property. Asian Pacific Journal of Tropical Biomedicine 2012; 320-330.

[35] Bonnefont-Rousselot D, Beaudeux JL, Thérond P, Peynet J, Legrand A, Delattre J. [Diabetes mellitus, oxidative stress and advanced glycation endproducts]. Annales Pharmaceutiques Francaises 2004; 62(3):147-157.

[36] Kavishankar GB, Lakshmidevi N, Mahadeva Murthy S, Prakash HS, Niranjana SR. Diabetes and medicinal plants-A review. International Journal of Pharmaceutical & Biomedical Sciences 2011; 2(3), 65-80.

[37] Akbarzadeh A, Norouzian D, Mehrabi MR, Jamshidi SH, Farhangi A, Verdi A. Allah, Mofidian SMA and Rad B. Lame. Induction of diabetes by streptozotocin in rats. Indian Journal of Clinical Biochemistry 2007; 22 (2) 60-64.

[38] Ali MM, Agha FG. Amelioration of streptozotocin-induced diabetes mellitus, oxidative stress and dyslipidemia in rats by tomato extract lycopene. Scandinavian Journal of Clinical Laboratory Investigation 2009; 69(3):371-379.

[39] Kade IJ, Ogunbolude Y, Kamdem JP, Rocha JB. Influence of gallic acid on oxidative stress-linked streptozotocin-induced pancreatic dysfunction in diabetic rats. Journal of Basic & Clinical Physiology & Pharmacology 2013; 26:1-11.

[40] Lenzen S. "The Mechanisms of Alloxan- and Streptozotocin-induced Diabetes". Diabetologia 2008; 51 (2): 216–226.

[41] Szkudelski T. The mechanism of alloxan and streptozotocin action in β cells of the rat pancreas. Physiological Research 2001; 50(6):537-546.

[42] Etuk EU, Bello SO, Isezuo SA, Mohammed. Ethnobotanical Survey of Medicinal Plants used for the Treatment of Diabetes Mellitus in the North Western Region of Nigeria. Asian Journal of Experimental Biology &. Sciences 2010; (1):55-59.

[43] Naik RG. Hypoglygemig Plants-Abstracts On Clinical Trials. [updated 1989 October;]. Available from: ttp://www.rssdi.org/1989_october/abstract.pdf.

[44] Herrera AA, Aguilar S L, Garc BH, Nicasio TP, Tortoriello J. Clinical trial of *Cecropia obtusifolia* and *Marrubium vulgare* leaf extracts on blood glucose and serum lipids in type 2 diabetics. Phytomedicine 2004; 11:561–566.

[45] Mohamed B, Abderrahim Z, Hassane M, Abdelhafid T, Abdelkhaleq L. Medicinal plants with potential antidiabetic activity – A review of ten years of herbal medicine research (1990-2000). International Journal of Diabetes Metabolism 2006; 14:1-25.

[46] Eddouks M, Maghrani M, Lemhadri A, Ouahidi ML, Jouad H. Ethnopharmacological survey of medicinal plants used for the treatment of diabetes mellitus, hypertension and cardiac diseases in the south-east region of Morocco. Journal of Ethnopharmacology 2002;.82:97-103

[47] Pulok KM, Kuntal M, Kakali M, Peter JH. Leads from Indian medicinal plantswith hypoglycemic potentials. Journal of Ethnopharmacology 2006; 106:1–28.

[48] Esmaeili MA, Yazdanparast R. Hypoglycaemic effect of *Teucrium polium*: studies with rat pancreatic islets. Journal of Ethnopharmacology 2004; 95:27-30.

[49] Miura T, Itoh C, Iwamoto N, Aato M, Kawai M, Park SR, Suziki I. Hypoglycemic activity of the fruit of the *Momordica charantia* in Type 2 diabetic mice. Journal of Nutrition Science & Vitaminology (Tokyo). 2001; 47:340-4.

[50] Kim MJ, Ryu GR, Chung JS, Sim SS, Min DS, Rhie DJ, Yoon SH, Hahn SJ, Kim MS, Jo YH.. Protective effects of epicatechin against the toxic effects of streptozocin on rat pancreatic islets: in vivo and in vitro. Pancreas 2003; 26:292-299.

[51] Gholap S, Kar A. Hypoglycaemic effects of some plant extracts are possibly mediated through inhibition in corticosteroid concentration. Pharmazie 2004; 59:876-878.

[52] Heidari R, Zareae S, Heidarizadeh M. Extraction, Purification, and Inhibitory Effect of Alpha-Amylase Inhibitor from Wheat (*Triticum aestivum* Var. *Zarrin)*. Pakistan Journal of Nutrition 2005; 4:101-105.

[53] Hideaki K, Taka-aki M, Yoshihisa N, Dan K, Munehide M, Yoshimitsu Y. Oxidative Stress and the JNK Pathway in Diabetes. Current Diabetes Reviews 2005; 65-72.

[54] Goycheva V, Gadjeva BP (2006). Oxidative stress and its complications in diabetes mellitus. Trakia Journal of Sciences 2006; 4:1-8.

[55] Pérez-Matute P, Zulet MA, Martínez JA. Reactive species and diabetes: counteracting oxidative stress to improve health. Current Opinion in Pharmacology 2009; 9:771-779.

[56] Dembinska-Kiec A, Mykkänen O, Kiec-Wilk B, Mykkänen H (2008). Antioxidant Diogo CV, Suski JM, Lebiedzinska M, Karkucinska-Wieckowska A, Wojtala A, Pronicki M, Duszynski J, Pinton P, Portincasa P, Oliveira PJ, Wieckowski MR. Cardiac mitochondrial dysfunction during hyperglycemia--the role of oxidative stress and p66Shc signaling. International Journal of Biochemistry & Cell Biology 2013; 45(1):114-22.

[57] Crespy V, Williamson G (2004). A review of the health effects of green tea catechins in in vivo animal models. J Nutr, 134:3431S–3440S.

[58] Uma MM, Sudarsanam D. Phytomedicine for Diabetes mellitus: An overview. Research in Pharmacy 2011; 1(4): 28-37.

[59] Grover JK, Yadav S, Vats V. Medicinal plants of India with anti-diabetic potential. Journal of Ethnopharmacology 2002; 81:81-100.

[60] Edwin J, Siddaheswar BJ, Dharam CJ. Diabetes and Herbal Medicines. Iranian Journal of Pharmacology & Therapeutics 2008; 7: 97-106.

[61] Akinkugbe OO, Yakubu AM, Johnson TO, Mabadaje AFB, Kaine WN, Ikeme AA, Akinyanju OO, Oli JM, Kuti JA, and Akintoye CO. Non communicable diseases in Nigeria. Spectrum Books Limited, Ibadan, 1992; pp. 2-47.

[62] Bakari AG, Onyemekwue GC, Sani BG, Hassan SS, Aliyu TM. Prevalence of diabetes mellitus in suburban Northern Nigeria; Results of public screening survey. Diabetes International 1990; 9:59-60.

[63] Aderibigbe AO, Emudianughe TS, Lawal BA. Antihyperglycaemic effect of *Mangifera indica* in rat. Phytotherapy Research 1999; 13(6):504-507.

[64] Aderibigbe AO, Emudianughe TS, Lawal BA. Evaluation of the antidiabetic action of Mangifera indica in mice. Phytotherapy Research 2001; 15(5):456-458.

[65] Ojewole JA. Antinociceptive, antiinflamatory and antidiabetic properties of Hypoxis hemerocallidea (hypoxidaceae) corm [African potato] aqueous extracts in mice and rats. Journal of Ethnopharmacology 2006; 103: 126-134

[66] Atangwho IJ, Ebong PE, Eyong EU, Asmawi MZ, Ahmad M. Synergistic antidiabetic activity of Vernonia amygdalina and Azadirachta indica: biochemical effectsand possible mechanism. Journal of Ethnopharmacology 2012; 141(3):878-887.

[67] Farombi EO, Owoeye O. Antioxidative and chemopreventive properties of Vernonia amygdalina and Garcinia biflavonoid. International Journal of Environment Research and Public Health 2011; 8(6):2533-2555.

[68] Etuk EU, Mohammed BJ. Informant consensus selection method: A reliability assessment on medicinal plants used in north western Nigeria for the treatment of diabetes mellitus. African Journal of Pharmacy and Pharmacology 2009; 3(10):496-500.

[69] Mukhtar HM, Ansari SH, Ali M, Naved T, Bhat ZA. Effect of water extract of *Psidium guajava* leaves on alloxan-induced diabetic rats. Pharmazie 2004; 59(9):734-735.

[70] Huang CS, Yin MC, Chiu LC. Antihyperglycemic and antioxidative potential of Psidium guajava fruit in streptozotocin-induced diabetic rats. Food and Chemical Toxicology 2011; 49(9):2189-2195.

[71] Campos KE, Diniz YS, Cataneo AC, Faine LA, Alves MJ, Novelli EL. Hypoglycaemic and antioxidant effects of onion, Allium cepa: dietary onion addition, antioxidant ac-

tivity and hypoglycaemic effects on diabetic rats. International Journal of Food Science and Nutrition 2003; 54(3):241-246.

[72] El-Demerdash FM, Yousef MI, El-Naga NI. Biochemical study on the hypoglycemic effects of onion and garlic in alloxan-induced diabetic rats. Food and Chemical Toxicology 2005; 43(1):57-63.

[73] Li F, Li Q, Gao D, Peng Y. The optimal extraction parameters and anti-diabetic activity of flavonoids from *Ipomoea batatas* leaf. African Journal of Traditional Complementary and Alternative Medicine 2009; 6(2):195-202.

[74] Niwa A, Tajiri T, Higashino H. *Ipomoea batatas* and *Agarics blazei* ameliorate diabetic disorders with therapeutic antioxidant potential in streptozotocin-induced diabetic rats. Journal of Clinical Biochemistry and Nutrition 2011; 48(3):194-202.

[75] Gbolade AA. Inventory of antidiabetic plants in selected districts of Lagos State, Nigeria. Journal of Ethnopharmacology 2009; 121:135-139.

[76] Saidu AN, Akanya HO, Dauda BEN, and Ogbadoyi EO. Antibacterial and comparative hypoglycemic effect of Anacardium occidentale leaves. International Research Journal of Biochemistry and Bioinformatics 2012; 2(1): 006-010.

Chapter 5

The Antidiabetic Activities of the Aqueous Leaf Extract of Phyllanthus Amarus in some Laboratory Animals

Adeolu Adedapo, Sunday Ofuegbe and
Oluwafemi Oguntibeju

Additional information is available at the end of the chapter

http://dx.doi.org/10.5772/57030

1. Introduction

Diabetes mellitus (DM), often simply referred to as diabetes, is a group of metabolic diseases in which a patient has high blood sugar, either because the body does not produce enough insulin, or because cells do not respond to the insulin that is produced. This high blood sugar produces the classical symptoms of polyuria (frequent urination), polydipsia (increased thirst) and polyphagia (increased hunger). It is characterized by hyperglycaemia due to defective insulin action, insulin secretion or both. Several medicinal plants are used in the management of diabetes mellitus (Akah et al., 2002). According to the World Health Organization (WHO), there are approximately 160,000 diabetics worldwide, the number of diabetics has double in the last few years and is expected to double once again in the year 2025 (Beretta, 2001). Due to its high prevalence and potential deleterious effect on a patient physical and psychological state, diabetes is a major medical concern (Macedo et al., 2002). The disease remains incurable and can only be controlled with drugs. The three main types of diabetes mellitus (DM) are: Type 1 DM results from the body's failure to produce insulin, and presently requires the administration of insulin for treatment (Lambert et al., 2002). It is also referred to as insulin-dependent diabetes mellitus (IDDM) or "juvenile" diabetes). Type 2 DM results from insulin resistance, a condition in which cells fail to use insulin properly, sometimes combined with an absolute insulin deficiency (Boussageon et al., 2011). It is formerly referred to as noninsulin-dependent diabetes mellitus (NIDDM) or "adult-onset" diabetes). Gestational diabetes occurs when pregnant patient, who have never had diabetes before, have a high blood glucose level during pregnancy. It may precede development of type 2 DM (Sattar et al., 2010).

Several plants have been used in folkloric medicine for the treatment and prevention of infectious and non-infectious diseases in man and his animals and this has led to renewed scientific interest in the use of plants for these purposes (Oridupa et al. 2011). There is global resurgence in the use of herbal preparations and in some developing countries like Nigeria; it is being gradually integrated into the primary and secondary health care systems. Nearly all societies have used herbal materials as sources of medicines and the development of these herbal medicines depended on local botanical flora (Adedapo et al., 2009).

Phyllanthus amarus belongs to the family Euphorbiaceae (the spurge family) of which the largest genus is the genus Euphorbia. The plant is known to originate from Malaysia. The species *Phyllanthus amarus* is a small tropical herb, which occurs widely as a rainy-season weed throughout the hotter parts of India (Bagchi et al., 1992). The widespread usage of this herb has prompted several investigations (Calixto et al., 1998; Odetola and Akojenu, 2000; Adeneye et al., 2006). The plant has a history of use in Ayurverdic medicine for over 2000 years as well as a wide variety of traditional applications. The plant is commonly found in Southern Nigeria, Sierra Leone and Equatorial Guinea. It also occurs in Ghana and other parts of tropical Africa (Irvine, 1930; Adedapo et al., 2005). It is a weed of cultivated land and in waste spaces, it is common to find it growing and spreading freely along the road sides, under flower beds and in many other places (Burkill, 1994). For this reason, grazing animals are prone to consuming this plant along with their feed particularly in drier tropical climates where lush green grass is not often available (Adedapo, 2002).

Many studies have thus been carried out on the plant in various parts of the world but there is a resurgence of interest in this plant as antidiabetic agent. The present study was therefore undertaken to investigate the phytochemical constituents, anti-diabetic and safety potentials of the aqueous leaf extract of *Phyllanthus amarus* Schum in experimental animals especially that diabetes has assumed a global dimension as a non-communicable disease.

2. Material and methods

2.1. Plant material and preparation of extracts

Fresh leaves of *Phyllanthus amarus* Schum were collected from the campus of the University of Ibadan, Nigeria in March 2012. The leaves were identified by botanists and a voucher specimen (UIH ADE/003/2012) deposited at the herbarium of the Department of Botany, University of Ibadan. The ground plant material (200 g) was shaken in 1 L distilled water for 48 h on an orbital shaker at room temperature of 24°C. The extract was filtered using a Buckner funnel and Whatman No 1 filter paper. The filtrate was concentrated to dryness under reduced pressure at 40ºC using a rotary evaporator. The thick solution was lyophilized using freeze drying system for biological investigations. The extract yield was 13.85%.

2.2. Animals

The animals used in this study were male Wistar rats weighing between 100 and 200g as well as mice weighing between 15 and 30g. They were maintained at the Experimental Animal House of the Faculty of Veterinary Medicine, University of Ibadan in rat cages and fed on commercial rabbit cubes (Ladokun and Son Livestock Feeds, Nigeria Ltd). The animals were allowed free access to clean fresh water in bottles *ad libitum*. All experimental protocols were in compliance with University of Ibadan Ethics Committee on Research in Animals as well as internationally accepted principles for laboratory animal use and care.

2.3. Chemicals

Alloxan used in this study was obtained from Sigma-Aldrich (Chemie Gmbh, Steinheim, Denmark). The standard drug used in the various experiments was glibenclamide. The chemical and drug used were of analytical grade. Normal saline and distilled water were also used in this study.

2.4. Phytochemical screening

The phytochemical analysis was performed on the ground (powered) leaf of *P. amarus* for identification of the constituents. The constituents tested for were alkaloids, tannins, saponins, anthraquinones, cardiac glycosides and flavonoids as described by Trease and Evans (1983); Abate (1989); Shale et al., (1999); Evans, (2002); Moody et al., (2006) and Sawadogo et al., (2006).

2.5. Acute toxicity test

The acute toxicity of *P. amarus* aqueous was determined in mice according to the method of Hilaly *et al.* (2004) with slight modifications. Mice fasted for 16 h were randomly divided into groups of six mice per group. Graded doses of the plant's extract (100, 200, 400, 800 and 1600 mg/kg p.o.) were separately administered to the mice in each of the groups by means of bulbed steel needle. All the mice in the groups were then allowed free access to food and water and observed over a period of 48 h for signs of acute toxicity. The number of deaths within this period of time was recorded.

3. Antidiabetic studies

3.1. Hypoglycaemic activity test

The hypoglycaemic effect of the aqueous extract was studied in alloxan-induced diabetic rats. The rats were fasted for 8 hours but allowed free access to water. At the end of the fasting period, the basal fasting blood glucose (FBG) level of the rats was determined. Subsequently, diabetes was induced by single intraperitoneal injection of alloxan monohydrate (70 mg/kg) (Aruna *et al.,* 1999) and normal feeding maintained thereafter. Five days later, blood was drawn from each rat and the blood glucose level was measured to establish diabetes. Animals with blood glucose level ≥225mg/dl was considered to be diabetic and used for this study. The diabetic animals were randomly divided into four groups (n=5) and received oral administration of aqueous extract (200 and 400 mg/kg), Distilled water (5ml/kg) and Glibenclamide (0.2 mg/kg) respectively. Aqueous extract was dissolved in distil water. Blood glucose was then measured before (i.e. 0 h) and at 0.5, 1, 2 and 4 h after treatment.

3.2. Normoglycaemic activity

Animals fasted overnight were randomly divided into four groups (n=5) and received oral administration of the extract (200 and 400mg/kg), glibenclamide (0.2mg/kg) and vehicle control (5ml/kg) respectively. The blood glucose level of each animal was measured prior to (pretreatment) and at 0.5, 1, 2 and 4hour after extract administration (Okoli et al., 2010).

3.3. Oral glucose tolerance test

Animals were fasted for 16h but with free access to water were randomly divided into four groups (n=5) and received oral administration of the aqueous extract (200 and 400mg/kg), glibenclamide (0.2mg/kg) and vehicle control (5ml/kg) respectively. Ninety minutes later, the rats were fed with glucose (4g/kg). The blood glucose level of animals in each group was then measured before (0) and at 30, 60, 90, 120, 150, 180 min after glucose load (Okoli et al., 2010).

3.4. Antidiabetic activity test

The antidiabetic effect of the plant extract was studied by evaluating the effect of its chronic administration on the blood glucose level of alloxan-induced diabetic rats. The basal fasting blood glucose (FBG) of the rats was determined and diabetes was induced as described before. 25 diabetic rats with glucose level ≥225 were selected and used for the study. The rats were fasted for 8h but allowed free access to water (Okoli et al., 2010). They were then divided randomly into five groups (n=5) and received oral administration of extract (200 and 400mg/kg), glibenclamide (0.2mg/kg, diabetic control), extract (200mg/kg) and the vehicle (5ml/kg) both of which serve as non diabetic control. The treatment was administered orally to the animals once daily for 28 days. Blood glucose level was then measured as described before (pretreatment) and on days 14 and 28 after commencement of the treatment. The body weight of each animal was also measured on these days.

3.5. Effects of the extract on lipid profile of diabetic rats

The effect of the extract on the lipid profile of treated diabetic rats was studied by monitoring the cholesterol and triglyceride levels. Blood samples were collected by ocular puncture, transferred into test tubes and centrifuged at 3000 rpm for 5 mins. The serum was collected and the total cholesterol and triglyceride levels of each sample were separately determined by enzymatic colorimetric method (Muller *et al.*, 1977) using reagent kits. Lipid levels of diabetic animals were measured before (Basal) and after the induction of diabetes (pre-treatment) as well as on days 14 and 28 after commencement of treatment. The absorbance of each sample containing the reaction mixture with or without serum was read at 540nm in a UV spectrophotometer. Total cholesterol or triglyceride is calculated using the formula: Total cholesterol (mg/dl) = SAod/STod x 200, where SAod = optical density of test sample and STod = optical density of standard.

3.6. Effects of the extract on haemoglobin and cell counts of diabetic rats

The effect of chronic administration of the extract on haemoglobin (Hb) and cell counts [white blood cells (WBC) and red blood cells (RBC)] of diabetic rats was also determined. Blood samples were collected by ocular puncture using haematocrit tubes, transferred into EDTA-containing test tubes and placed in a haematology analyzer (Abacus Junior®, Budapest-Hungary) for determination of the parameters. Measurements were taken before (basal) and after the induction of diabetes (Pre-treatment) as well as on days 14 and 28 after the commencement of treatment (Post-treatment).

3.7. Estimation of haemoglobin

Cyanohaemoglobin method was used for this purpose (Coles, 1986). Four mls of Drabkin′s solution (diluents) was placed in a tube, 0.02ml of the collected blood sample was put in the tube using pipette and the pipette was rinsed for more than three times. The mixture was stirred well and allowed to stand for 10minutes. This was read in a colorimeter at 540nm wavelength. The equivalent haemoglobin was read from a calibration curve or table. The haemoglobin value of the blood sample was calculated as:

Photometer reading of unknown x g% Hb value of standard x DF/Photometer reading of standard

DF = dilution factor and it was calculated as:

Volume of the whole blood used + volume of diluent/volume of whole blood used.

It is expressed in gram percent.

3.8. Determination of erythrocyte (rbc) count

Erythrocyte diluting pipette marked 101 above the bulb was used to draw the blood sample up to exactly 0.5mark. The tip of the pipette was then inserted into the erythrocyte diluting fluid - Gower′s solution and through a steady suction; the pipette was filled with the fluid to the 101 line above the bulb, rotating it gently while filling. The pipette was brought to a horizontal position and finger tip was placed over the tip before removing the rubber tubing. The pipette was shaken for more than 30minutes in a mechanical shaker; the haemocytometer was then filled with the diluted blood and then allowed to stand for a few minutes for the cells to settle. The erythrocytes were then counted under microscope lens (x 40 objective) counting all the erythrocytes in the 5 of the 25 small squares in the central area. Each of the 5 small squares to be counted was bordered by double or triple lines and was divided into 16 smaller squares. A total of 80 of these small squares were counted. The cells were counted beginning at the left of the top row of small squares, then from right to left for the next row and so on.

Calculation

Cells counted x 10(0.1mm depth) x 5(1/5 of sqmm) x 200(1:200) dilution = erythrocytes per cu mm.

OR

The sum of the cells in the five small squares multiplied by 10,000 = total erythrocytes per cu mm (Coles, 1986)

3.9. Determination of leucocyte (wbc) count

Leucocyte diluting pipetting was used to draw the blood sample to a point marked 0.5 and filled with leucocyte diluting fluid up to the 11mark above the bulb. The mixture was shaken for 3minutes until well mixed. Two to three drops from the pipette was discarded before filling the counting chamber of haemocytometer. The leucocytes were allowed to settle for 1minute. The leucocytes in the larger squares of haemocytometer chamber were counted and multiplied by 50 to obtain the total number of white blood cells (Coles, 1986).

Calculation:

Cells counted x 20 (1:20 dilution) x 10(0.1mm depth)/4 (no of sq mm counted)

= WBC/cubic mm

OR

The sum of the cell counted in the 4 corner squares multiplied by 50 = total leucocytes per cubic mm.

4. Histological studies on the liver, kidney and pancreas

The effect of the extracts on tissue architecture of the pancreas of treated diabetic rats was evaluated by histological studies of tissue sections obtained from the animals. On day 28 of the experiment, one animal was randomly selected from the different groups and sacrificed by over-dose of chloroform anaesthesia. The whole pancreas from each animal was removed and placed in 10% formalin in normal saline for histological studies. The isolated organ was placed in an automatic tissue processor for 24 hrs. After 24 hrs, the tissues were solidified in molten wax and sectioned using automatic tissue sectioner. The tissue sections were then fixed on slides with haematoxylin and eosin. The stained slides were fixed with mountant, allowed to dry and viewed under the microscope (x400). This procedure was repeated for the liver and kidney collected from the sacrificed animals.

4.1. Statistical analysis

Data was analyzed using graph pad prism 5 and the results expressed as mean ± SD. The results were further subjected to one way ANOVA for comparisons and differences between means were considered significant at $P< 0.05$.

5. Results and discussion

Phytochemical screening of the leaves of *P. amarus* showed the presence of alkaloids, tannin, flavonoids, saponin, anthraquinones and cardiac glycosides. Flavonoids and tannins are phenolic compounds and plant phenolics are also a major group of compounds that act as primary antioxidants or free radical scavengers (Adedapo et al., 2008a, 2008b, Ayoola et al., 2008). Tannins and saponins are also found to be effective antioxidants, antimicrobial, and anti-carcinogenic agents (Lai et al., 2010). Polyphenolic compounds are ubiquitous in foods of plant origin, and thus they constitute an integral part of the human diet (Bravo 1998). Interest in polyphenols has greatly increased recently because these phytochemicals are known to suppress rates of degenerative processes such as cardiovascular disorders and cancer (Bravo 1998, Duthie 2000, Huang et al., 2007; Jimoh et al., 2010). Some of these potential health benefits of polyphenolic substances have been related to the action of these compounds as antioxidants, free radical scavengers, quenchers of singlet and triplet oxygen and inhibitors of peroxidation (Li-Chen et al., 2005). As a group, phenolic compounds have been found to be strong antioxidants against free radicals and other reactive oxygen species, the major cause of many chronic human diseases (Kyung-Hee et al., 2005, Chen and Yen 2007).

In the acute toxicity test, no death was recorded in all the groups. All the mice appeared to be normal and none of them showed any visible signs of toxicity. Acute oral administration of *Phyllanthus amarus* to mice indicated that the plant is non toxic even at the dose of 1600mg/kg body weight. It thus showed that this plant is safe for medicinal use at this dose.

The aqueous extract caused a significant ($P<0.05$) dose related reduction in the fasting blood glucose (FBG) of normoglycaemic rats. Maximum reduction occurred within 2hr post- treatment with 400mg/kg dose of the extract (Table 1). In this study, experimental evaluation of the antidiabetic potentials of *P. amarus* has shown that single oral administration of the extract to normal rats reduced fasting blood glucose which suggests an inherent hypoglycaemic effect (Table 2). The extract also suppressed the postprandial rise in blood glucose in normal rats following a heavy glucose meal with maximum suppressive effect coinciding with the time of peak blood glucose level after the meal (Table 3). Chronic hyperglycaemia in DM is a risk factor constantly fuelled by postprandial elevation of blood glucose. Control of postprandial hyperglycaemia in diabetes is of great importance due to its close relation to the risk of micro and macro-vascular complications and death (Balkau, 2000; Ceriello, 2005).

Treatment	Dose mg/kg	Fasting Blood Glucose level (mg/dl)				
		Pretreatment	0.5hr	1hr	2hr	4hr
Control	2ml/kg	72.4±5.5	71.2±6.0	70.6±5.6	70±5.1	70±4.7
Glibenclamide	0.2	72.2±4.1	66.6±3.4[b] (7.7)	62.0±6.9[b] (14.1)	54.0±3.4[ab] (25.2)	49.0±3.9[ab] (32.1)
Aqueous Extract	200	73.0±4.0	69.6±4.0 (4.7)	64.0±4.2[b] (12.3)	56.0±4.9[ab] (23.3)	50.6±5.8[ab] (30.7)

[ab]P< 0.05 compared to control and pre-treatment values respectively (t-test). Values in parenthesis represent reduction (%) in fasting blood levels glucose levels of normoglycaemic rats calculated relative to pre-treatment values.

Table 1. Effects of Aqueous extract of *P. amarus* on blood glucose of normoglycaemic rats (n=5; mean ± SD.).

Treatment	Dose mg/kg	Blood Glucose level (mg/dl)						
		0 min	30min	60min	90min	120min	150min	180min
Control	2ml/kg	61.4±1.9	74.4±4.6 (21.2)	78.0±7.0 (27.0)	73.2±5.8 (19.2)	69.8±5.5 (13.7)	63.2±7.1 (2.9)	59.6±5.1 (2.9)
Glibenclamide	0.2	65.0±2.8	67.8±2.7 (4.3)	70.2±4.0[a] (8.00)	66.8±4.1 (2.8)	64.2±7.8(1. 2)	62.4±1.5(4. 00)	61.8±1.8(4.9)
Aqueous Extract	200	62.6±6.7	73.2±7.5[a] (16.9)	80.2±6.7[a] (28.1)	72.8±4.5[a] (16.3)	64.2±3.5 (2.6)	55.4±5.8 (11.5)	49.4±4.6[a] (21.1)
Aqueous Extract	400	62.0±9.0	65.4±6.2 (5.5)	67.0±5.4 (8.1)	63.4±4.7 (2.3)	59.6±3.8 (3.9)	54.0±2.3 (12.9)	50.6±2.2[a] (12.4)

[a]P< 0.05 compared to 0 minute values (t-Test). Superscripted items ([a]) indicate significant values when compared to 0 min values. Values in parenthesis represent change (%) in blood glucose level calculated relative to 0 min.

Table 2. Effects of aqueous extract of *Phyllanthus amarus* on oral glucose tolerance in rats (n=5; mean ± SD.)

Treatment	Dose mg/kg	Blood Glucose level (mg/dl)				
		Pretreatment	0.5hr	1hr	2hr	4hr
Control	2ml/kg	311.0±33.8	298.0±34.3	282.0±31.2	268.0±24.8	256.0±24.2
Glibenclamide	0.2	290.0±26.1	268.0±27.7 (7.6)	252.0±27.1 (13.1)	228.0±17.2[ab] (21.4)	208.0±16.3[ab] (28.3)
Aqueous Extract	200	296.0±39.3	276.0±32.2 (6.8)	256.0±35.1 (13.5)	230.0±36.9[b] (22.3)	204.0±43.1[ab] (31.1)
Aqueous Extract	400	276.0±24.2	256.0±20.6[a] (7.3)	236.0±20.6[ab] (14.5)	217.0±24.4[ab] (21.4)	200.0±18.7[ab] (27.5)

[ab]P< 0.05 compared to control and pre-treatment values respectively (t-Test). Superscripted items ([ab]) indicate significant values when compared to control and pre-treatment values respectively. Values in parenthesis represent reduction (%) in blood glucose level calculated relative to pre treatment values.

Table 3. Hypoglycaemic effects of aqueous extract of *P. amarus* on diabetic rats (n=5; mean ± SD.)

Following oral administration of glucose, postprandial blood glucose levels of the control rats increased to the peak at 60min. Pre-treatment with aqueous extract (200 and 400mg/kg) suppressed the rise in blood glucose by 28.1 and 8.1% respectively. The aqueous extract used in this study evoked a progressive dose-dependent decrease in blood glucose level up to 180mins. Chronic oral administration of aqueous extract caused a significant (P<0.05) dose-related reduction in blood glucose of diabetic rats. The extract at dose of 400mg/kg reduced the blood glucose of the treated rats better than glibenclamide; while the extract at 200mg/kg exerts almost the same effect as glibenclamide. The highest reduction in the blood glucose was 60.9% and this was obtained with the 400mg/kg on 28th day (Table 4). In this study, daily oral administration of the extract for 28 days produced a gradual but sustained reduction in blood glucose levels in diabetic rats. Alloxan causes hyperglycaemia and glucose intolerance or syndromes similar to either type 1 or type 2 DM (Lenzen et al., 1996: Frode and Medeiros, 2008). Effective and sustained reduction in blood glucose levels of treated diabetic rats by the extract indicates that the plant may be useful in overt cases of DM. Effective control of blood glucose level is a key step in preventing and reversing diabetic complications, and improving the quality of life of diabetic patients (Bavarva and Narasimhacharya, 2008).

Treatment	Dose mg/kg	Blood glucose concentration (mg/dl)			
		Pre-Diabetic (Basal)	Diabetic (Pretreatment)	Diabetic Post-Rx	
				Day 14	Day 28
Control (NDNT)	2ml/kg	57.4±6.2	58.8±5.8	69.2±4.6[a]	86.6±4.6[a]
Control (NDT)	200	54.8±8.4	56.8±8.7	70.8±7.4[a]	90.2±5.5[a]
Glibenclamide	0.2	56.2±5.2	290±26.1	148.0±13.3a (49.0)	122.0±9.3a (57.9)
Aqueous Extract	200	55.0±5.0	296.0±32.3	140.0±20.7a (52.7)	126±19.9a (57.4)
Aqueous Extract	400	53.4±3.3	276.0±24.2	132.0±17.2a (52.2)	107.8±5.0a (60.9)

[a]P< 0.05 compared to diabetic pre-treatment values (t-Test). Superscripted items ([a]) indicate significant values when compared to diabetic pre-treatment values. NDNT= Non-diabetic non-treated was a non-diabetic control and received the vehicle; NDT= Non-diabetic treated was a non-diabetic control and received AE (200mg/kg). Values in parenthesis represent reduction (%) in blood glucose level calculated for treatment groups relative to diabetic pre-treatment values.

Table 4. Effect of Aqueous extract of *P. amarus* on blood glucose of diabetic rats (n=5; mean ± SD.)

Treatment	Dose mg/kg	Parameters	Total Cholesterol (mg/dl); Triglycerides (mg/dl); Haemoglobin (g%)			
			PreDiabetic (Basal)	Diabetic (Pre-Rx)	Diabetic Post-Rx	
					Day 14	Day 28
Control (NDNT)	2ml/kg	Cholesterol	122.4±7.3	124.6±5.20	124.0±9.7 (0.5)	126.2±4.6 (-1.3)
		Triglycerides	114.0±5.7	115.8±7.4	126.4±14.7 (-9.2)	117.6±13 (-1.6)
		Hb	14.6±0.5	13.8±0.6	14.0±1.3	13.3±1.2
Control (NDT)	200	Cholesterol	117.2±7.8	111.0±9.9	109.6±8.5 (1.3)	105.8±7.9^{a} (4.7)
		Triglycerides	106.4±9.0	109.6±6.5	92.6±11.6^{b} (15.5)	85.4±9.5^{ab}(22.1)
		Hb	14.4±1.1	14.0±0.9	15.5±1.1	14.1±2.3
Glibenclamide	0.2	Cholesterol	120.8±8.3	115.0±14.1	118.8±8.6 (-3.3)	110.6±5.2^{a} (3.8)
		Triglycerides	104.2±11.2	119.4±7.5	111.2±5.0 (6.0)	104.0±4.3^{b} (12.9)
		Hb	14.8±1.0	13.9±0.8	15.4±1.0^{b}	14.3±0.4
Aqueous Extract	200	Cholesterol	118.6±4.7	128.0±2.8	95.0±7.1^{ab} (25.8)	88.4±7.1^{ab} (30.9)
		Triglycerides	114.2±6.1	142.0±9.0	124.8±5.2ab (12.1)	109.6±7.6^{b} (22.8)
		Hb	15.4±2.0	14.8±1.8	15.4±0.7	15.2±1.1
Aqueous Extract	400	Cholesterol	115.0±7.1	123.2±9.1	100.0±7.1^{ab} (18.8)	87.0±5.1^{ab} (29.4)
		Triglycerides	114.0±9.2	121.0±8.8	115.2±7.8 (4.8)	105.6±9.4^{b} (12.7)
		Hb	15.8±1.5	14.6±1.8	15.2±0.8	14.7±0.8

$^{ab}P<0.05$ compared to Basal and Diabetic pre-treatment values respectively (t-Test); Superscripted items (^{ab}) indicate significant values when compared to control and pre-treatment values respectively. NDNT=Non diabetic non treated was a non diabetic control and received the vehicle, NDT = Non diabetic treated was a non diabetic control and received aqueous extract (200mg/kg). Values in parenthesis represent reduction (%) of total cholesterol and triglycerides calculated for treatment groups relative to diabetic pre-treatment values.

Table 5. Effect of Aqueous extract of *P. amarus* on Cholesterol, triglycerides and haemoglobin levels of diabetic rats (n=5; mean ± SD.)

Chronic administration of aqueous extract reduced total cholesterol level of diabetic rats. The aqueous extract caused a significant (P<0.05) reduction in the total cholesterol of treated diabetic rats. The magnitude of reduction was greater than that evoked by glibenclamide. Chronic administration of aqueous extract reduced triglyceride concentration of the diabetic rats. The aqueous extract caused a significant (P<0.05) reduction in the triglyceride level of treated diabetic rats. The magnitude of reduction was greater than that evoked by glibenclamide. The haemoglobin level of all the animals was increased initially on day 14 with no significant difference except for the glibenclamide-treated animals. Subsequently, there was reduction in the haemoglobin level on day 28 (Table 5). Diabetic dyslipidaemia is marked by elevated triglycerides, cholesterol and low density lipoprotein (LDL) particles of altered composition and decreased high density lipoprotein (HDL), and constitutes an important cardiovascular risk factor in diabetics (Agrawal et al., 2006). Reduction in total cholesterol and triglycerides through dietary or drug therapy has been found beneficial in preventing diabetic complications as well as improving lipid metabolism in diabetic patients (Brown et al., 1993; Ahmed et al., 2001). Experimentally, alloxan-induced diabetic hyperglycaemia is accompanied by increase in serum cholesterol and triglyceride levels (Choi et al., 1991;

http://dx.doi.org/10.5772/57030

Ahmed et al., 2001; Okoli et al., 2010) and mimics overt diabetes disease. Thus, in addition to glycaemic control, extract of this plant may further reduce mortality from complications of the disease by ameliorating diabetes-induced dislipidaemia. The RBC count of all the animals was reduced on day 14 with all the groups showing significant difference except the 400mg/kg dose of the aqueous extract. Subsequently, there was increase in the RBC count on day 28 with all the groups showing significant difference with the exception of the 400mg/kg dose of the aqueous extract. The white blood cell (WBC) count of all the control and glibenclamide- treated animals was reduced initially on day 14 with no significant difference; while there was increase in the WBC count of the extract-treated group on day 14 and the increase continued on day 28 with the 400mg/kg dose of the extract showing significant difference. Likewise, there was subsequent increase in the control (both NDT and NDNT) groups and glibenclamide-treated group on day 28 with no significant difference (Table 6). Again, assessment of the effect of chronic administration of the extracts on haemoglobin level as well as white blood cell and red blood cell counts revealed an increase following an initial reduction in most cases of the experiment. It is not clear if it would progress to a return to basal levels and how long it may take.

Treatment	Dose mg/kg	Parameters	RBC ($X10^6/\mu L$); WBC ($X10^3/\mu L$)			
			PreDiabetic (Basal)	Diabetic (Pre-Rx)	Diabetic Post-Rx	
					Day 14	Day 28
Control (NDNT)	2ml/kg	RBC	5.2±0.1	4.9±0.1	4.6±0.1^{ab}	6.8±0.7^{ab}
		WBC	4.8±0.3	4.8±0.3	4.8±0.3	4.9±0.3
Control (NDT)	200	RBC	5.2±0.1	5.1±0.03	4.9±0.1^{ab}	5.0±0.2a
		WBC	5.0±0.3	4.9±0.3	4.8±0.3	5.1±0.03
Glibenclamide	0.2	RBC	5.6±0.2	5.3±0.3	4.8±0.3ab	5.4±0.2
		WBC	4.7±0.6	5.0±0.5	4.7±0.2	4.8±0.1
Aqueous Extract	200	RBC	5.2±0.1	5.1±0.1	4.8±0.2ab	5.4±0.1ab
		WBC	4.8±0.3	4.8±0.3	5.0±0.3	5.1±0.3
Aqueous Extract	400	RBC	4.8±0.4	4.6±0.3	4.6±0.1	4.8±0.1
		WBC	4.9±0.2	4.8±0.2	5.0±0.1	5.2±0.1^{ab}

$^{ab}P<0.05$ compared to Basal and Diabetic pre-treatment values respectively (t-Test); Superscripted items (^{ab}) indicate significant values when compared to control and pre-treatment values respectively. NDT = Non diabetic treated was a non diabetic control and received aqueous extract (200mg/kg); NDNT = Non diabetic non treated was a non diabetic control and received the vehicle.

Table 6. Effect of Aqueous extract of *P. amarus* on the Red Blood Cell (RBC) and White Blood Cell (WBC) counts of diabetic rats (n=5; mean ± SD.)

There was increase in the body weight of all the groups on day 14 and the increase continued on day 28 with the 400mg/kg dose of aqueous extract showing significant difference (P<0.05). The weight increase occurred most in the NDT control group followed by the NDNT control group and then the 400mg/kg dose of aqueous extract (Table 7). Due to the association of obesity with DM, weight control is an important aspect of diabetes management. Poor glycaemic control usually results in weight loss. The results showed that all the animals used gained weight during the study. The weight gain was highest in the nondiabetic treated control while glibenclamide-treated control has modest weight gain. In some cases however, adequate glycaemic control by some agents may lead to increase in body weight such as that observed with the thiazolidinediones (Monnier et al., 2003; Bhat et al., 2007). The result showed that at 400mg/kg dose, aqueous extract showed a significant increase in body weight. It is also important to note that chronic administration of the extracts did not inhibit the natural growth process of these animals with or without diabetes.

Treatment	Dose mg/kg	Body weight (g)			
		Pre-Diabetic (Basal)	Diabetic (Pre-Rx)	Diabetic Post-Rx	
				Day 14	Day 28
Control (NDNT)	2ml/kg	214.0±11.2	209.0±14.1	226.6±10.4 (8.4)	231.8±7.68 (10.91)
Control (NDT)	200	135.0±36.9	137.0±35.9	150.0±37.5 (8.7)	157.0±38.43 (14.60)
Glibenclamide	0.2	191.0±34.6	188.0±37.9	196.0±33.9 (4.3)	200.0±32.6 (6.4)
Aqueous Extract	200	196.0±18.1	192.0±18.2	206.6±20.9 (7.6)	211.0±22.2 (9.9)
Aqueous Extract	400	214.0±15.0	212.0±13.0	228.0±7.8^{b} (7.6)	234.0±5.8^{ab} (10.4)

$^{ab}P<0.05$ compared to Basal and Diabetic pre-treatment values respectively (t-Test); Superscripted items (^{ab}) indicate significant values when compared to control and pre-treatment values respectively. NDT = Non diabetic treated was a non diabetic control and received AE (200mg/kg); NDNT = Non diabetic non-treated was a non diabetic control and received the vehicle. Value in parenthesis represents percentage increase (%) of body weight calculated for treatment groups relative to diabetic pre-treatment values.

Table 7. Effect of chronic administration of aqueous extract of *Phyllanthus amarus* on body weight of diabetic rats (n=5; mean ± SD.).

Histological examination of the pancreas shows the necrosis of the islet tissues with the alveolar cells moderately destroyed; there was also moderate congestion of the blood vessels (Figure 1) in the diabetic non-treated group. In the extract-treated group, the architecture of the pancreas appeared intact. The interlobular, intralobular and the alveolar granules were seen (Figure 2). There was slight necrosis of the pancreas around the islet tissues in the glibenclamide-treated group (Figure 3). Microscopical examination of liver section of diabetic non-treated group (Figure 4) showed various degrees of pathological changes such as centrilobular fatty degeneration, cloudy swelling, and vacuolar change of the hepatocytes as well as necrosis of hepatic cells. Microscopical examination of liver section of diabetic extract-treated control group (Figure 5) showed normal arrangement of hepatocytes with clear broad of central vein at portal layer. The histopathological study showed recovery of the damaged liver cells in the extract- treated group. The liver of the glibenclamide-treated group showed widespread vacuolar change of the hepatocytes (figure 6). Microscopical ex-

http://dx.doi.org/10.5772/57030

amination of the kidney section of diabetic non-treated control showed moderate loss of renal tubules and congestion of renal blood vessels in the medulla (figure 7). There was no visible lesion seen in the extract-treated (figure 8). There was no visible lesion seen in the glibenclamide-treated group (Figure 9). Several factors such as oxidative stress (Hayden et al., 2005), chronic hyperglycaemia (Leung and Leung, 2008) and autoimmune (Yoshida et al., 1995) or fibrocalculous (Mohan et al., 2008) types of chronic pancreatitis damage the pancreas and impair insulin secretion and hence glycaemic control. Results of histological studies on pancreas isolated from treated diabetic rat showed that the extract may have repaired the pancreas damaged by alloxan. Alloxan causes diabetes by destruction of ß-cells of the islet (Szudelski, 2001; Frode and Medeiros, 2008) which consequently impairs insulin secretion and gives rise to hyperglycemia. Treatment with the extract may have restored the integrity and perhaps, functions of the damaged pancreatic tissues. Also, the extract was able to restore the damaged kidney and liver to their normal architecture. Glibenclamide used as a reference hypoglycemic agent did not cause such effect to the same extent as the extract (Figures 1-9). The precise mechanism of this tissue repair is not known. However, due to the large implication of oxidative stress (Hayden et al., 2005; Leung and Leung, 2008) in damage to the pancreas, it seems reasonable to suggest that the antioxidant (Tasaduq et al., 2003) and radical scavenging (Jagetia and Baliga, 2004) effects of this plant may play a key role in protecting pancreatic tissues from oxidants including that generated by alloxan. Alloxan destroys insulin-producing pancreatic ß-cells through the formation of reactive oxygen species that cause tissue damage (Lee et al., 2008).

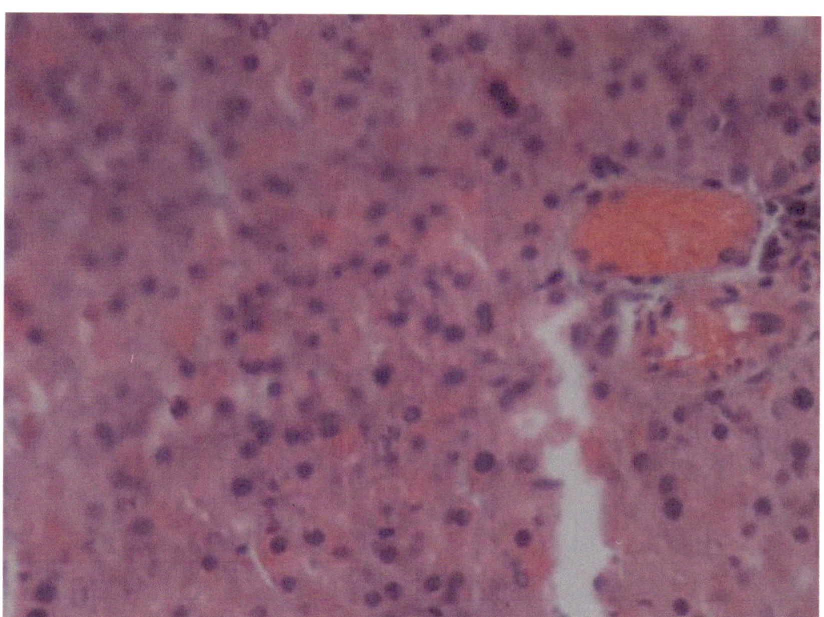

Figure 1. Pancreas of diabetic non-treated rat (X400)

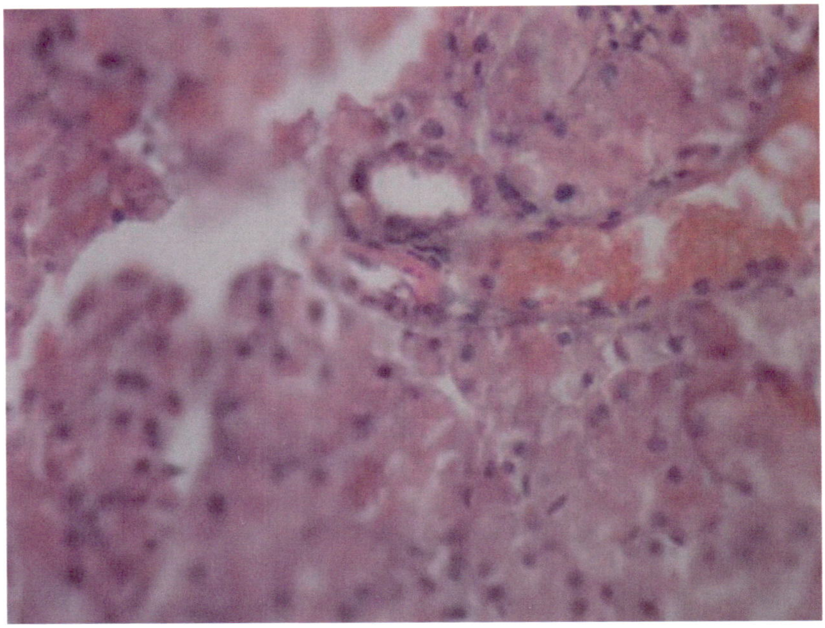

Figure 2. Effect of *P. amarus* extract on the pancreas of alloxan-induced diabetic rats (X400)

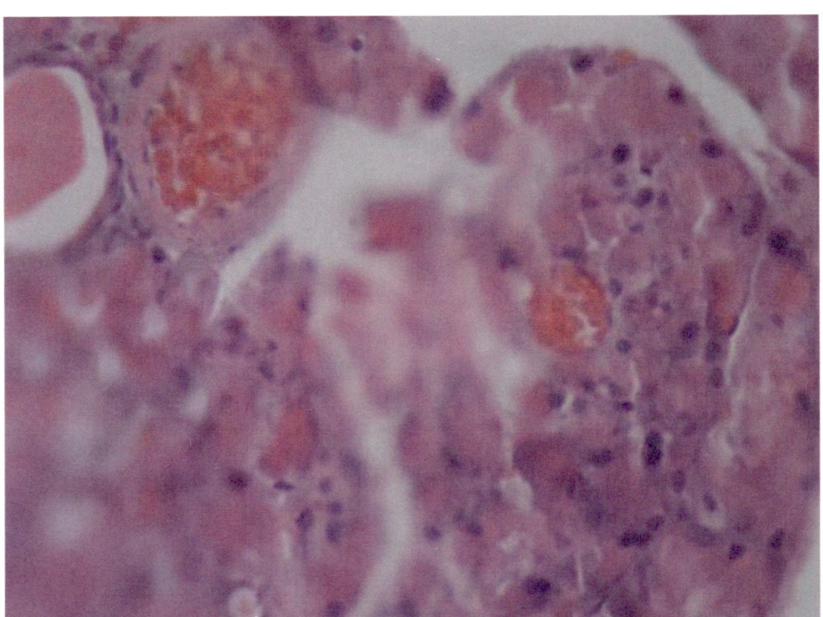

Figure 3. Effect of glibenclamide on the pancreas of alloxan-induced diabetic rat (X400)

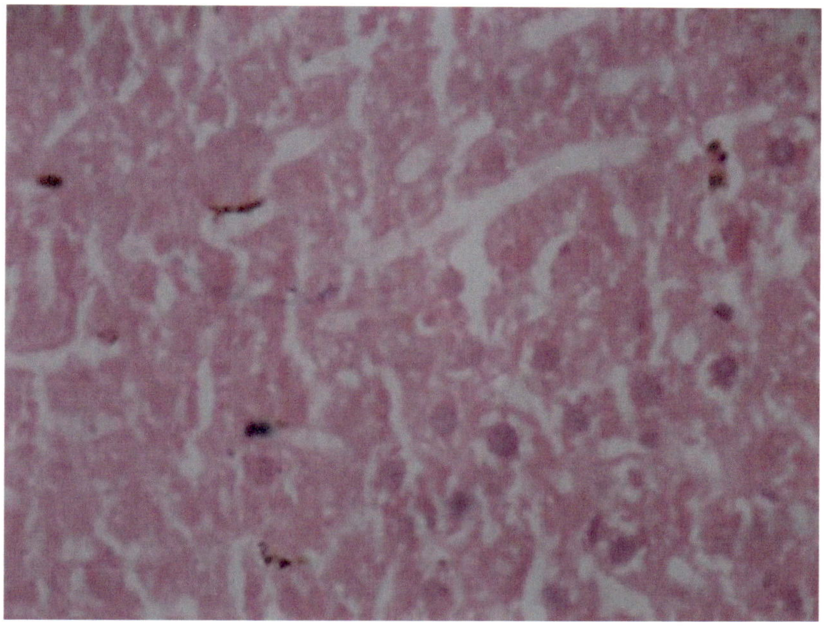

Figure 4. Liver section of diabetic non-treated group (X400)

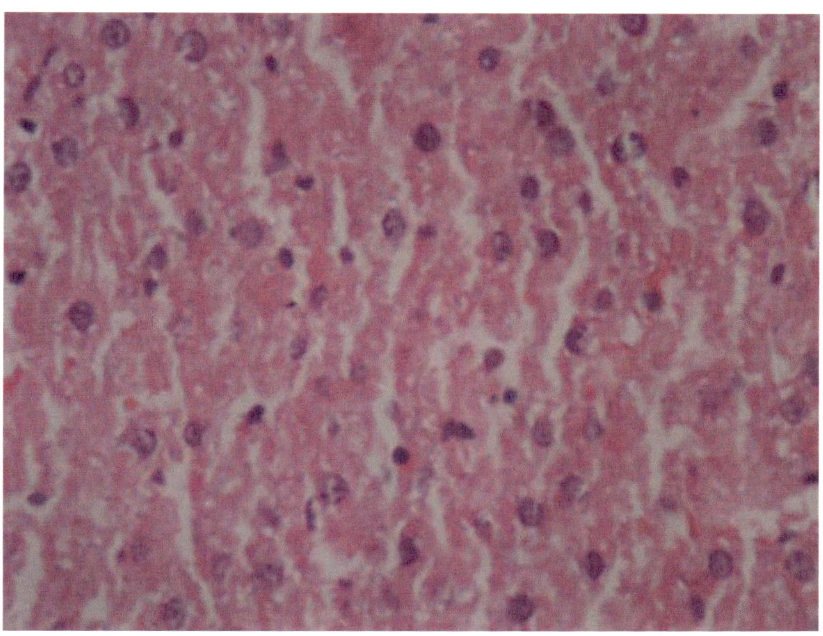

Figure 5. Effect of *P. amarus* extract on the liver of alloxan-induced diabetic rats (X400)

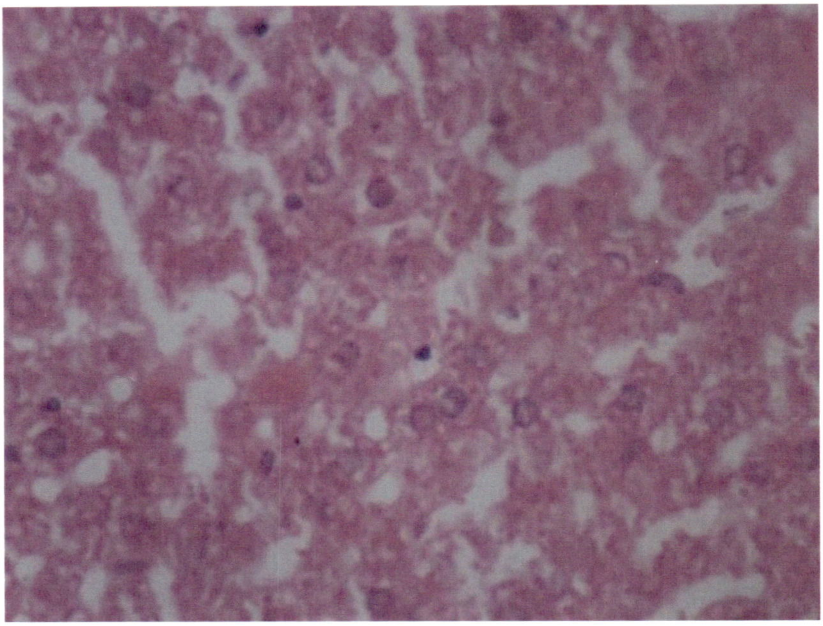

Figure 6. Effect of glibenclamide on the Liver of alloxan-induced diabetic rat (X400)

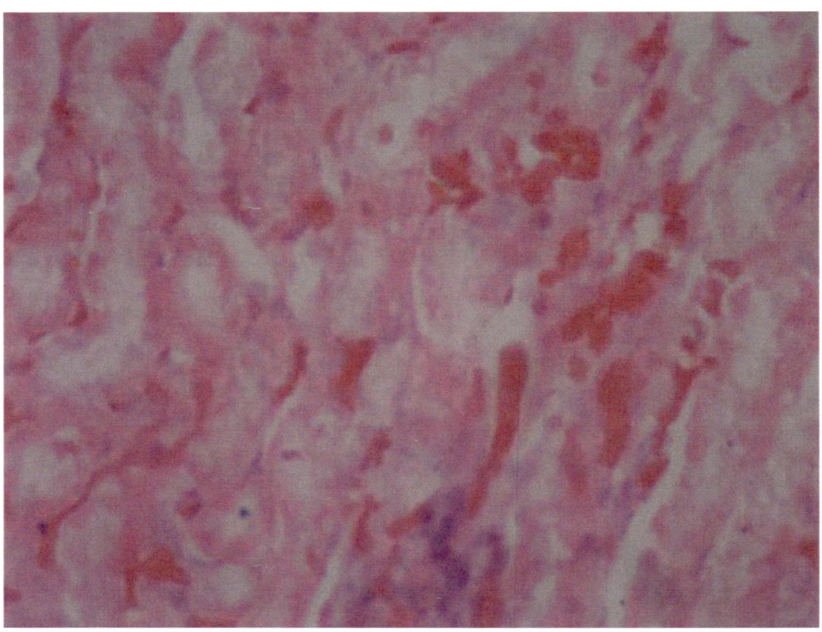

Figure 7. Kidney section of diabetic non-treated group (X400)

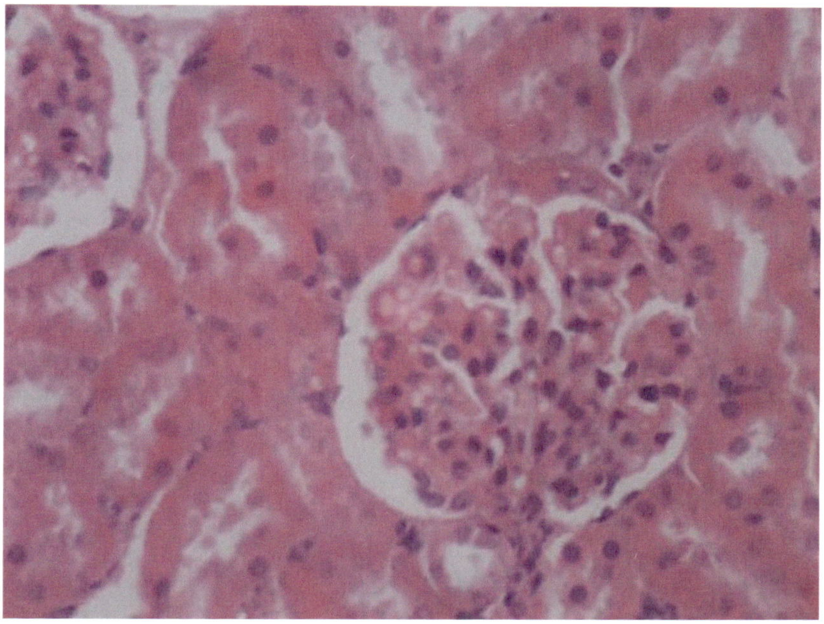

Figure 8. Effect of *P. amarus* extract on the kidney of alloxan-induced diabetic rats (X400)

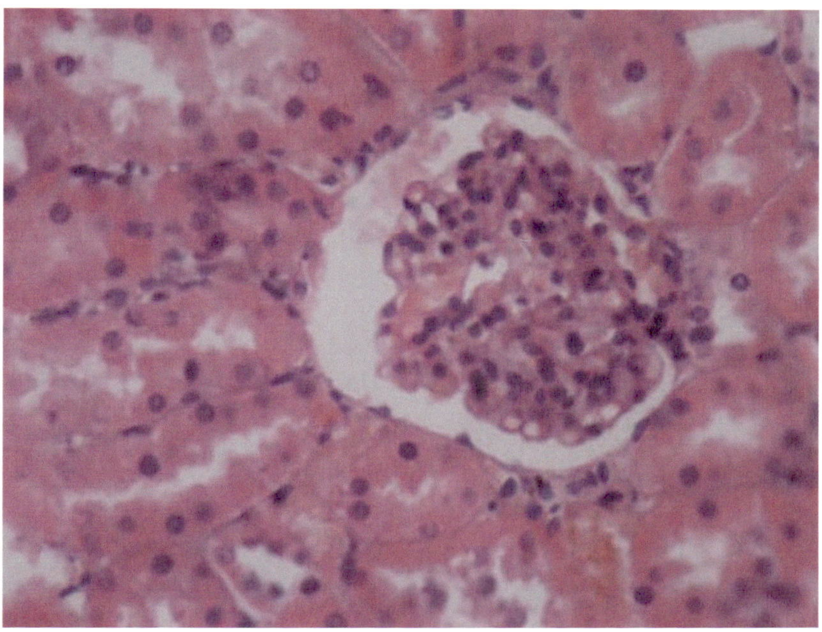

Figure 9. Effect of glibenclamide on the kidney of alloxan-induced diabetic rat (X400)

6. Conclusion

While the antidiabetic effect of the extract may derive from its hypoglycaemic effect, the mechanisms of the hypoglycaemic effect are yet to be elucidated. The hypoglycaemic effect in normal and diabetic rats suggests an insulin-like effect probably mediated via peripheral glucose consumption (De Sousa et al., 2004; Zanatta et al., 2007). Also, postprandial hyperglycemia is related to postprandial hyperinsulinemia (Wang et al., 2004) and its suppression by the extract suggests an insulin-like effect. Phytochemical analysis of the extract revealed the presence of flavonoids, alkaloids, glycosides and tannins which are typical plant constituents. Thus there are chances that any of these constituents may possess anti-diabetic properties. The histological studies also indicated that 0.2mg/kg of glibenclamide produced some histological changes whereas the 200 and 400 mg/kg doses of the plant extracts did not produce any histological change. This showed that this plant is not only effective as medicinal agent but also has high safety margin.

Acknowledgements

This study was carried out with the University of Ibadan Senate Research Grant (SRG/FVM/2010/10[A]) awarded to Dr. Adedapo A.A.

Author details

Adeolu Adedapo[1], Sunday Ofuegbe[1] and Oluwafemi Oguntibeju[2]

*Address all correspondence to: aa.adedapo@ui.edu.ng; adedapo2a@yahoo.com

1 Department of Veterinary Physiology, Biochemistry and Pharmacology, Faculty of Veterinary Medicine, University of Ibadan, Nigeria

2 Department of Biomedical Sciences, Faculty of Health & Wellness Sciences, Cape Peninsula University of Technology, Bellville Campus, South Africa

The authors declare that we have no conflict of interest to declare

References

[1] Abate, G: In: Demissew, S. (Ed.), Este Debdabe.(1989). Ethiopian Traditional Medicine. Department of Biology, Science Faculty, Addis Ababa University pp: 3-5.

[2] Adedapo, A.A. (2002). Toxicological studies of some plants in the family Euphorbiaceae in rats, Ph.D Thesis, University of Ibadan.

[3] Adedapo, A.A., Adegbayibi, A.Y., Emikpe, B.O. (2005). Some Clinico-pathological Changes associated with the Aqueous Extract of the Leaves of Phyllanthus amarus in Rats. Phytother. Res. 19, 971–976.

[4] Adedapo, A.A., Koduru, S. Jimoh, F.O., Masika, P.J., Afolayan, A.J. (2008a). Evaluation of the medicinal potentials of the methanol extracts of the leaves and stem of Halleria lucida. Bioresource Tech 99(10), 4158-4163.

[5] Adedapo, A.A., Jimoh, F.O., Afolayan, A.J., Masika, P.J. (2008b). Antioxidant activities and phenolic contents of the methanol extracts of the stems of Acokanthera oppositifolia and Adenia gummifera. BMC Complement. Alternat. Med. 8:54 doi: 10.1186/1472-6882-8-54.

[6] Adedapo, A.A., Jimoh, F.O., Afolayan, A.J., Masika, P.J. (2009). Antioxidant activities of the methanol extracts of the leaves and stems of Celtis africana. Rec. Nat. Prod. 3 (1), 23-31.

[7] Adeneye, A.A., Benebo, A.S., Agbaje, E.O. (2006). Protective effect of the Aqueous Leaf and seed Extract of Phyllanthus amarus on alcohol–induced hepatotoxicity in rats. West Afr. J. Pharmacol. Drug Res. 22&23, 42-50.

[8] Agrawal, R.P., Sharma, P., Pal, M., Kochar, A., Kochar D.K. (2006). Magnitude of dyslipidemia and its association with micro and macro vascular complications in type 2 diabetes: A hospital based study from Bikaner (Northwest India). Diabetes Res. Clin. Pract 73, 211-214.

[9] Ahmed, I., Lakhani, M.S. Gillet, M., John, A., Raza, H. (2001). Hypotriglyceridemic and hypocholesterolemic effects of antidiabetic Momordica charantia (Karela) fruit extract in streptozotocin-induced diabetic rats. Diabetes Res. Clin. Pract. 51, 151-161.

[10] Akah, P.A., Okoli, C.O., Nwafor, S.V. (2002). Phytotherapy in the management of diabetes mellitus. J. Nat. Rem. 2, 1-10.

[11] Aruna, R.V., Ramesh. B., Kartha, V.N. (1999). Effect of beta carotene on protein glycosylation in alloxan induced diabetic rats, Indian J. Exp. Biol. 32, 399-401.

[12] Ayoola, G.A., Coker, H.A.B., Adesegun, S.A., Adepoju-Bello, A.A., Obaweya, K., Ezennia, E.C., Atangbayila, T.O. (2008). Phytochemical Screening and Antioxidant Activities of Some Selected Medicinal Plants Used for Malaria Therapy in Southwestern Nigeria. Trop. J. Pharm. Res. 7 (3), 1019-1024.

[13] Bagchi, G.D., Srivastava, G.N., Singh, S.C. (1992). Distinguishing features of medicinal herbaceous species of Phyllanthus occuring in Lucknow District (U.P) India, Int. J. Pharmacogno. 30(3), 161-168.

[14] Balkau, B. (2000). The DECODE study, Diabetes epidemiology: collaborative analysis of diagnostic criteria in Europe. Diabetes Metab. 26, 282-286.

[15] Bavarva, J.H., Narasimhacharya, A.V.R.L. (2008). Antihyperglycemic and Hypolipidemic Effects of Costus speciosus in alloxan induced Diabetic rats. Phytother. Res. Clin.Pract. 78, 349-354.

[16] Beretta, A. (2001). Campanha de prevencao e diagnostico do diabetes realizada pela UNIARARAS.

[17] Bhat, R., Bhansali, A., Bhadada, S., Sialy, R. (2007). Effect of pioglitazone therapy in lean type 1 diabetes mellitus Diabetes. Res. Clin. Pract. 78, 349-354.

[18] Boussageon, R., Bejan-Angoulvant, T., Saadatian-Elahi, M. (2011). "Effect of intensive glucose lowering treatment on all cause mortality, cardiovascular death, and microvascular events in type 2 diabetes: meta-analysis of randomized controlled trials". BMJ 343: d4169. DOI:10.1136/bmj.d4169.

[19] Bravo, L. (1998). Polyphenols: chemistry, dietary sources, metabolism, and nutritional significance. Nutr. Rev. 56, 317-333.

[20] Brown, G.B., Xue-Qiao, Z., Sacco D.E., Alberts, J.J. (1993). Lipid lowering and plaque regression. New insights into prevention of plaque disruption and clinical events in coronary disease. Circ. 87, 1781-1791.

[21] Burkill, H.M. (1994). The Useful Plants of West Tropical Africa. Vol. II. Royal Botanical Gardens: Kew.

[22] Calixto, J.B., Beirith, A., Ferreira, J., Santos, A.R., Cechinel Filho, V., Yunes R.A. (2000). Naturally occurring antinociceptive substances from plants. Phytother. Res. 14, 401-18.

[23] Ceriello, A. (2005). Postprandial hyperglycemia and diabetes complications; is it time to treat? Diabetes, 54, 1-7.

[24] Chen, H.Y., Yen, G.C. (2007). Antioxidant activity and free radical-scavenging capacity of extracts from guava (Psidium guajava L.) leaves. Food Chem. 101, 689-694.

[25] Choi, J.S., Yokozawa, T., Oura, H. (1991). Improvement of hyperglycemia and hyperlipemia in streptozotocin-diabetic rats by a methanolic extract of Prunus daidiana stems and its main component, pruning. Planta Med. 57, 208-211.

[26] Cole, E.H. (1986). Veterinary Clinical Pathology 4th edition W.B. Saunders Publishing Company.

[27] De Sousa, E., Zanatta, L., Seifriz, I., Creczynski-Pasa, T.B., Pizzolatti, M.G., Szpoganicz, B., Silva, F.R.M.B. (2004). Hypoglycemic effect and antioxidant potential of kaempferol-3, 7-O-(_)-dirhamnoside from Bauhinia forficate leaves. J. Nat. Prod. 67, 829-832.

[28] Duthie, M. (2000). Plant polyphenols in cancer and heart disease: Implications as nutritional antioxidants, Nutr. Res. Rev. 13, 79-106.

[29] Evans, W.C. (2002). Pharmacognosy: London, W.B. Saunders.

[30] Fröde, T.S., Medeiros, Y.S. (2008). Animal models to test drugs with potential antidiabetic activity. J. Ethnopharmacol. 115, 173-183.

[31] Hayden, M.R., Tyagi, S.C., Kerklo, M.M., Nicolls, M.R. (2005). Type 2 Diabetes Mellitus as a conformational Disease. J. Pancreas (Online), 6(4), 287-302

[32] Hilaly, J.E., Israili, Z.H., Lyoussi, B. (2004). Acute and chronic toxicological studies of Ajuga iva in experimental animals. J. Ethnopharmacol. 91, 43-30.

[33] Huang, Z., Wang, B., Eaves, D.H., Shikany, J.M., Pace, R.D. (2007). Phenolic compound profile of selected vegetables frequently consumed by African Americans in the southeast United States. Food Chem. 103, 1395-1402.

[34] Irvine, F.R. (1930). Plants of the Gold Coast. Oxford University Press.

[35] Jagetia, G.C., Baliga, M.S. (2004). The evaluation of nitric oxide scavenging activity of certain Indian medicinal plants in vitro: a preliminary study. J. Med. Food, 7(3), 343-348.

[36] Jimoh, F.O., Adedapo, A.A., Afolayan, A.J. (2010). Assessing the polyphenolic, nutritive and biological activities of acetone, methanol and aqueous extracts of Rumex sagittatus Thunb. Afric. J. Pharm. Pharmacol. 4(9), 629-635.

[37] Kyung-Hee, K., Rong, T., Yang, R., Steve, W.C. (2005). Phenolic acid profiles and antioxidant activities of wheat bran extracts and the effect of hydrolysis conditions. Food Chem. 95, 466-473.

[38] Lai, F.R., Wen, Q.B., Li, L., Wu, H., Li, X.F. (2010). Antioxidant activities of water-soluble polysaccharide extracted from mung bean (Vigna radiata L.) hull with ultrasonic assisted treatment. Carbohyd. Polym. 81(2), 323-329.

[39] Lambert, P., Bingley, P.J. (2002). "What is Type 1 Diabetes?" Medicine 30: 1–5. DOI: 10.1383/medc.30.1.1.28264

[40] Lee J.H., Park, J.W., Kim, J.S., Park, B.H., Rho, H.W. (2008). Protective Effect of Amomi Semen Extract on Alloxan-induced Pancreatic ß-Cell Damage. Phytother. Res. 22, 86-90.

[41] Lenzen, S., Tiedge, M., Jorns, A., Munday, R. (1996). Alloxan derivatives as a tool for the elucidation of the mechanism of the diabetogenic action of alloxan. In: Shafrir, E. (ed.) Lessons from Animal Diabetes, Birkhauser, Boston, pp. 113-122.

[42] Leung, K.K., Leung, P.S. (2008). Effects of Hyperglycemia on the Angiotensin II Receptor Type 1 Expression and Insulin Secretion in an INS-1E Pancreatic Beta-Cell Line. JOP. J. Pancreas (Online) 9(3), 290-299.

[43] Li-Chen, W., Hsiu-Wen, H., Yun-Chen, C., Chih-Chung, C., Yu-In, L., Ja-an, A.H. (2005). Antioxidant and antiproliferative activities of red pitaya. Food Chem. 17, 341-346.

[44] Macedo, C.S., Capelletti, S.M., Mercadante, M.C.S., Padovani, C.R., Spadella, C.T. (2002). Role of metabolic control on diabetic nephropathy. Acta Cir. Bras. 17(6), 37 –5.

[45] Mohan, V., Farooq, S., Deepa, M. (2008). Prevalence of Fibrocalculous Pancreatic Diabetes in Chennai in South India. J. Pancreas (Online) 9(4), 489-492.

[46] Moody, J.O., Robert, V.A., Connolly, J.D., Houghton, P.J. (2006). Anti-inflammatory activities of the methanol extracts and an isolated furanoditerpene constituent of Sphenocentrum jollyanum

[47] Pierre (Menispermaceae). J. Ethnopharmacol. 104, 87-91.

[48] Monnier, L., Lapinski, H., Colette, C. (2003). Contributions of fasting and postprandial plasma glucose increments to the overall diurnal hyperglycemia of type2 diabetes patients. Diabetes Care. 26, 881-885.

[49] Muller, P.H., Schmulling, R.M., Eggstein, M. (1977). A fully enzymatic triglyceride determination. J. Clin. Chem. 15, 457-504.

[50] Odetola, A.A., Akkojenu, S.M. (2000). Antidiarrhoeal and gastrointestinal potentials of the aqueous extracts of Phyllanthus amarus (Euphorbiaceae). Afri. J.Med. Sci. 29, 119-122.

[51] Okoli, C.O., Ibiam, F.A., Ezike, A.C., Akah, P.A., Okoye, T.C. (2010). Evaluation of antidiabetic potentials of Phyllanthus niruri in alloxan diabetic rats. Afric. J. Biotech. 9 (2), 248-259.

[52] Oridupa, O.A., Saba, A.B., Sulaiman, L.K. (2011). Preliminary report on the antiviral activity of the ethanolic fruit extract of Lagenaria breviflora Roberts on Newcastle Disease virus. Trop. Vet. 29 (1), 22-33.

[53] Sawadogo, W.R., Boly, R., Lompo, M., Some, N. (2006). Anti-inflammatory, analgesic and antipyretic activities of Dicliptera verticillata. Intl. J. Pharmacol. 2 (4), 435-438.

[54] Sattar, N., Preiss, D., Murray, H.M., Welsh, P., Buckley, B.M., de Craen, A.J., Seshasai, S.R., McMurray, J.J., Freeman, D.J. (2010). "Statins and risk of incident diabetes: a collaborative meta-analysis of randomised statin trials". The Lancet. 375 (9716), 735–42.

[55] Shale, T.L., Stirk, W.A., Van Staden, J. (1999). Screening of medicinal plants used in Lesotho for antibacterial and anti-inflammatory activity. J. Ethnopharmacol. 67, 347-354.

[56] Szudelski, T. (2001). The mechanism of alloxan and streptozotocin action B cells of the rat pancreas. Physiol. Res. 50, 536-546.

http://dx.doi.org/10.5772/57030

[57] Tasaduq, S.A., Singh, K., Sethi, Sharma, S., Bedi, S.C., Singh, K.L.J., Jaggi, B.S., Johri, R.K. (2003). Hepatocurative and antioxidant profile of HP-1, a polyherbal phytomedicine. Hum. Exp. Toxicol. 22(12), 639-645.

[58] Trease, G.E., Evans, W.C. (1983). Trease and Evans Pharmacognosy. Low English Book Edition, London.

[59] Wang, J.J., Qiao, Q., Miettinen, M.E., Lappalainen, J., Hu, G., Tuomilehto, J. (2004). The metabolic syndrome defined by factor analysis and incident type 2 diabetes in a Chinese population with high postprandial glucose. Diabetes Care, 27, 2429-2437.

[60] Yoshida, K., Toki, F., Takeuchi, T., Watanabe, S., Shiratori, K., Hayashi, N. (1995). Chronic pancreatitis caused by an autoimmune abnormality. Proposal of the concept of autoimmune pancreatitis. Dig. Dis. Sci. 40, 1561-1568.

[61] Zanatta, L., De Sousa, E., Cazarolli, L.H., Cunha Jr., A., Pizzolatti, A.M.G., Szpoganicz, B., Silva, F.R.M.B. (2007). Effect of crude extract and fractions from Vitex megapotamica leaves on hyperglycemia in alloxan-diabetic rats. J. Ethnopharmacol. 109, 151-155.

Chapter 6

Antidiabetic Botanicals and their Potential Benefits in the Management of Diabetes Mellitus

Afolabi Clement Akinmoladun,
Ebenezer Olatunde Farombi and
Oluwafemi Omoniyi Oguntibeju

Additional information is available at the end of the chapter

http://dx.doi.org/10.5772/57339

1. Introduction

1.1. Diabetes: Definition, aetiology and classification

The term "diabetes", when used alone, generally refers to diabetes mellitus (DM) and not a rare, unrelated disease called diabetes insipidus. DM is a metabolic disorder resulting from a defect in insulin secretion, insulin action, or both. Insulin deficiency in turn leads to chronic hyperglycaemia with disturbances of carbohydrate, fat and protein metabolism [1,2]. The magnitude of the challenge that diabetes presents to health services is enormous [3].

DM was traditionally classified based on whether or not the patient is insulin dependent or independent [4]. However, there has been a paradigm shift in the classification of DM from one based on the need for insulin therapy to maintain glycaemic control and prevent ketosis to that based on the underlying aetiopathogenetic mechanisms [5]. The current classes of DM and their aetiopathogenetic mechanisms are (i) Type 1A (auto-immune), (ii) Type 1B (non-auto immune or idiopathic) [6], (iii) Type 2 (insulin resistance), (iv) Gestational (diagnosed for the first time in pregnancy but usually characterized by insulin resistance) and (v) other specific aetiologies (secondary to other diseases and identified gene mutations) [5]. Once considered a disease of acute onset, it is now generally accepted that the 1A subtype is a genetically determined chronic immune-mediated disorder that leads to selective loss of pancreatic insulin-secreting β-cells [6]. The classic point of view regarding type I diabetes mellitus (T1DM) pathogenesis was that, in genetically predisposed individuals, some environmental factors may trigger an autoimmune process that leads to β-cell destruction; but despite considerable progress over recent years, the autoimmune process underlying T1DM is still poorly understood [6].

The high blood glucose level (hyperglycaemia) that accompanies T1DM and type 2 diabetes mellitus (T2DM) can cause serious health complications including ketoacidosis, kidney failure, heart disease, stroke, and blindness. Patients are often diagnosed with diabetes when they see a physician for clinical signs such as excessive thirst, urination, and hunger [7]. The direct symptoms of type-2 diabetes can be mild and may cause minimal interruption to activities of daily living. However, it is the complications of the disease which lead to damage to vital organs, and consequently, to substantial morbidity and mortality.

Diabetes in the young is often categorized as Type 1 and this comprises the auto-immune Type 1A and non-auto immune Type 1B. T2DM which is mainly diagnosed in adults is increasingly being reported in young people. The increased prevalence of T2DM in young people is associated with the increasing rates of obesity in young people. Type 2 diabetes accounts for 90% to 95% of all cases of diabetes [8-10].

2. Prevalence, global burden and increasing incidence of diabetes

Several statistics from various scientific studies on the incidence, prevalence and global burden of diabetes mellitus are available. While there might be minor discrepancies in these statistics, the consensus is that they are ominous and call for urgent and definitive action on this disease [11,12].

DM is estimated to affect 2.8% of the world's population at present and projected to cross 5.4% mark by 2025 [13]. Over the last decades, the prevalence of diabetes mellitus has reached epidemic proportions in Western societies, and is even higher in some developing countries [14 -16]. According to Shaw *et al.* [17], the world's prevalence of diabetes among adults (aged 20–79 years) will be 6.4%, affecting 285 million adults, in 2010, and will increase to 7.7%, and 439 million adults by 2030 and, between 2010 and 2030, there will be a 69% increase in numbers of adults with diabetes in developing countries and a 20% increase in developed countries. More recently, the International Diabetes Federation (IDF) estimated that in 2011 there were 366 million people with diabetes and this was expected to rise to 552 million by 2030 [18]. The International Diabetes Federation (IDF) reported that 151 million people had diabetes in the 172 IDF member countries with a forecast that 334 million people will have the disease in 2025 [19]. The human cost of diabetes has been put at one death every 10 seconds [20].

Zhang *et al.*[21] estimated that global health expenditures to prevent and treat diabetes and its complications would be at US dollar (USD) 376 billion in 2010 and that by 2030, this number will exceed USD490 billion. In addition, diabetes leads to loss in productivity and economic growth. The American Diabetes Association estimated that the US economy lost USD58 billion, equivalent to about an half of the direct health care expenditure on diabetes in 2007, as a result of lost earnings due to lost work days, restricted activity days, lower productivity at work, mortality and permanent disability caused by diabetes [21]. Diabetes and its complications place huge burdens upon individuals, their careers and families and have crippling effects upon national health services [20].

http://dx.doi.org/10.5772/57339

3. Pathological complications of diabetes mellitus

Persistent hyperglycaemia and the development of diabetes-specific microvascular (retinopathy, neuropathy and nephropathy) and macrovascular (heart attack, stroke and peripheral arterial disease) complications are the main characteristics of all forms of diabetes mellitus. The importance of protecting the body against persistent elevation of blood glucose cannot be overemphasized because its direct and indirect effects on the human vascular system are the major cause of morbidity and mortality in both T1DM and T2DM [22]. Hospitalisations for complications account for more than half of the healthcare costs of T2DM and three-quarters of people with diabetes die from cardiovascular disease. Research has shown that the risk of development of both microvascular and macrovascular complications associated with elevated blood glucose increases with the length of time blood glucose is uncontrolled [23,24].

As a result of the association of diabetes with accelerated atherosclerotic macrovascular disease affecting arteries that supply the heart, brain and lower extremities, patients with diabetes have a much higher risk of myocardial infarction, stroke and limb amputation [25]. Lower limb amputations are at least 10 times more common in people with diabetes than in non-diabetic individuals in developed countries; more than half of all non-traumatic lower limb amputations are due to diabetes [26].

Diabetes is one of the leading causes of visual impairment and blindness in developed countries [27]. Retinopathy may begin to develop as early as 7 years before the diagnosis of diabetes in patients with T2DM [28]. Osmotic stress from sorbitol accumulation has been postulated as an underlying mechanism in the development of diabetic microvascular complications, including diabetic retinopathy [22]. According to Massin *et al* [29] lens opacification leading to cataract is a frequent comorbidity of diabetes, as adults with T2DM are five times more often affected than the general population. They also reported that while juvenile diabetic cataract is rare, adult-onset, mostly cortical cataract in T2DM patients is similar to age-related cataract in the general population, except for an earlier onset and greater prevalence [29,30]. Major risk factors for cataract in T2DM include hyperglycaemia, diabetes duration and the presence of diabetic retinopathy, although specific risk factors or markers may differ according to cataract subtype. Smoking, for example, is associated with nuclear opacities, whereas ultraviolet radiation increases the risk for cortical opacities, and high blood pressure and corticosteroids raise the odds for subcapsular cataract [31]. Various pathophysiological mechanisms are involved in cataract formation, including osmosis-driven lens overhydration triggered by the polyol pathway (mostly ascribed to juvenile cataract), lens protein glycation and an excess of free radicals, with the latter being particularly associated with the nuclear subset of age-related cataract [32,33].

Studies have shown an increased incidence of erectile dysfunction (ED) in diabetes patients. In addition, ED appears to arise about 10 years earlier in diabetic patients than in the general population [34] and is more severe, decreasing health-related quality of life. ED is most often a forewarning of cardiovascular disease; thus, the treatment of ED among diabetics is a priority. Diabetic ED is multifactorial in aetiology and more resistant to treatment compared with non-diabetic ED [35]

Diabetic neuropathy is the presence of symptoms and/or signs of peripheral nerve dysfunction in people with diabetes after the exclusion of other causes [36]. More than 80% of amputations occur after foot ulceration or injury, which can result from diabetic neuropathy [37].

Diabetic nephropathy has been defined by proteinuria > 500 mg in 24 hours in the setting of diabetes, which is however preceeded by lower degrees of proteinuria, or "microalbuminuria." Microalbuminuria is defined as albumin excretion of 30–299 mg/24 hours. Without intervention, diabetic patients with microalbuminuria typically progress to proteinuria and overt diabetic nephropathy [22]. This progression occurs in both type1 and type 2 diabetes. As many as 7% of patients with type 2 diabetes may already have microalbuminuria at the time they are diagnosed with diabetes [38]. In the European Diabetes Prospective Complications Study, the cumulative incidence of microalbuminuria in patients with type 1 diabetes was ~ 12% during a period of 7 years. In the U.K. Prospective Diabetes Study (UKPDS), the incidence of microalbuminuria was 2% per year in patients with type 2 diabetes, and the 10-year prevalence after diagnosis was 25% [38-40]. Diabetic nephropathy can progress to end-stage renal disease. Diabetes is the leading cause of renal failure in the United States accounting for nearly 44 percent of new cases [40].

Diabetes increases the risk that an individual will develop cardiovascular disease (CVD) [22]. Although the precise mechanisms through which diabetes increases the likelihood of atherosclerotic plaque formation are not completely defined, the association between the two is profound. CVD is the primary cause of death in people with either type 1 or type 2 diabetes and accounts for the greatest component of health care expenditures in people with diabetes [41,42]. Among macrovascular diabetes complications, coronary heart disease has been associated with diabetes in numerous studies beginning with the Framingham study [43]. More recent studies have shown that the risk of myocardial infarction (MI) in people with diabetes is equivalent to the risk in non-diabetic patients with a history of previous MI [44]. These discoveries have led to new recommendations by the American Diabetes Association (ADA) and American Heart Association (AHA) that diabetes be considered a coronary artery disease risk equivalent rather than a risk factor. Patients with type 1 diabetes bear a disproportionate burden of coronary heart disease. Studies have shown that these patients have a higher mortality from ischemic heart disease at all ages compared to the general population [45].

Diabetes is also a strong independent predictor of risk of stroke [46]. Patients with type 2 diabetes have a much higher risk of stroke, with an increased risk of 150–400%. Risk of stroke-related dementia and recurrence, as well as stroke-related mortality, is elevated in patients with diabetes [47]. In addition, the risk of tuberculosis is three times higher among people with diabetes [48].

Insulin resistance and glucose intolerance are components of metabolic syndrome, a group of metabolic risk factors that predisposes people to diseases related to fatty buildups in artery walls such as coronary heart disease, which can lead to heart attack, stroke and peripheral vascular disease [49]. People with this syndrome are also more likely to develop type 2 diabetes. Other components of metabolic syndrome are abdominal obesity, atherogenic dyslipidemia, raised blood pressure, proinflammatory state and prothrombotic state [49]. The term pre-diabetes has been used to describe the condition of individuals with a high risk of developing diabetes in the future and already showing a glycaemic abnormality [50,51].

People with diabetes require at least two to three times the health-care resources compared to people who do not have diabetes, and diabetes care may account for up to 15% of national health care budgets [52].

Many authors agreed that hyperglycaemia causes tissue damage through the following clearly defined mechanisms [25, 53]: increased flux of glucose and other sugars through the polyol pathway, increased intracellular formation of advanced glycation end products (AGEs), increased expression of the receptor for AGEs and its activating ligands, activation of protein kinase (PK) C isoforms, and overactivity of the hexosamine pathway.

3.1. Increased polyol pathway flux

Aldose reductase (alditol:NAD(P)$^+$ 1-oxidoreductase, EC 1.1.1.21) is the first enzyme in the polyol pathway. It is a cytosolic, monomeric oxidoreductase that catalyses the reduced nicotinamide adenine dinucleotide phosphate (NADPH)-dependent reduction of a wide variety of carbonyl compounds, including glucose [54]. At the normal glucose concentrations found in non-diabetics, metabolism of glucose by this pathway is a very small percentage of total glucose use. But in a hyperglycaemic environment, increased intracellular glucose results in its increased enzymatic conversion to the polyalcohol sorbitol, with concomitant decreases in NADPH [25,55,56]. In the polyol pathway, sorbitol is oxidized to fructose by the enzyme sorbitol dehydrogenase, with NAD$^+$ reduced to NADH. Flux through this pathway during hyperglycaemia varies from 33% of total glucose use in the rabbit lens to 11% in human erythrocytes [25]. Thus, the contribution of this pathway to diabetic complications may be very much species, site and tissue dependent [25]. It has also been proposed that reduction of glucose to sorbitol by NADPH consumes NADPH [25]. As NADPH is required for regenerating reduced glutathione (GSH), this could induce or exacerbate intracellular oxidative stress. Decreased levels of GSH have in fact been found in the lenses of transgenic mice that overexpress aldose reductase, and this is the most likely mechanism by which increased flux through the polyol pathway has deleterious consequences [57]. This conclusion is further supported by recent experiments with homozygous knockout mice deficient in aldose reductase, which showed that, in contrast to wild-type mice, diabetes neither decreased the GSH content of sciatic nerve nor reduced motor nerve conduction velocity [25].

3.2. Increased intracellular formation of advanced glycation end-products

AGEs are found in increased amounts in diabetic retinal vessels and renal glomeruli and intracellular hyperglycaemia appears to be the primary initiating event in the formation of both intracellular and extracellular AGEs [23]. AGEs contribute to diabetic complications via three principal mechanisms: the modification of intracellular proteins including, most importantly, proteins involved in the regulation of gene transcription [58,59]; diffusion of these AGE precursors out of the cell and their modification of extracellular matrix molecules nearby, which changes signaling between the matrix and the cell and causes cellular dysfunction [60,

61]; and diffusion of AGE precursors out of the cell and their modification of circulating proteins in the blood, such as albumin, which can then bind to AGE receptors and activate them thereby causing the production of inflammatory cytokines and growth factors, which in turn cause vascular pathology [62-65].

3.3. Activation of protein kinase C (PKC)

PKCs are a family of at least 11 isoforms that are widely distributed in mammalian tissues. The enzyme phosphorylates various target proteins. The activity of the classic isoforms is dependent on both Ca^{2+} ions and phosphatidylserine and is greatly enhanced by diacylglycerol (DAG) [53]. Intracellular hyperglycaemia increases the *de novo* synthesis of DAG from the glycolytic intermediate dihydroxyacetone phosphate by reducing it to glycerol-3-phosphate and stepwise acylation [66]. Hyperglycaemia may also activate PKC isoforms indirectly through both ligation of AGE receptors[67] and increased activity of the polyol pathway [68], presumably by increasing reactive oxygen species. One significant effect of PKC activation is seen in the decrease in the vasodilator producing endothelial nitric oxide (NO) synthase (eNOS), while the vasoconstrictor endothelin-1 is increased. Transforming growth factor- β and plasminogen activator inhibitor-1 are also increased [69].Abnormal activation of PKC has been implicated in the decreased glomerular production of nitric oxide induced by experimental diabetes [70], and in the decreased production of nitric oxide in smooth muscle cells that is induced by hyperglycaemia [71]. Activation of PKC also contributes to increased microvascular matrix protein accumulation by inducing expression of TGF-b1, fibronectin and type IV collagen both in cultured mesangial cells [72] and in glomeruli of diabetic rats [66].

3.4. Increased flux through the hexosamine pathway

Glucose is one of the most largely used energy substrate in living cells. A fraction (2–3%) of the glucose entering the cell is converted into UDP–N-Acetyl Glucosamine (UDP-GlcNAc), through the hexosamine biosynthetic pathway (HBP). The level of UDPGlcNAc in the cell thus reflects the flux of glucose through this pathway [73]. In this pathway, fructose-6-phosphate is diverted from glycolysis to provide substrates for reactions that require UDP-*N* acetylglucosamine, such as proteoglycan synthesis and the formation of *O*-linked glycoproteins [23]. O-GlcNAcylation may affect the phosphorylation status of a protein, by regulating the phosphorylation of adjacent residues or by competing for the same serine or threonine residue (the so-called Yin-Yang mechanism), in which modification of a serine or threonine residue by either phosphorylation or O-GlcNAcylation differently affects the protein's function [73]. O-GlcNAcylations also regulate insulin signaling and seem to play an important part in the development of diabetes and its complications [74,75]. Inhibition of the rate-limiting enzyme in the conversion of glucose to glucosamine, glutamine:fructose-6-phosphate amidotransferase (GFAT), blocks hyperglycaemia-induced increases in the transcription of TGF-α, TGF-β1. This pathway has been shown to play a role both in hyperglycaemia-induced abnormalities of glomerular cell gene expression and in hyperglycemia-induced cardiomyocyte dysfunction in cell culture [25,76].

http://dx.doi.org/10.5772/57339

4. Management of diabetes mellitus

Diabetes mellitus is a syndrome implying that efforts targeted at its management should be multifaceted. Adequate consideration should be given to all the accompanying comorbidities and all symptomatic and asymptomatic features. Efforts should be geared towards the attainment of normal or near normal glucose levels. The general objective of diabetes management include to (i) relieve symptoms (ii) correct associated health problems and reduce morbidity, mortality and economic costs of diabetes (iii) prevent as much as possible acute and long-term complications (iv) monitor the development of such complications and provide timely intervention and, (v) improve the quality of life and productivity of the individual with diabetes [77]. The orthodox approach to the management of diabetes mellitus has always included lifestyle modification and dietary therapy, administration of oral antidiabetic drugs, and insulin therapy.

4.1. Diet and lifestyle modification

Weight reduction and an increase in daily energy expenditure decrease insulin resistance and increase glucose tolerance [78]. Advice on diet and exercise are an important part of the treatment of T2DM and overweight patients are normally advised to restrict calorie intake, consume food with low total (especially saturated) fat content and high (predominately unrefined) carbohydrate content.

Dietary and lifestyle modifications are regarded as the mainstay of treatment and management for T2DM. The majority of people with T2DM are overweight and usually have other metabolic disorders of the insulin resistance syndrome. Therefore, the major aims of dietary and lifestyle changes are to reduce weight, improve glycaemic control and reduce the risk of coronary heart disease (CHD), which accounts for 70- 80% of deaths among those with diabetes [79]. Even modest weight reduction is associated with a reduction in insulin resistance, a reduction in hepatic glucose production, and perhaps, an improved islet β-cell function [80,81]. Several studies have demonstrated the effectiveness of diet and exercise in reducing the progression of diabetes [82-85].

Fat is the most energy-rich of all nutrients and reduction of fat intake helps to reduce total energy intake, which is important for many people with type 2 diabetes and some with type 1 diabetes. Results from several research studies suggest that populations consuming a low saturated fat diet have lower incidence and mortality from CHD compared with those living in countries with a high intake of saturated fat and that reduced saturated fat intake is associated with reduced levels of low-density lipoprotein (LDL) – cholesterol [86,87].

4.2. Oral antidiabetic drugs

Oral antidiabetic drugs (OADs) are normally introduced when lifestyle modifications fail to adequately control glycaemia. They are very useful for managing hyperglycaemia, especially in the early stages of disease. However, there are several limitations that prevent OADs from reaching their potentials [88]. Sulfonylureas cause hypoglycaemia by stimulating insulin release from pancreatic β -cells. They bind to sulfonylurea (SUR) receptors on the β -cell plasma membrane, causing closure of adenosine triphosphate (ATP)-sensitive potassium channels, leading to depolarization of the cell membrane. This in turn opens voltage-gated channels, allowing influx of calcium ions and subsequent secretion of preformed insulin granules [89]. Acute administration of sulfonylureas T2DM patients increases insulin release from the pancreas and also may further increase insulin levels by reducing hepatic clearance of the hormone. Initial studies showed that a functional pancreas was necessary for the hypoglycaemic actions of sulfonylureas [90]. With chronic administration, circulating insulin levels decline to those that existed before treatment. But, despite this reduction in insulin levels, reduced plasma glucose levels are maintained [89].

Metformin, the popular antidiabetic drug has its origin in the plant *Galega officinalis.* It is one of the major success stories of the reward of prospecting for drugs from botanical sources. Metformin is antihyperglycaemic, not hypoglycaemic [91]. Clarke *et al.*reported that metformin does not cause insulin release from the pancreas and does not cause hypoglycaemia, even in large doses [92]. Metformin has been shown to increase peripheral uptake of glucose and to reduce hepatic glucose output by approximately 20-30% when given orally but not intravenously [93,94]. Impaired absorption of glucose from the gut has also been suggested as a mechanism of action, but has not been shown to have clinical relevance. Metformin has also been shown to decrease serum triglycerides and fatty acid concentrations and slows the rate of lipid oxidation. These actions indirectly inhibit gluconeogenesis [95].

The meglitinide analogues act on β-cell receptors to stimulate insulin secretion by binding to the sulfonylurea receptor subunit and closing the K^+ ATP channel but probably at a site distinct from that of the sulfonylurea receptor [96,97]. Closure of the potassium channel leads to depolarization of β-cell plasma membrane, which promotes influx of calcium ions through voltage-gated calcium channels, resulting in exocytosis of insulin granules [89]. α-Glucosidase inhibitors competitively block small intestine brush border enzymes that are necessary to hydrolyze oligo and polysaccharides to monosaccharides [98]. Inhibition of this enzyme slows the absorption of carbohydrates and the postprandial rise in plasma glucose is blunted in both normal and diabetic subjects [99].

4.3. Insulin

Insulin has proven to be the therapy with the highest potential to achieve glycaemic target in diabetics. It is typically prescribed after OADs have failed, and often later than is ideal [88]. The physiological plasma insulin profile in healthy individuals displays low but constant insulin levels in fasting conditions, with sharp prandial peaks shortly (within 30 minutes) after meals followed by a slow return to basal levels when increased insulin secretion is no longer necessary. In order to avoid glycaemic excursions, exogenously administered insulin would ideally closely mimic the healthy physiological pharmacokinetic insulin profile [88].

Although all patients with T2DM become relatively insulinopenic late in the course of their disease, some patients with T2DM may have insufficient insulin secretion early in the course of the disease. This difference arises from the heterogeneity in the metabolic expression of the diabetic state and the difference in the extent to which different abnormalities contribute to

http://dx.doi.org/10.5772/57339

the hyperglycaemic state. In lean patients with T2DM, impaired insulin secretion is a common defect, and insulin resistance tends to be less severe than in obese patients with T2DM [100].

5. Limitations of orthodox approaches in the treatment of diabetes mellitus

Despite the significant improvements recorded from the administration of the currently available therapies in the treatment of diabetes, several undesirable side effects have been observed in the course of treatment using these therapies. Reports have shown that the success of OADs is limited by their mechanisms of action, which often address the symptoms of diabetes rather than its underlying pathophysiology. For instance, up to 2.5% and 17.5% of sulfonylurea (SU)-treated patients experience major and minor hypoglycaemia, respectively, while gastrointestinal (GI) problems affect up to 63% of metformin, and 30% of acarbose-treated patients. These side effects can have a negative impact on patient adherence to treatment, resulting in higher HbA1c levels and increased risk for all-cause hospitalization and all-cause mortality [101].

Another limitation that hinders the efficacy of OADs is the tendency of health professionals to delay initiation and intensification of therapy. OADs are frequently initiated too late in the progression of the disease and intensification is delayed and thus exposes the patient to hyperglycemia [88]. According to the recent American Association of Clinical Endocrinologists (AACE) road map guidelines, combination therapy is to be initiated when continous titration of OAD monotherapy fails to achieve target HbA1c levels (ie, ≤ 6.5%) [102].

Although insulin is the most effective antihyperglycemic agent, its initiation is also delayed to an excessive degree. Brown *et al.* estimated that the average patient accumulated HbA1c- which contribute to excess glyacemic burden (HbA1c > 8%) from diagnosis until insulin initiation, thereby increasing the prevalence of complications [103]. The economic burden of managing diabetes is also a limitation to the use of oral antidiabetic drugs especially in less developed countries where the people can scarcely afford orthodox treatment. There is therefore the need to investigate the antidiabetic effects of indigenous plants and their continuous role in the management of diabetes mellitus with a view to developing new and more effective drugs to stem the tide of the ravaging epidemic of diabetes.

6. Therapeutic and chemoprophylactic potentials of botanicals

Terrestrial plants have been used as medicines in Egypt, China, India and Greece from ancient time and an impressive number of modern drugs have been developed from them [104]. According to the World Health Organization (WHO), a medicinal plant is any plant which, in one or more of its organs contains substances that can be used for therapeutic purposes, or which are precursors for chemo-pharmaceutical semi synthesis. Such a plant will have its parts including leaves, roots, rhizomes, stems, barks, flowers, fruits, grains or seeds, employed in the control or treatment of a disease condition and therefore contains chemical components that are medically active. These non-nutrient plant chemical compounds or bioactive components are often referred to as phytochemicals ('phyto-' from Greek - *phyto* meaning 'plant') or phytoconstituents.

Phytochemicals have been isolated and characterized from fruits such as grapes and apples, vegetables such as broccoli and onion, spices such as turmeric, beverages such as green tea and red wine, as well as many other sources [105]. The WHO estimates that approximately 80% of the world's inhabitants rely on traditional medicine for their primary health care [106].

7. Botanicals and their antidiabetic property

Many medicinal plants have ethnomedical claims of usefulness in the treatment of diabetes worldwide and have been employed empirically in antidiabetic and antihyperlipidemic remedies. Hundreds of plants with antidiabetic and hypoglycaemic activities have also been reported in literature. Despite this, studies on plants with these activities are still necessary. This is because a large percentage of plants are yet to be explored for their medicinal properties. Also, successful antidiabetic drug development from investigated plants is still largely absent although numerous dietary supplements have been formulated. Plants contain glycosides, alkaloids, terpenoids, anthocyanins, tocopherols, flavonoids, carotenoids, polyphenols, peptidoglycans, steroids, coumarins and other constituents that are frequently implicated as having antidiabetic activities [107]. The antidiabetic activities could be obtained from several parts of the plants - aerial parts, bark, flower, root, seeds, leaves, bulb, tubers and/or whole plant [108].

Many studies have confirmed the benefits of medicinal plants with hypoglycaemic effects in the management of diabetes mellitus. The plant families most studied for their hypoglycaemic effects include: Leguminoseae, Lamiaceae, Liliaceae, Cucurbitaceae, Asteraceae, Moraceae, Rosaceae, Euphorbiaceae and Araliaceae [109]. The effects of these plants may delay the development of diabetic complications and correct the metabolic abnormalities. During the past few years, efforts at the study of antidiabetic medicinal plants have culminated in the isolation and characterization of single bioactive compounds and the preparation of herbal extracts and multiherbal products. Interestingly, some of these extracts and herbal preparations have shown significant insulinomimetic and antidiabetic activities with more efficacy than conventional hypoglycemic agents [13]. For this paper, we shall briefly consider the antidiabetic potential of few of these botanicals.

7.1. Fenugreek

Leaves, seeds or the entire plant of *Trigonella foenum-graecum* L. (fenugreek) are used for the treatment of diabetes in many countries of the world and several human studies have confirmed the efficacy of the plant. The beneficial effect of the plant has been partly attributed to the high fibre content. The proposed mechanism of action was related to the inhibition of diffusion or transport of glucose independent of hormonal mechanisms [110].

7.2. *Gymnema sylvestre*

Extracts of *G. syvestre* have been reported to demonstrate antidiabetic activity possibly via reduction in insulin requirement by enhancing endogenous insulin availability, improving vitiated blood glucose homeostasis, better control of hyperlipidemia associated with diabetes, reduction in amylase activity in serum and, increase in β-cell function as shown by higher levels of serum C peptide. Extract of the leaves of the plant produced a significant reduction in blood glucose, glycosylated haemoglobin and glycosylated plasma proteins, with a decrease in conventional drug dosages. Some patients were able to discontinue conventional drugs and even maintain their blood glucose homeostasis with extracts alone in T2DM patients [111,112].

7.3. *Morinda lucida*

Alcoholic and aqueous extracts of roots and leaves of *Morinda lucida* Benth (Rubiaceae) have been reported to possess remarkable antidiabetic property in alloxan- and streptozotocin (STZ)-induced diabetic rats. Suggested mechanisms of action include the stimulation of beta cells to release insulin [113, 114].

7.4. *C. chinensis* Franch, *Astragalus membranaceus*, and *Lonicera japonica*

Using scientifically validated animal models in a study, a multicomponent berberine-containing remedy comprising *C. chinensis* Franch, *Astragalus membranaceus*, and *Lonicera japonica* was used to treat male Zucker diabetic fatty rats. The three-herb medicine showed sustained glucose-lowering effects for 1 week after a single-dose treatment. Two-week treatment attenuated insulin resistance and fatty degeneration, with hepatocyte regeneration lasting for 1 month posttreatment. The beneficial effects were found to have persisted for 1 year after 1-month treatment and were associated with activation of AMPK, Akt, and insulin-like growth factor-binding protein (IGFBP)1 pathways, with downregulation of miR29-b and expression of a gene network implicated in cell cycle, intermediary, and NADPH metabolism with normalization of CYP7a1 and IGFBP1 expression. Authors concluded that the pluripotent effects of the medicine in altering gene expression, in part through changes in miRNA, explained its sustained beneficial effects on glucose metabolism, fatty liver, and cellular repair [115].

7.5. *Pterocarpus marsupium*

A crude extract (water decoction) of *P. marsupium* was reported to have protective and restorative effect on β-cells in alloxan-induced diabetic rats. The results were substantiated by histological observations. Various active principles responsible for the antidiabetic activity have been isolated [116,117].

7.6. Kolaviron

Kolaviron, a biflavonoid complex isolated from *Garcinia kola* possesses multiple biological activities. Kolaviron demonstrated significant hypoglycaemic effect when administered to alloxan diabetic rabbits. The blood sugar was lowered from 506 mg/100 mL to 285 mg/100 mL at 12 h after the administration of 100 mg/kg kolaviron. Kolaviron also inhibited rat lens aldose reductase (RLAR) activity, with an IC_{50} value of 5.4 x 10^{-6} [118]. Adaramoye and Adeyemi reported that fractions obtained from kolaviron reduced blood sugar levels in STZ-diabetic rats within 4 h of oral administration and showed favourable effect on the plasma lipid profile of diabetic animals [119]. In addition to its antidiabetic property, kolaviron showed remarkable protective effects on cardiac, renal and hepatic tissues of STZ-diabetic rats. Many antidiabetic drugs do not offer significant tissue-protective effect in diabetic animals [120].

7.7. *Aloe barbadensis*

Aloe barbadensis (*Aloe vera*), the acclaimed "miracle plant" has been documented to ameliorate the diabetic condition in human subjects and experimental animals and to probably prevent the onset of hyperglycemia in alloxan intoxicated rabbits [121]. Reports of studies on the effect of aloe vera in experimental and clinical diabetes are available. In general, these reports agreed on the antidiabetic efficacy of *Aloe vera*. Oral administration of *Aloe vera* gel extract at a dose of 300 mg/kg bodyweight per day to STZ-induced diabetic rats for a period of 21 days resulted in a significant reduction in fasting blood glucose, hepatic transaminases (aspartate amino-transferase and alanine aminotransferase), plasma and tissue (liver and kidney) cholesterol, triglycerides, free fatty acids and phospholipids and a significant improvement in plasma insulin [122]. Can *et al.* concluded from their study that Aloe gel extract has a protective effect comparable to glibenclamide against hepatotoxicity produced by diabetes if used in the treatment of T2DM [123]. Another research finding showed that orally ingested aloe sterols altered the expressions of genes related to glucose and lipid metabolism, and ameliorated obesity- and diabetes-associated disorders in rats [124].

7.8. *Vernonia amygdalina*

Alcohol extract of *V. amygdalina* was found to significantly improve glucose tolerance in STZ-diabetic rats, decrease fasting blood glucose, show protective effect over pancreatic β-cells and cause a slight increase in insulin level in STZ-induced diabetic rats [125]. The same authors found that *V. amygdalina* increased the expression of GLUT 4 in rat skeletal muscle and its translocation to plasma membrane as well. *V. amygdalina* was also found to significantly inhibit the key hepatic gluconeogenic enzyme, glucose-6-phosphatase. Investigation of the synergistic antidiabetic effect of *V. amygdalina* and other medicinal plants yielded positive results. A study on the synergistic antidiabetic activity of *V. amygdalina* and *Azadirachta indica* [126] showed that compared with single extracts, the combined extract of *V. amygdalina* and *A. indica* promptly lowered blood glucose and maintained a relatively steady level over the study period, in tandem with insulin. The features of diabetic pathology, indicated in the histology of the liver and pancreas, were reversed. The extent of recovery was partial with *V. amygdalina*, better with *A. indica*, and distinct and total with *V. amygdalina* and *A. indica* combined. The beneficial synergistic effect was postulated to be exerted via oxidative stress attenuation, insulin mimetic action and β-cell regeneration. The synergistic postprandial blood glucose modulatory properties of *V. amygdalina, Gongronema latifolium* and *Occimum gratissimum* aqueous decoctions has also been reported [127]. It was concluded from the study that the decoction containing the three vegetables was superior in activity to any one or blends of only two, of the three decoctions.

7.9. *Moringa oleifera*

Moringa oleifera is a popular food plant with multiple medicinal uses including treatment of diabetes [128]. Various parts of the plant have been shown to have antidiabetic potential in several studies. In severely diabetic animals, 200 mg/kg aqueous leaf extract of *M. oleifera* reduced fasting blood sugar by 69.2% after 21 days of treatment and also significantly reduced urine sugar [129]. The progression of diabetes was significantly reduced in STZ-diabetic rats treated with methanol extract *M. oleifera* pods for 21 days with treated animals showing a significant reduction in serum glucose and nitric oxide, with concomitant increases in serum insulin and protein levels [130]. It has also been shown that extracts of the bark of the plant prevented dexamethasone-induced insulin resistance in peripheral tissues [131].

7.10. Pinitol (3-O-methyl-D-chiro-inositol)

In a study which assessed the effects of pinitol supplementation on glucose tolerance and insulin sensitivity, investigators found that a single dose of pinitol, from a naturally-occurring food ingredient, administered acutely influences indices of whole-body glucose tolerance and insulin sensitivity in healthy subjects. The study showed that consumption of a pinitol-enriched beverage, containing a dose of 6.0 g, reduced the increase in glycaemia and insulinaemia provoked by oral carbohydrate over-load when compared with a placebo. They remarked that this dietary intervention would be an effective first-step strategy for treating hyperglycaemia and related insulin resistance states, although future research is warranted to evaluate whether chronic doses of pinitol are effective in subjects with altered glucose metabolism [132]. Inositol phosphoglycans (IPG) have been reported to be important post-receptor mediators of insulin action [133,134] and it was suggested that by acting as insulin's second messenger, pinitol could increase insulin sensitivity.

8. Mechanisms of action of antidiabetic botanicals

Antidiabetic botanicals have been reported to foster protection via several mechanisms. These include amelioration of oxidative stress, anti-inflammatory and antiatherogenic effects; control of metabolic fluxes among various organs and energy metabolism within individual tissues and cells leading to the maintenance of glucose and lipid homeostasis and stable levels of energy stores; cytoprotection of pancreatic β-cells; inhibition of aldose reductase; improvement of endothelial dysfunction; inhibition of angiogenesis and the regulation of the expression of genes relevant for the development of T2DM A number of candidate genes have been identified in humans and many phytochemicals/extracts from traditional medicinal plants that can target diabetogenic genes have also been identified [135,136].

Medicinal plants can delay or inhibit glucose absorption, facilitate the entry of glucose into cells such as muscle cells, or stimulate insulin secretion by the pancreas. It was reported that oral administration of the ethanolic extract of *Allium sativum* showed significant antidiabetic effect in normal and alloxan-induced diabetic rats and that this effect was probably mediated through the stimulation of insulin secretion from the pancreas [137]. Oral administration of *Gymnena sylvestre* to diabetic rats was reported to increase the number of pancreatic islet cells as well as insulin levels suggesting a possible repair or regeneration of the pancreas [138]. *In vitro* and *in vivo* studies showed that water soluble extracts of *Gymnena sylvestre* released insulin probably due to the regeneration of pancreatic beta cells [139].

Aqueous extract of unripe fruit of *Momordica charantia* showed partial stimulation of insulin release from isolated beta cells of obese hyperglycaemic mice which is an indication of its insulin releasing action as a result of perturbations of membrane functions [140]. *Parinari excelsa* showed hypoglycaemic effects due to its insulin secretory activity in diabetic animal models [141]. Epicatechin which is the active principle isolated from the bark of *Pterocarpus maruspium* showed protective and restorative effect on beta cells of diabetic subjects. This may be due to its ability to regenerate beta cells [139].

Aqueous extract of *Citrullus colocynths* showed a dose dependent increase in insulin released from isolated islets [142]. Immunohistochemistry studies [143] showed that the amount of insulin in beta cells of the islet of Langerhans is greater in *Citrullus colocynthis* treated rats when compared with the control group.

A report on *in vitro* assays on some medicinal plants showed that they possess inhibitory activity on alpha glucosidase enzyme. In a study, thirty seven of forty-five samples examined showed IC_{50} values of between 2.33 μg/mL and 112.02 μg/mL, which were lower than that of acarbose (117.20 μg/mL) [144]. Also, 80% ethanol extract from *Garcinia daedalanthera* Pierre. leaves (Clusiaceae), *Antidesma celebicum* leaves (Euphorbiaceae), *Amaracarpus pubescens,* (Rubiaceae), and *Willughbeia tenuiflora* leaves (Apocynaceae) had the highest α-glucosidase inhibiting activity with IC_{50} of 2.33 μg/mL, 2.34 μg/mL, 3.64 μg/mL, and 8,16 μg/mL respectively. Meanwhile, types of enzyme inhibition mechanism from *Garcinia kydia* leaves (Clusiaceae), *Antidesma celebicum* leaves (Euphorbiaceae), and *Amaracarpus pubescens* leaves (Rubiaceae) were non-competitive inhibitor, competitive inhibitor, and mixed inhibitor respectively.

12. Conclusion

Diabetes mellitus and all its comorbidities constitute major causes of high economic loss which can in turn pose significant challenges to the economic development of developing

http://dx.doi.org/10.5772/57339

nations [145]. Despite efforts aimed at containing the disease, no definite cure has been found. Although the current available therapies have yielded appreciable improvements in the quality of life of diabetics, several reports have indicated that such improvements are not without the associated side effects. Studies have confirmed the benefits of medicinal plants with hypoglycaemic effects in the management of diabetes mellitus and many phytomedical preparations and compounds have been touted as candidates for antidiabetic drug development. However, the rate of developing these drugs is very slow, with only one clinical drug being reported to have gone from plant to pharmacy [110]. Therefore, there should be a focus on developing effective drugs from potent antidiabetic botanicals already identified while further research continues with new plants for the discovery of novel candidates for antidiabetic drugs. Also, potent herbal extracts should be standardized and made commercially available as many of these extracts often lack the drawbacks associated with single compounds.

Antidiabetic plants do not always have the same mechanism of actions because activities relate to their effects on the pancreatic β cells, the protective/inhibitory effect against insulinase and the increase of insulin sensitivity or the insulin-like activity of the plant extracts. Other mechanisms may involve improved glucose homeostasis, inhibition of intestinal glucose absorption, reduction of glycaemic index of carbohydrates. The mechanisms of action of antidiabetic botanicals need to be properly delineated so that different cases of diabetes can be specifically addressed.

Further research studies on the antidabetic potentials of botanicals, especially in developing countries, are suggested. The aims of such studies should be to find the botanicals with the most effective antidiabetic activities and to examine the possibilities of developing these active ingredients into antidiabetic drugs for the effective management and treatment of diabetes.

Author details

Afolabi Clement Akinmoladun[1*], Ebenezer Olatunde Farombi[2] and Oluwafemi Omoniyi Oguntibeju[3]

*Address all correspondence to: akinmoladunfc@yahoo.com; acakinmoladun at futa.edu.ng

1 Phytomedicine, Drug Metabolism and Toxicology Unit, Department of Biochemistry, School of Sciences, The Federal University of Technology, Akure, Nigeria

2 Drug Metabolism and Toxicology Research Unit, Department of Biochemistry, College of Medicine, University of Ibadan, Nigeria

3 Oxidative Stress Research Centre, Department of Biomedical Sciences, Faculty of Health & Wellness Sciences, Cape Peninsula University of Technology, South Africa

References

[1] Kumar PJ, Clark M. Textbook of Clinical Medicine. London: Saunders; 2002.

[2] Beverley B, Eschwège E. The diagnosis and classification of diabetes and impaired glucose tolerance. In: Textbook of Diabetes 1 John C Pickup and Gareth Williams Third edition; pp 2.1-2.11, 2003.

[3] McGill M, Felton AM. New global recommendations: A multidisciplinary approach to improving outcomes in diabetes. Prim Care Diabetes. 2007; 1(1):49-55

[4] World Health Organization. Diabetes mellitus: report of a WHO study group Geneva. WHO; 1985, Technical Report Series 727.

[5] American Diabetes Association. Diagnosis and classification of diabetes mellitus. Diabetes Care 2012; 35 (Suppl. 1):S64–71.

[6] Vlad A, Timar R. Pathogenesis of Type 1 diabetes mellitus: a brief overview. Romanian Journal of Diabetes Nutrition and Metabolic Diseases. 2012; 19(1): 67–72.

[7] van Belle TL, Coppieters KT, von Herrath MG. Type 1 Diabetes: Etiology, immunology, and therapeutic strategies. Physiol Rev. 2011; 91(1): 79-118.

[8] Ehtisham S, Barrett TG, Shaw NJ. Type 2 diabetes mellitus in UK children-an emerging problem. Diabet Med. 2000; 17(12): 867-71.

[9] Field AE, Coakley EH, Must A, Spadano JL, Laird N, Dietz WH, et al. Impact of overweight on the risk of developing common chronic diseases during a 10-year period. Arch Intern Med. 2001; 161(13): 1581-1586.

[10] Bloomgarden ZT. Type 2 diabetes in the young: the evolving epidemic. Diabetes Care. 2004; 27(4):998-1010.

[11] Amos AF, McCarty DJ, Zimmet P. The rising global burden of diabetes and its complications: estimates and projections to the year 2010. Diabetic Med 1997; 14: S1-S85.

[12] Zimmet P. Globalization, coca-colonization and the chronic disease epidemic: can the Doomsday scenario be averted? J Intern Med 2000; 247: 301-310.

[13] Patel DK, Prasad SK, Kumar R, Hemalatha S. An overview on antidiabetic medicinal plants having insulin mimetic property. Asian Pacific Journal of Tropical Biomedicine 2012; 320-330.

[14] Zimmet P, Alberti KG, Shaw J. Global and societal implications of the diabetes epidemic. Nature 2001;414:782– 7.

[15] Beran D, Yudkin JS. Diabetes care in sub-Saharan Africa. Lancet 2006;11(368):1689–95

[16] Wang Y, Mi J, Shan XY, Wang QJ, Ge KY. Is China facing an obesity epidemic and the consequences? The trends in obesity and chronic disease in China. Int J Obes (Lond) 2007; 31:177–88.

[17] Shaw JE, Sicree RA, Zimmet PZ. Global estimates of the prevalence of diabetes for 2010 and 2030. Diabetes Res Clin Pract. 2010; 87(1):4-14.

[18] Whiting DR, Guariguata L, Weil C, Shaw J. IDF Diabetes Atlas: global estimates of the prevalence of diabetes for 2011 and 2030. Diabetes Res Clin Pract 2011; 94:311–21.

[19] International Diabetes Federation. Diabetes Atlas (Second edition). Brussels, 2003

[20] Hirst MW, Felton, A. The UN Resolution on Diabetes and World Diabetes Day. Primary Care Diabetes 2008; 2: 95-96

[21] Zhang P, Zhang X, Brown JB, Vistisen D, Sicree RA, Shaw J, Nichols GA.. Economic impact of Diabetes. Diabetes Atlas 2010, IDF, 4.

[22] Fowler MJ. Microvascular and Macrovascular Complications of Diabetes. Clinical Diabetes 2008; 26(2) 77-82.

[23] Gray RP, Yudkin JS. Cardiovascular disease in diabetes mellitus. In: Pickup JC, Williams G (Eds.), Textbook of diabetes, Blackwell Sciences Ltd., Oxford, 1997.

[24] Stratton IM, Adler AI, Neil HA, Matthews DR, Manley SE, Cull CA, Hadden D, Turner RC, Holman RR. Association of glycaemia with macrovascular and microvascular complications of type 2 diabetes (UKPDS 35): prospective observational study. Br Med J 2000; 321: 405–412.

[25] Brownlee M. Biochemistry and molecular cell biology of diabetic complications. Nature 2001; 414:813-820.

[26] Icks A, Haastert B, Trautner C, Giani G, Glaeske G, Hoffmann F. Incidence of lower-limb amputations in the diabetic compared to the non-diabetic population. Findings from nationwide insurance data, Germany, 2005-2007. Experimental and Clinical Endocrinology & Diabetes, 2009, 117:500–504.

[27] Resnikoff S, Pascolini D, Etya'ale D, Kocur I, Pararajasegaram R, Pokharel GP, Mariotti SP. Global data on visual impairment in the year 2002. Bulletin of the World Health Organization, 2004; 82:844.

[28] Fong DS, Aiello LP, Ferris FL 3rd, Klein R. Diabetic retinopathy. Diabetes Care 2004; 27:2540– 2553.

[29] Massin P., Angioi-Duprez K., Bacin F., Cathelineau B., Cathelineau G., Chaine G., and al. Detection, monitoring and treatment of diabetic retinopathy. Recommendations of ALFEDIAM. Committee of above-mentioned experts and validated by the board of directors and scientific board of ALFEDIAM Diabetes Metab 1996 ; 22 : 203-209

[30] Hermans MP, Ahn SA, Rousseau MF. Statin therapy and cataract in type 2 diabetes. Diabetes Metab. 2011 37(2):139-43].

[31] Klein BE, Klein R, Lee KE, Grady LM. Statin use and incident nuclear cataract. JAMA 2006; 295:2752–8.

[32] Dodson PM. Diabetes and the eye. In: Dodson PM, editor. Diabetic retinopathy. Oxford, Oxford University Press; 2009.

[33] Feldman HA, Goldstein I, Hatzichristou DG, Krane RJ, McKinlay JB; Impotence and its medical and psychosocial correlates: results of the Massachusetts Male Aging Study. J Urol 1994;151:54–61.

[34] Malavige LS, Levy JC. Erectile dysfunction in diabetes mellitus. J Sex Med. 2009; 6(5): 1232-47.

[35] American Diabetes Association: Standards of medical care in diabetes—2007 [Position Statement]. *Diabetes Care* 30:S4–S41, 2007

[36] Boulton AJ, Vinik AI, Arezzo JC, Bril V, Feldman EL, Freeman R, Malik RA, Maser RE, Sosenko JM, Ziegler D: Diabetic neuropathies: a statement by the American Diabetes Association. Diabetes Care 2005; 28: 956–962,

[37] Gross JL, de Azevedo MJ, Silveiro SP, Canani LH, Caramori ML, Zelmanovitz T.Diabetic nephropathy: diagnosis, prevention, and treatment. Diabetes Care 2005; 28:164–176. complications in patients with type 2 diabetes (UKPDS 33). Lancet 1998;352:837–53.

[38] Chaturvedi N, Bandinelli S, Mangili R, Penno G, Rottiers RE, Fuller JH: Microalbuminuria in type 1 diabetes: rates, risk factors and glycemic threshold. Kidney Int 2001; 60:219– 227, 2001.

[39] Adler AI, Stevens RJ, Manley SE, Bilous RW, Cull CA, Holman RR. Development and progression of nephropathy in type 2 diabetes: the United Kingdom Prospective Diabetes Study (UKPDS 64). Kidney Int 2003; 63:225–232.

[40] United States Renal Data System. USRDS 2007 Annual Data Report. Bethesda, MD: National Institute of Diabetes and Digestive and Kidney Diseases, National Institutes of Health, U.S. Department of Health and Human Services; 2007.

[41] Laing SP, Swerdlow AJ, Slater SD, Burden AC, Morris A, Waugh NR, Gatling W, Bingley PJ,Patterson CC: Mortality from heart disease in a cohort of 23,000 patients with insulin-treated diabetes. Diabetologia 2003; 46:760–765.

[42] Paterson AD, Rutledge BN, Cleary PA, Lachin JM, Crow RS: The effect of intensive diabetes treatment on resting heart rate in type 1 diabetes: The Diabetes Control and Complications Trial/Epidemiology of Diabetes Interventions and Complications study. 2007; 30:2107– 2112.

[43] Kannel WB, McGee DL: Diabetes and cardiovascular disease: the Framingham study. 1979; 241:2035–2038.

[44] Haffner SM, Lehto S, Ronnemaa T, Pyorala K, Laakso M: Mortality from coronary heart disease in subjects with type 2 diabetes and in nondiabetic subjects with and without prior myocardial infarction. N Engl J Med 1998; 339:229–234.

[45] Buse JB, Henry RR, Han J, Kim DD, Fineman MS, Baron AD. Effects of exenatide (exendin-4) on glycemic control over 30 weeks in sulfonylurea-treated patients with type 2 diabetes. Diabetes Care. 2004; 27(11):2628-2635.

[46] Lehto S, Ronnemaa T, Pyorala K, Laakso M: Predictors of stroke in middle-aged patients with non-insulin-dependent diabetes. Stroke 1996; 27:63–68.

[47] Beckman JA, Creager MA, Libby P: Diabetes and atherosclerosis: epidemiology, pathophysiology, and management. JAMA 2002; 287:2570– 2581.

[48] Jeon CY, Murray MB. Diabetes mellitus increases the risk of active tuberculosis: a systematic review of 13 observational studies. PLoS Medicine 2008; 5(7):e152.doi: 10.1371/journal.pmed.0050152)

[49] Grundy SM, Brewer HB Jr, Cleeman JI, Smith SC Jr, Lenfant C Grundy SM, Brewer HB Jr, Cleeman JI, Smith SC Jr, Lenfant C. Definition of metabolic syndrome: Report of the National Heart, Lung, and Blood Institute/American Heart Association conference on scientific issues related to definition. Arterioscler Thromb Vasc Biol. 2004; 24(2):e13-8

[50] Lefèbvre P. Prediabetes or what's in a name? Diabetes Metab 2005;31:519.

[51] Valensi P, Schwarz EH, Hall M, Felton AM, Maldonato A, Mathieu C. Pre-diabetes essential action: a European perspective. Diabetes Metab 2005; 31(6):606-20.

[52] Zhang SX, Sun H, Sun WJ, Jiao GZ and Wang XJ. Proteomic study of serum proteins in a type 2 diabetes mellitus rat model by Chinese traditional medicine Tianqi Jiangtang Capsule administration. J Pharm Biomed Anal *2010*; 53: 1011-1014.

[53] Giacco F, Brownlee M. Oxidative Stress and diabetic complications. Circ Res 2010; 107(9):1058-70.

[54] Bohren KM, Bullock B, Wermuth B, Gabbay KH. The aldo-keto reductase superfamily. cDNAs and deduced amino acid sequences of human aldehyde and aldose reductases. J Biol Chem. 1989 Jun 5;264(16):9547-51

[55] Lee AY, Chung SK, Chung SS. Demonstration that polyol accumulation is responsible for diabetic cataract by the use of transgenic mice expressing the aldose reductase gene in the lens. Proc Natl Acad Sci USA 1995; 92:2780 –2784.

[56] Engerman RL, Kern TS, Larson ME: Nerve conduction and aldose reductase inhibition during 5 years of diabetes or galactosaemia in dogs. Diabetologia 1994; 37:141–144.

[57] Lee AY, Chung SS: Contributions of polyol pathway to oxidative stress in diabetic cataract. FASEB J 1999; 13:23–30.

[58] Giardino I, Edelstein D, Brownlee M: Nonenzymatic glycosylation in vitro and in bovine endothelial cells alters basic fibroblast growth factor activity: a model for intracellular glycosylation in diabetes. J Clin Invest 1994; 94:110 –117.

[59] Shinohara M, Thornalley PJ, Giardino I, Beisswenger P, Thorpe SR, Onorato J, Brownlee M: Overexpression of glyoxalase-I in bovine endothelial cells inhibits intracellular advanced glycation endproduct formation and prevents hyperglycemia-induced increases in macromolecular endocytosis. J Clin Invest 1998; 101:1142–1147.

[60] McLellan AC, Thornalley PJ, Benn J, Sonksen PH: Glyoxalase system in clinical diabetes mellitus and correlation with diabetic complications. Clin Sci (Lond) 1994; 87:21–29.

[61] Charonis AS, Reger LA, Dege JE, Kouzi-Koliakos K, Furcht LT, Wohlhueter RM, Tsilibary EC: Laminin alterations after in vitro nonenzymatic glycosylation. Diabetes 1990; 39:807– 814.

[62] Doi T, Vlassara H, Kirstein M, Yamada Y, Striker GE, Striker LJ: Receptorspecific increase in extracellular matrix production in mouse mesangial cells by advanced glycosylation end products is mediated via platelet derived growth factor. Proc Natl Acad Sci U S A 89:2873–2877, 1992.

[63] Neeper M, Schmidt AM, Brett J, Yan SD, Wang F, Pan YC, Elliston K, Stern D, Shaw A: Cloning and expression of a cell surface receptor for advanced glycosylation end products of proteins. J Biol Chem 1992; 267:14998 –15004.

[64] Li YM, Mitsuhashi T, Wojciechowicz D, Shimizu N, Li J, Stitt A, He C, Banerjee D, Vlassara H: Molecular identity and cellular distribution of advanced glycation endproduct receptors: relationship of p60 to OST-48 and p90 to 80K-H membrane proteins. Proc Natl Acad Sci USA 1996; 93:11047–11052.

[65] Abordo EA, Thornalley PJ. Synthesis and secretion of tumour necrosis factor-alpha by human monocytic THP-1 cells and chemotaxis induced by human serum albumin derivatives modified with methylglyoxal and glucose-derived advanced glycation endproducts. Immunol Lett 1997; 58:139 –147.

[66] Koya, D. & King, G. L. Protein kinase C activation and the development of diabetic complications. Diabetes 1998; 47:859–866.

[67] Portilla, D. *et al.* Etomoxir -induced PPARalpha-modulated enzymes protect during acute renal failure. Am J Physiol Renal Physiol 2000; 278, F667–F675.

[68] Keogh, R. J., Dunlop, M. E. & Larkins R.. G. Effect of inhibition of aldose reductase on glucose flux, diacylglycerol formation, protein kinase C, and phospholipase A2 activation. Metabolism 1997; 46:41–47.

[69] Brownlee M. The Pathobiology of Diabetic Complications A Unifying Mechanism. Diabetes 2005; 54(6):1615-1625.

[70] Craven PA, Studer RK, DeRubertis FR. Impaired nitric oxide-dependent cyclic guanosine monophosphate generation in glomeruli from diabetic rats. Evidence for protein kinase C-mediated suppression of the cholinergic response. J Clin Invest 1994; 93: 311–320.

[71] Ganz MB, Seftel A. Glucose-induced changes in protein kinase C and nitric oxide are prevented by vitamin E. Am J Physiol 2000; 278: E146–E152.

[72] Studer, R. K., Craven, P. A. & DeRubertis, F. R. Role for protein kinase C in the mediation of increased fibronectin accumulation by mesangial cells grown in high-glucose medium. Diabetes 1993; 42:118–126.

[73] Issad T, Massona E, Pagesy P. O-GlcNAc modification, insulin signaling and diabetic complications. Diabetes Metab 2010; 36(6 Pt 1):423-35.

[74] Lefebvre T, Dehennaut V, Guinez C, Olivier S, Drougat L, Mir AM, et al. Dysregulation of the nutrient/stress sensor O-GlcNAcylation is involved in the etiology of cardiovascular disorders, type-2 diabetes and Alzheimer's disease. Biochim Biophys Acta 2009;1800: 67–79.

[75] Issad T, Kuo M. O-GlcNAc modification of transcription factors, glucose sensing and glucotoxicity. Trends Endocrinol Metab 2008;19: 380–9.

[76] Clark RJ, McDonough PM, Swanson E, Trost SU, Suzuki M, Fukuda M, Dillmann WH: Diabetes and the accompanying hyperglycemia impairs cardiomyocyte calcium cycling through increased nuclear O-GlcNAcylation. J Biol Chem 2003; 278:44230–44237.

[77] Alwan AAS. Management of diabetes mellitus standards of care and clinical practice guidelines; noncommunicable diseases WHO, Alexandria, 1994.

[78] Stoffers DA, Ferrer J, Clarke WL, Habener JF. Earlyonset type-II diabetes mellitus (MODY) linked to IPF- 1. Nature Genet 1997; 17: 138-139.

[79] National Institutes of Health. Diabetes in America, 2nd edn. Bethesda, MD: National Institutes of Health, 1995. (NIH Publication no. 95-1468.)

[80] Goldstein, D. J. (1992) Beneficial health effects of modest weight loss.Int J Obes Relat Metab Disord 1992; 16: 397-415.

[81] Franz MJ, Monk A, Barry B, McClain K, Weaver T, Cooper N, Upham P, Bergenstal R, Mazze RS: Effectiveness of medical nutrition therapy provided by dietitians in the management of non-insulin-dependent diabetes mellitus: a randomized, controlled clinical trial. 1995; 95:1009–1017.

[82] Hamman RF, Wing RR, Edelstein SL, Lachin JM, Bray GA, Delahanty L, Hoskin M, Kriska AM, Mayer-Davis EJ, Pi-Sunyer X, Regensteiner J, Venditti B, Wylie-Rosett J.

Effect of weight loss with lifestyle intervention on risk of diabetes. Diabetes Care. 2006; 29(9):2102-7.

[83] Tuomilehto J, Schwarz P, Lindström J. Long-term benefits from lifestyle interventions for type 2 diabetes prevention: time to expand the efforts. Diabetes Care. 2011; 34 Suppl 2:S210-4.

[84] Knowler WC, Barrett-Connor E, Fowler SE, Hamman RF, Lachin JM, Walker EA, Nathan DM; Diabetes Prevention Program Research Group. Reduction in the incidence of type 2 diabetes with lifestyle intervention or metformin. N Engl J Med. 2002 Feb 7;346(6):393-403.

[85] Eriksson K, Lindgrade F. Prevention of type 2 (non-insulin-dependent) diabetes mellitus by diet and physical exercises. Diabetologia 1991; 34: 891-898.

[86] Jean Ferrières The French paradox: lessons for other countries. Heart. 2004 January; 90(1): 107–111.

[87] Kromhout D, Menotti A, Kesteloot H, Sans S. Prevention of coronary heart disease by diet and lifestyle: evidence from prospective cross-cultural, cohort, and intervention studies. Circulation. 2002 Feb 19;105(7):893-8.

[88] Philis-Tsimikas A. Type 2 diabetes: limitations of current therapies. Consultant 2009; 49(Suppl.): S5–11.

[89] Bastaki S. Diabetes mellitus and its treatment. Int J Diabetes & Metabolism 2005; 13:111-134.

[90] Levine R. Sulfonylureas: background development of the field. Diabetes Care 1984; 7 (suppl 1): 3-7.

[91] Bailey CJ. Biguanides and NIDDM. Diabetes Care 1992; 15: 755-772. metformin and a sulfonylurea. Diabetes Care. 2005; 28(5):1083-1091.

[92] Clarke BF, Duncan LJP; Biguanide treatment in the management of insulin dependent (maturity-onset) diabetes: clinical experience with metformin. Res Clin Forums 1979; 1: 53-63.

[93] Perriello G, Misericordia P, Volpi E, Santucci A, Santucci C, Ferrannini E, Ventura MM, Santeusanio F, Brunetti P & Bolli GB 1994 Acute antihyperglycemic mechanisms of metformin in NIDDM: evidence for suppression of lipid oxidation and hepatic glucose production.

[94] Sum CF, Webster JM, Johnson AB, Catalano C, Cooper BG, Taylor R. The effect of intravenous metformin on glucose metabolism during hyperglycaemia in type 2 diabetes. Diabet Med. 1992; 9(1):61-5.

[95] Wu MS, Johnson P, Sheu WH, et al. Effect of metformin on carbohydrate and lipoprotein metabolism in NIDDM patients. Diabetes care 1990; 13: 1-8.

http://dx.doi.org/10.5772/57339

[96] Hu S, Wang S, Fanelli B, et al. Pancreatic beta-cell K (ATP) channel activity and membrane-binding studies with nateglinide: a comparison with sulfonylureas and repaglinide. J Pharmacol Exp Ther 2000; 293: 444-452.

[97] Fuhlendorff J, Rorsman P, Kofod H, et al. Stimulation of insulin release by repaglinide and glibenclamide involves both common and distinct process, diabetes 1998; 47: 345-451.

[98] Bischoff H. The mechanism of a-glucosidase inhibition in the management of diabetes. Clin Invest Med 1995; 18: 303-311.

[99] Reabasa-Lhoret R, Chiasson J-L. Potential of alphaglucosidase inhibitors in elderly patients with diabetes mellitus and impaired glucose tolerance. Drug Aging 1998; 13: 131-143.

[100] Caro JF: Insulin resistance in obese and nonobese man (clinical review 26). J Clin Endocrinol Metab 73:691-702, 1991.

[101] . Ho MP, Rumsfeld JS, Masoudi FA, et al. Effect of medication nonadherence on hospitalization and mortality among patients with diabetes mellitus. Arch Intern Med 2006;166:1836-1841.

[102] Jellinger PS, Davidson JA, Blonde L, Einhorn D, Grunberger G, Handelsman Y, Hellman R, Lebovitz H, Levy P, Roberts VL; ACE/AACE Diabetes Road Map Task Force. Road maps to achieve glycemic control in type 2 diabetes mellitus: ACE/AACE Diabetes Road Map Task Force. Endocr Pract. 2007; 13(3):260-8.

[103] Brown JB, Nichols GA, Perry A. The burden of treatment failure in type 2 diabetes. *Diabetes Care.* 2004;27:1535-1540.

[104] Samuelsson G. Drugs of natural origin. A textbook of pharmacognosy. 4th ed., Stockholm,

[105] Doughari JH. Human IS, Bennade S, Ndakidemi PA. Phytochemicals as chemotherapeutic agents and antioxidants: Possible solution to the control of antibiotic resistant verocytotoxin producing bacteria. Journal of Medicinal Plants Research 2009; 3(11): 839-848.

[106] Farnsworth N.R, Akerele O, Bingel AS, Soejarto D.D, Guo Z. Medicinal plants in therapy. Bull World Health Organization 1985; 63: 965-81.

[107] Malviya N, Jain S, Malviya S. Antidiabetic potential of medicinal plants. Acta Pol Pharm 2010; 67(2): 113-118.

[108] Maroo J, Vasu VT, Aalinkeel R, Gupta S. Glucose lowering effect of aqueous extract of *Enicostemma littorale* Blume in diabetes: a possible mechanism of action. J Ethnopharmacol 2002; 81(3): 317-320.

[109] Bnouham M, Ziyyat A, Mekhfi H, Tahri A, Legssyer A. Medicinal plants with potential antidiabetic activity - A review of ten years of herbal medicine research (1990-2000). Int J Diabetes & Metabolism 2006; 14: 1-25.

[110] Gunn J, Che C-T, Farnsworth N. Diabetes and natural products. In: Bioactive food as dietary interventions for diabetes. Watson R and Preedy B (Eds) 2013. pp 381-394.

[111] Shanmugasundaram ER, Rajeswari G, Baskaran K, Rajesh Kumar BR, Radha Shanmugasundaram K, Kizar Ahmath B. Use of *Gymnema sylvestre* leaf extract in the control of blood glucose in insulin-dependent diabetes mellitus. J. Ethnopharmacol 1990; 30, 281–294.

[112] Siddiqui AA, Ahmed B and Dogra AJ. Med. Aromat. Plant Sci., 2000; 22, 223–231.

[113] Kamanyi A, Nijamen D, Nkeh B. Hypoglycaemic properties of the aqueous root extract of *Morinda lucida* (Benth) (Rubiaceae). Studies in the mouse. Phytotherapy Research 1994; 8, 369–371.

[114] Olajide O, Awe S, Makinde J, Morebise O. Evaluation of the anti-diabetic property of *Morinda lucida* leaves in streptozotocin-diabetic rats. Journal of Pharmacy and Pharmacology 1999; 51, 1321–1324.

[115] Zhao HL, Sui Y, Qiao CF, Yip KY, Leung RK, Tsui SK, Lee HM, Wong HK, Zhu X, Siu JJ, He L, Guan J, Liu LZ, Xu HX, Tong PC, Chan JC. Sustained antidiabetic effects of a berberine-containing Chinese herbal medicine through regulation of hepatic gene expression. Diabetes 2012; 61(4):933-43.

[116] Chakravarty BK, Gupta S, Gambheer SS and Gode KD. Indian J. Pharmacol 1980, 12, 123–127

[117] Tiwari AK and Rao JM. Diabetes mellitus and multiple therapeutic approaches of phytochemicals: Present status and future prospects. Current Science 2002; 83 (1) 30-38

[118] Iwu MM, Igboko OA, Okunji CO, Tempesta MS. Antidiabetic and aldose reductase activities of biflavanones of *Garcinia kola.* J Pharm Pharmacol 1990; 42(4):290-2.

[119] Adaramoye OA, Adeyemi EO. Hypoglycaemic and hypolipidaemic effects of fractions from kolaviron, a biflavonoid complex from *Garcinia kola* in streptozotocin-induced diabetes mellitus rats. J Pharm Pharmaco 2006; 58(1):121-8.

[120] Adaramoye OA. Antidiabetic effect of kolaviron, a biflavonoid complex isolated from *Garcinia kola* seeds, in Wistar rats. Afr Health Sci 2012; 12(4):498-506.

[121] Akinmoladun AC, Akinloye O. Prevention of the onset of hyperglycaemia by extracts of *Aloe barbadensis* in rabbits treated with alloxan. African Journal of Biotechnology 2007; 6 (8):1028-1030.

[122] Rajasekaran S, Ravi K, Sivagnanam K, Subramanian S. Beneficial effects of *Aloe vera* leaf gel extract on lipid profile status in rats with streptozotocin diabetes. Clin Exp Pharmacol Physio. 2006; 33(3):232-7.

[123] Can A, Akev N, Ozsoy N, Bolkent S, Arda BP, Yanardag R, Okyar A. Effect of *Aloe vera* leaf gel and pulp extracts on the liver in type-II diabetic rat models. Biol Pharm Bull 2004; 27(5):694-8.

[124] Misawa E, Tanaka M, Nomaguchi K, Nabeshima K, Yamada M, Toida T, Iwatsuki K. Oral ingestion of *Aloe vera* phytosterols alters hepatic gene expression profiles and ameliorates obesity-associated metabolic disorders in zucker diabetic fatty rats. J Agric Food Chem 2012; 60(11):2799-806.

[125] Ong KW, Hsu A, Song L, Huang D, Tan BK. Polyphenols-rich *Vernonia amygdalina* shows anti-diabetic effects in streptozotocin-induced diabetic rats. J Ethnopharmacol 2011; 133(2):598-607.

[126] Atangwho IJ, Ebong PE, Eyong EU, Asmawi MZ, Ahmad M. Synergistic antidiabetic activity of *Vernonia amygdalina* and *Azadirachta indica*: biochemical effects and possible mechanism. J Ethnopharmacol 2012; 141(3):878-87.

[127] Ejike CE, Awazie SO, Nwangozi PA, Godwin CD. Synergistic postprandial blood glucose modulatory properties of *Vernonia amygdalina* (Del.), *Gongronema latifolium* (Benth.) and *Occimum gratissimum* (Linn.) aqueous decoctions. J Ethnopharmacol 2013; 149(1):111-6

[128] Anwar F, Latif S, Ashraf M, Gilani AH. *Moringa oleifera*: a food plant with multiple medicinal uses. Phytother Res 2007; 21(1):17-25.

[129] Jaiswal D, Kumar Rai P, Kumar A, Mehta S, Watal G. Effect of *Moringa oleifera* Lam. leaves aqueous extract therapy on hyperglycemic rats. J Ethnopharmacol 2009; 123(3):392-6.

[130] Gupta R, Mathur M, Bajaj VK, Katariya P, Yadav S, Kamal R, Gupta RS. Evaluation of antidiabetic and antioxidant activity of *Moringa oleifera* in experimental diabetes. J Diabetes. 2012; 4(2):164-71.

[131] Sholapur HN, Patil BM. Effect of *Moringa oleifera* bark extracts on dexamethasone-induced insulin resistance in rats. Drug Res (Stuttg). 2013; [Epub ahead of print]

[132] Hernández-Mijares A, Bañuls C, Peris JE, Monzó N, Jover A, Bellod L, Victor VM, Rocha M. A single acute dose of pinitol from a naturally-occurring food ingredient decreases hyperglycaemia and circulating insulin levels in healthy subjects. 2013; 141(2):1267-72.

[133] Larner J, Allan G, Kessler C, Reamer P, Gunn R, Huang LC. Phosphoinositol glycan derived mediators and insulin resistance. Prospects for diagnosis and therapy. J Basic Clin Physiol Pharmacol 1998;9(2-4):127-37.

[134] Larner J, Brautigan DL, Thorner MO. D-chiro-inositol glycans in insulin signaling and insulin resistance. Mol Med. 2010; 16(11-12):543-52.

[135] Dembinska-Kiec A, Mykkänen O, Kiec-Wilk B, Mykkänen H. Antioxidant phytochemicals against type 2 diabetes. Br J Nutr. 2008; E Suppl 1:ES109-17.

[136] Anuradha CV. Phytochemicals targeting genes relevant for type 2 diabetes. Can J Physiol Pharmacol. 2013 Jun;91(6):397-411.

[137] Chauhan A, Sharma PK, Srivastava P, Kumar N, Duehe R. Plants having potential antidiabetic activity: a review. Der Pharm Lett 2010; 2(3): 369-387.

[138] Kaczmar T. Herbal support for diabetes management. Clin Nutr Insights 1998; 6(8): 1-4.

[139] Saxena A, Vikram NK. Role of selected Indian plants in management of type 2 diabetes: a review. J Altern Complement Med 2004; 10(2): 369-378.

[140] Grover JK, Yadav S, Vats V. Medicinal plants of India with antidiabetic potential. J Ethnopharmacol 2002; 81(1): 81-100.

[141] Rao MU, Sreenivasulu M, Chengaiah B, Reddy KJ, Chetty CM. Herbal medicines for diabetes mellitus: a review. Int J PharmTech Res 2010; 2(3): 1883-1892.

[142] Singh LW. Traditional medicinal plants of Manipur as antidiabetics. J Med Plant Res 2011; 5(5): 677-687.

[143] Dallak M, Al-Khateeb M, Abbas M, Elessa R, Al-Hashem F, Bashir N, et al. In vivo, acute, normo-hypoglycemic, antihyperglycemic, insulinotropic actions of orally administered ethanol extract of *Citrullus colocynthis* (L.) Schrab pulp. Am J Biochem Biotechnol 2009; 5(3): 119-126.

[144] Berna E, Katrin B, AbdulMun'im,Wulan Y, Anastasia B, and Eva K. S: Screening of α-Glucosidase Inhibitory Activity from Some Plants of Apocynaceae, Clusiaceae, Euphorbiaceae, and Rubiaceae: Journal of Biomedicine and Biotechnology Volume 2012.

[145] Narayan KMV, Zhang P, Kanaya AM, Williams DE, Engelgau MM, Imperatore G, Ramachandran A, "Diabetes: The Pandemic and Potential Solutions." 2006. Disease Control Priorities in Developing Countries (2nd Edition), ed., 591-604. New York: Oxford University Press.

Section 2

Antioxidant Natural Products

Chapter 7

Antioxidant-Rich Natural Grain Products and Human Health

Afam I.O. Jideani, Henry Silungwe,
Thakhani Takalani, Tonna A. Anyasi,
Henry Udeh and Adewale Omolola

Additional information is available at the end of the chapter

http://dx.doi.org/10.5772/57169

1. Introduction

Over the years, several definitions have been used to describe whole grains. Though these definitions exist, a harmonized definition is yet to be agreed upon with many nations rather adopting the definition of whole grains as used by the American Association of Cereal Chemist (AACC) international due primarily to its comprehensiveness [1]. Accordingly in 1999, the AACC defined whole grains as grains that consist of an intact, milled, cracked or flaked caryopsis whose primary components; starchy endosperm, germ and bran are present in the same relative proportions as they exist in the intact caryopsis. Plant produce that can be classified as whole grains include amaranth, brown and coloured rice, sorghum, teff, wheat, faro, wild rice, triticale, millet, quinoa, oats, buckwheat, whole rye, barley, corn (including popcorn) and bulgur. According to the Food and Drug Administration (FDA) of the United States, foods such as soybeans, oilseeds (sunflower seeds), roots and corn flour or corn meal without the pericarp and other essential fractions cannot be classified as whole grains [1,2]. The term grains can also be used as a collective name given to seeds of cereals (wheat, barley, oats, corn/maize and sorghum) and legumes like peanuts and cowpea (*Cajanus cajan*) [2].

Whole grains are rich in phytochemicals and provide unique bioactive compounds that are complementary to those in fruits and vegetables when consumed together. The additive and synergistic effects of phytochemicals in fruits, vegetables and whole grains are responsible for their health benefits [3]. Important groups of phytochemicals with great beneficial nutritional and health effects are phenolics, carotenoids, vitamin E compounds, lignans, β-glucan and insulin. Phenolic compounds are the most common antioxidants in whole grains and are generally categorized as phenolic acids, flavonoids, stilbenes, coumarines and tannins [4]. The most abundant phenolic compounds found in whole grains are phenolic acids and flavonoids (Figure 1).

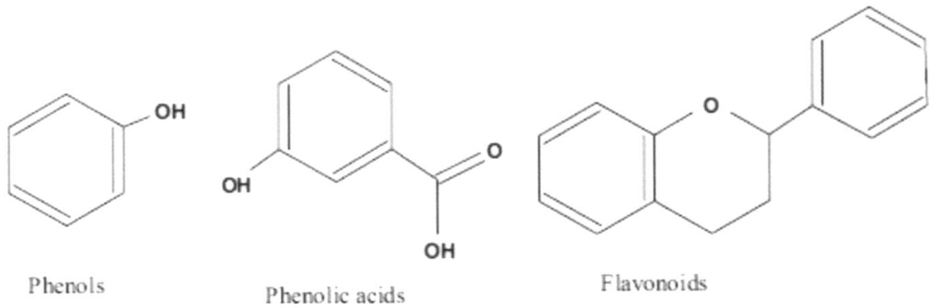

Figure 1. Structures of common phenolic compounds

Minerals mg/kg	Whole grains								
	Wheat	**Rye**	**Barley**	**Corn**	**Oats**	**Rice**	**Buckwheat**	**Millet**	**Sorghum**
Phosphorus	1170	3010	2460	990	4110	1030	1550	2400	350
Potassium	1550	4380	3290	1200	4000	1500	2420	2200	240
Magnesium	250	930	670	470	1170	350	1010	1000	188
Calcium	170	330	270	60	530	60	110	100	27
Sodium	20	50	40	10	40	20	10	NA	5
Zinc	8	28	13	5	30	17	25	34	3
Iron	12	28	24	11	38	12	15	48	11
Manganese	5	22	13	NA	58	9	15	7	1
Copper	1	3	1	NA	2	2	6	5	0.2

NA not available. Source: [8,9].

Table 1. Mineral content of whole grains

According to the FDA, a whole grain food is said to meet the whole grain health claim when it contains 51% whole grain flour by weight of its final product. It is also said to meet the whole grain health claims when it contains all components of the intact grain, has about 1.7 g of dietary fibre and also contains 16 g whole grain per serving [5]. *In vitro* minerals (Table 1) and phytochemicals in grains can act as antioxidants and used as nutraceuticals when consumed, by providing the body with protection against cardiovascular, anticancer, antidiabetics and antiobese agents, immune boosters, chronic inflammatory disorders and degenerative diseases [6]. Epidemiological studies have also revealed that regular consumption of whole grains and their products have been associated with reduced risk of developing chronic diseases [7]. Therefore, dietary modification by increasing the consumption of a wide variety of fruits, vegetables and whole grains daily, is said to be a practical strategy for consumers to optimize their health and reduce the risk of chronic diseases.

2. High antioxidant grains

Whole cereal grains contain a wide range of bioactive components with antioxidant effect [10] such as dietary fibre (DF) and phytochemicals [11,12] that are beneficial against diabetes, colon cancer and cardiovascular disease (CVD) [13,6,14]. Antioxidants present in whole grain cereals act in defense to remove the reactive oxygen species (ROS) thereby preventing and curing oxidative stress-related diseases. In [15], it was reported that vitamin E, folates, polyphenols, minerals, trace elements, carotenoids, phytic acid, lignin and alkylresorcinols are the bioactive compounds available in cereal grains. Polyphenols that are predominant in cereals are hydroxycinnamic, ferulic, gallic, vanillic and ϱ-coumaric acids, of which, ferulic acid is the most potent. Phenolic compounds [16] are said to be present in cereal grains in free and bound form, as conjugates with sugars, fatty acids or as proteins. These polyphenols have several biological functions such as antioxidant, anti-inflammatory and anti-cancer activities that can protect the human body, which is constantly exposed to endogenous and exogenous free radicals [17]. Plant sterols, also called phytosterols, found in plants, have been clinically shown to lower low-density lipoprotein (LDL) cholesterol by about 8 to 15% as part of a heart-healthy diet. Also, wholegrains that serve as source of DF are useful in the prevention and treatment of constipation, CVD and hypertension [8,12].

Grains can be classified as typical and pseudo-cereals. Typical cereals include sorghum, wheat, rice, barley, millet, rye, oat, maize, buckwheat, triticale, fonio, canary grass. Pseudo-cereals include amaranth, buckwheat, quinoa, kaniwa, and pitseed. Cereals reported with high antioxidant capacity include sorghum, wheat, barley, millet and amaranth. It has also been reported that bioactive substances occur in grains at different concentrations and identities depending on genotypes and phenotypes [9]. Sorghum, millet and barley adapted to the UAE environment, were found to contain reasonable levels of DF and antioxidant properties [9]. Experimental evidence has shown that certain cereals such as sorghum are rich in antioxidants that are comparable to those in fruits and vegetables [19]. Varieties of sorghum such as black sorghum, have been shown to contain significant amount of antioxidants; condensed tannins, anthocyanins (Figure 2 and 3) and other phytochemicals with properties that complement the phytochemicals present in fruits and vegetables [19]. Whole wheat and wheat bran-based ready-to-eat breakfast cereals have also been reported to be an important source of dietary antioxidants [20]. It has been shown [21] that buckwheat constitutes high amount of total phenolics, with the highest DPPH radical scavenging activity and capacity for Fe^{3+} reduction. Phenolic acids from breakfast cereals exhibit strong antioxidant activity *in vitro* at concentrations that can be obtained from a normal serving of whole wheat cereal [20]. Available data from the literature also reveals that sorghum is a significant source of phytosterols (tocopherols, tocotrienols) and policosanol, while rice has been shown to be rich in oryzanols [22].

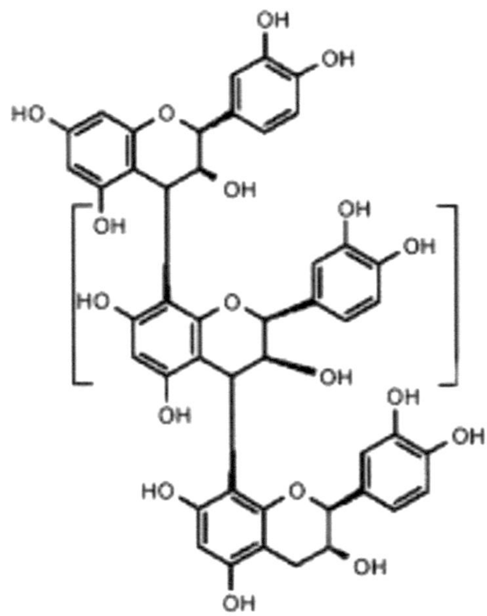

Figure 2. Condensed tannin

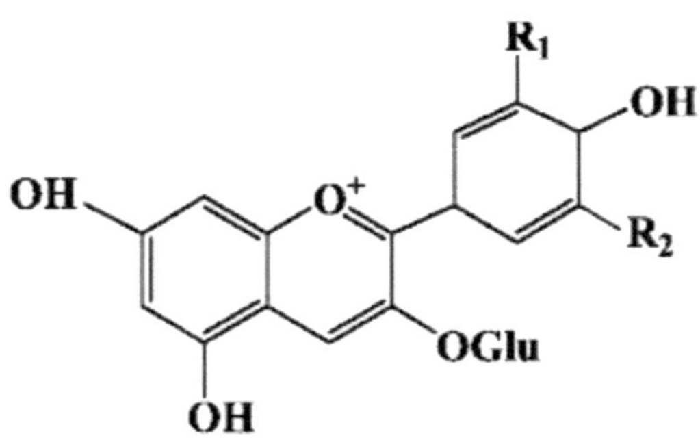

Figure 3. Chemical structure of anthocyanin

Cereals naturally contain a wide variety of polyphenols such as the hydroxycinnamic, ferulic, vanillic, and ϱ-coumaric acids [20], which show a strong antioxidant power and may help to protect oxidative stress thus decreasing the risk of contracting several diseases [23,24]. Whole grains including wheat, contains several essential compounds that impact on the oxidative stability of cells. These compounds include selenium, β-carotene, vitamins C and E, phytate, proteins, polysaccharides, phenolics, lignans and tocopherols [20]. Phytic acid can protect tissues against oxidative reactions through its ability to sequester and inactivate pro-oxidative transition metals [25,20]. In addition, acid conditions and enzymic hydrolysis has been reported to increase the solubility and activity of wheat phenolics, suggesting that the digestive process could be important in altering the antioxidant potential of wheat-based foods [20]. Simulated gastrointestinal pH treatment and enzymatic hydrolysis also increase the antioxidant activity of wheat and wheat-based breakfast cereal extracts, suggesting that the digestive process could be important in further enhancing the antioxidant potential of wheat-based foods [20]. However, it is still unclear if the consumption of cereal causes better health or whether it is a case of health status influencing food choice [26,27,23].

Processed products from cereals contain different antioxidant contents at varying amounts (Table 2). The cereals containing most antioxidants include barley, millet, maize and oats. Notably, polished rice and refined wheat, which are the main cereals eaten by humans globally are among the cereals with the lowest content of antioxidants [28]. In contrast, common millet and sorghum, which are important in particular regions in sub-Saharan Africa, South America and Asia, contains medium to high concentrations of antioxidants. The predominant types of antioxidants in corn are ferulic acid, anthocyanins, catechin and ϱ-caomaric acid. Wheat is high in β-glucan, β-cryptoxanthin, catechins, lutein, zeaxanthin and phytosterols. Barley is rich in tocopherols, tocotrienols and ferulic acids. Millet is high in tricin, luteolin and serotonin, whilst buckwheat contains rutin and catechins. Oats and rice are rich in avertramidin, catechins, proanthocyanidins and anthocyanins [3].

In the case of whole grains, corn, wheat, rice and oats are regarded as grains with high antioxidant activities. Corn has the highest total antioxidant activity compared to the other three grain types, followed by wheat and then oats. Rice has the lowest antioxidant activity compared to corn, wheat and oats [29]. Corn shows the highest total phenolic content at 1560 ± 60 μmol gallic acid equivalents/100 g, followed by wheat at 800 ± 40 μmol gallic acid equivalents/100 g, oats at 650 ± 20 μmol gallic acid equivalents/100 g and rice at 560 ± 20 μmol gallic acid equivalents/100 g. A study designed to investigate the complete phytochemical profiles in free, soluble conjugated, and insoluble bound forms, as well as their antioxidant activities in uncooked whole grains [30] showed that corn had the highest total antioxidant activity (181.42 ± 0.86 μmol of vitamin C equivalent/g of grain), followed by wheat (76.70 ± 1.38 μmol of vitamin C equivalent/g of grain), oats (74.67 ± 1.49 μmol of vitamin C equivalent/g of grain), and rice (55.77 ± 1.62 μmol of vitamin C equivalent/g of grain). Bound phytochemicals were the major contributors to the total antioxidant activity; 90% in wheat, 87% in corn, 71% in rice and 58% in oats. Bound phytochemicals can survive stomach and intestinal digestion to reach the colon. This may partly explain the mechanism of grain consumption in the prevention of colon cancer, other digestive cancers, breast cancer and prostate cancer as supported by epidemiological studies. Antioxidant activity of methanolic extracts from some grains consumed in Korea [31] revealed that the methanolic extracts prepared from red sorghum and black rice showed significantly higher antioxidant activities and contained higher polyphenolic contents than other grains such as white rice, brown rice, mungbean, foxtail millet, prosomillet, barley and adlay. Polyphenolic compounds were found to be the major naturally occurring antioxidants in grains. Antioxidant activity of small grain cereals

Cereals	Botanical name	Family	Amount present in cereals mmol/100 g
Barley, whole meal flour	*Hordeum vulgare*	*Poaceae*	1.09
Common millet, wholemeal flour	*Pennisetum glaucum*	*Poaceae*	0.82
Maize, white flour	*Zea mays*	*Poaceae*	0.62
Oats, rough oatmeal	*Avena sativa*	*Poaceae*	0.59
Barley, white flour	*Hordeum vulgare*	*Poaceae*	0.58
Rye, wholemeal flour	*Secale cereal*	*Poaceae*	0.47
Wheat, wholemeal flour	*Triticum aestivum*	*Poaceae*	0.33
Oats, white flour	*Avena sativa*	*Poaceae*	0.32
Bulgur wheat, wholemeal flour	*Triticum aestivum*	*Poaceae*	0.31
Sorghum, wholemeal flour	*Sorgum bicolor*	*Poaceae*	0.30
Common millet, white flour	*Pennisetum glaucum*	*Poaceae*	0.25
Rye, white flour	*Secale cereal*	*Poaceae*	0.23
Rice, grains	*Oryza sativa*	*Poaceae*	0.17
Wheat, white flour	*Triticum aestivum*	*Poaceae*	0.13
Durum wheat, white flour	*Triticum durum*	*Poaceae*	0.05
Rice, white flour	*Oryza sativa*	*Poaceae*	0.04
Pseudo-cereals			
Buckwheat, wholemeal flour	*Fagopyrum esculentum*	*Polygonaceae*	1.99
Buckwheat, white flour	*Fagopyrum esculentum*	*Polygonaceae*	1.23

Adapted from [28].

Table 2. Total antioxidant concentration of cereals.

caused by phenolics and lipid soluble antioxidants as investigated in [32] showed a general considerable variation in antioxidant activities and phytochemical contents between cereals. A higher DPPH radical scavenging ability and reducing power were detected in hull-less barley, followed by rye and hull-less oat and durum and bread wheat, indicating that small grain species have different major antioxidants with different properties. Hull-less barley was found to have the highest content of total free phenols, flavonoids, PVPP bound phenolics and contained flavan-3-ols, not found in other species. Hull-less oat had the highest content of tocopherols, very high content of yellow pigments and PVPP bound phenolics. Ferulic acid was the major free phenolic acid in small grain cereals tested. A study designed to determine the composition in hydroxycinnamic acids and the antioxidant properties of soluble extracts from wheat, rye and buckwheat [33] revealed that the highest levels of total hydroxycinnamic acids and derivatives were found in the wheat bran and rye bran fractions whereas the buckwheat flours had only trace quantities of these compounds. The most abundant com-

http://dx.doi.org/10.5772/57169

Grains	Tocopherols				Tocotrienols			
	α	β	γ	δ	α	β	γ	δ
Wheat	10	7	NA	NA	4	28	NA	NA
Rye	16	4	NA	NA	15	8	NA	NA
Barley	8.6	0.9	5.6	0.7	40.3	8.7	10.4	0.9
Oats	14.9	3.0	0.4	NA	56.4	5.4	NA	NA
Maize	3.7	0.2	45.0	1.0	5.3	NA	11.3	0.4
Rice	14.6	1.0	1.3	0.1	8.7	NA	11.9	0.5

NA = not available. Source: [35-37].

Table 3. Vitamin E content of whole grains flour mg/kg dry matter

pound present in the wheat and rye fractions was ferulic acid but small quantities of diferulic acids, sinapic acid, ϱ-coumaric acid and benzoic acid derivatives were also present. The largest proportions of these phenolic compounds were found as covalently bound (esters) in the insoluble pellet but between 10% and 30% of the total compounds were solubilized, mostly in water. Most of the antioxidant capacity was found in the water extracts from all the cereal fractions. Overall, buckwheat and wheat germ products exhibited the highest antioxidant capacity whereas the rye products had the lowest antioxidant values, an indication that the consumption of buckwheat and wheat germ could be an important source of antioxidants required for healthy living.

The phytochemical content and antioxidant activity of six diverse varieties of whole wheat as reported in [34] showed free phenolic content ranging from 255 (KanQueen) to 499 (Roane) 1mol gallic acid equivalents/100 g DW. The bound phenolic content ranged from 582 (Roane) to 662 (Cham1) 1mol gallic acid equivalents/100 g DW. The bound fraction contributed 53.8 - 69.7% of the total phenolic content of the wheat varieties analysed. Ferulic acid was the predominant phenolic acid found in whole wheat. Total ferulic acid content ranged from 310.8 (Caledonia) to 496.1 (KanQueen) 1mol ferulic acid/100 g DW. The percentage of ferulic acid found in the insoluble-bound fraction ranged from 87.4% (Caledonia) to 97.2% (KanQueen). Other phenolic acids, ϱ-coumaric acid, syringic acid, vanillic acid, and caffeic acid were also detected. Lutein was the predominant carotenoid found in the whole wheat varieties analysed. Zeaxanthin, β-carotene, and β-cryptoxanthin were also detected. Mainly α- and β-tocopherols and α- and β-tocotrienols were found in all varieties of whole wheat though δ-tocopherol was detected in all but two varieties. β-tocotrienol was the predominant form of vitamin E found in all varieties of whole wheat (Table 3). The antioxidant activity was assessed using the oxygen radical absorbance capacity (ORAC) assay. The ORAC of the free fraction ranged from 1958 to 3749 1mol Trolox equivalents/100 g DW. The ORAC of the bound fraction ranged from 3190 to 5945 1mol Trolox equivalents/100 g DW. Total phenolic content correlated with oxygen radical absorbance capacity ($R^2 = 0.810$; $p < 0.001$). They concluded that phytochemicals found in whole grains may be responsible for the health benefit derived from whole grain consumption.

Rice is rich in phytochemicals that are present in lipophilic, hydrophilic and insoluble forms. In reference [38], it was indicated that tocopherols, tocotrienols (Figure 4) and γ-oryzanol, are major lipophilic fractions of whole grain rice and are beneficial to human health. It also contains tricin, ferulic acid, caffeic acid and methoxycinnamic acid which are hydrophilic phenolic compounds reported to have cancer protective potential. Barley grains contain DFs, β-glucans, arabinoxylans and polyphenols [39,40]. β-glucans and arabinoxylans present in barley are critical nutrients that determine wort viscosity, foam stability and beer filtration rates, thus playing a significant role in beer brewing process [41,42]. Barley β-glucans also plays health beneficial roles in the reduction of blood cholesterol level, glucose level and helps in weight loss by increasing satiety, thereby reducing susceptibility to heart disease and type-2 diabetes [40]. Oats and psyllium husk which contains fibres have also been implicated in the reduction of homocysteine, cholesterol and risk of CVD [43]. Millets are rich source of DF, phytochemicals, micronutrients, nutraceuticals, and could be rightly termed as nutricereals.

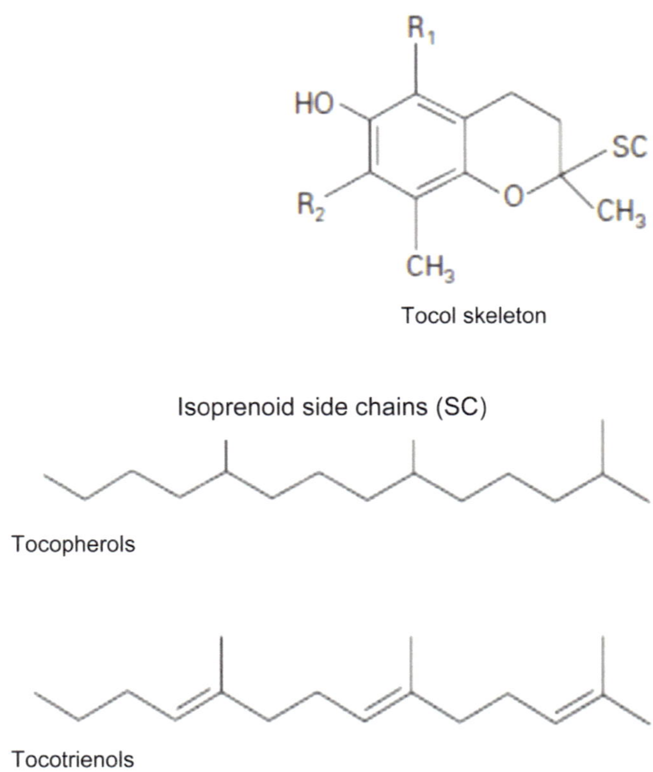

α-Tocopherol $R_1 = R_2 = CH_3$
β-Tocopherol $R_1 = CH_3$; $R_2 = H$
γ-Tocopherol $R_1 = H$; $R_2 = CH_3$
δ-Tocopherol $R_1 = R_2 = H$

Figure 4. Tocopherols and tocotrienols in grains

3. Grains and human health

Dietary antioxidants are food compounds that impede the deleterious effects of reactive oxygen species, reactive nitrogen species, or both, on the normal physiological function in humans [44,27]. Dietary antioxidants include ascorbate, tocopherols, carotenoids and bioactive plant phenols. ROS; oxygen ions, free radicals, and peroxides and reactive nitrogen species (RNS); nitrous anhydride, peroxynitrite, and nitrogen dioxide radicals, causes oxidation, nitration, halogenation and deamination of biomolecules of all types, including lipids, proteins, carbohydrates, and nucleic acids, with the resultant formation of toxic and mutagenic products [45,46]. Biological systems control these oxidative factors by a variety of antioxidative mechanisms that restrict the reactivity of ROS and RNS and oxidation catalysts [20]. In human cells, *de novo* antioxidant production is much more limited and oxidative damage resulting from excess production of free radicals has been reported to initiate the pathogenesis of most chronic degenerative diseases such as brain stroke, diabetes mellitus, rheumatoid arthritis, Parkinson's disease, Alzheimer's disease, and cancer [27,28]. The production of ROS and RNS are speedily formed in cells as a consequence of disease processes (e.g. inflammation), tobacco smoke, environmental pollutants, ingestion of oxidized foods, ischemia, drugs, ethanol and radiations. If unchecked, such cellular event can promote a chain of chemical reactions that form free radicals, peroxides and secondary oxidation breakdown products which in turn reacts with and cause damage to cellular membranes, proteins and nucleic acids [20,23].

Phenolic compounds present in whole grains are known to be effective in protecting against CVDs and some cancer (Table 4). This protective effect is thought to be mediated through their action as antioxidants to prevent oxidative damage induced by ROS to some biomolecules (DNA, lipids and proteins) under pathological conditions [47]. In reference [48], it was reported that phenolic compounds could be responsible for chelating metals as well as inhibiting the free radicals capitation by limiting the action of the lipoxygenase enzyme. Phytate compounds on the other hand may exert antioxidant activity by complexing with iron, reducing the formation of free radicals and peroxidation of membranes, which could provide anticarcinogenic power. Lignans on their part are a group of dietary phytoestrogen found in a variety of plant foods like corn, oats, rye, wheat, flaxseeds, legumes, fruits and vegetables. These plant lignans when consumed are converted to the mammalian lignans, enterodiol and enterolactone which have strong antioxidant activity. β-glucan is mostly found in cell walls of oats, barley and wheat. Its major biological effects include lowering of blood cholesterol level, controlling blood sugar, promotion of weight management, encouraging the growth of beneficial gut microflora and enhancing the immune system. This is probably due to its high viscosity property as a soluble fibre to bind cholesterol and bile acids and facilitate their elimination from the body. It has been [93] indicated that β-glucan had an effect in controlling blood sugar in diabetes subjects, and was helpful in reducing the elevation in blood sugar levels after a meal. The authors further indicated that this is probably as a result of delaying gastric emptying, allowing dietary sugar to be absorbed more gradually, as well as by possibly increasing the tissue sensitivity to insulin. The United States Food and Drug Administration (FDA) is allowing whole grain barley products that can supply β-glucan at levels of 0.75 g per serving or 3 g per day to carry a claim that they reduce the risk of coronary heart disease [49].

Compounds	Cereals/Parts Found	Method of Determination	Effects on Humans	References
Vitamins (Tocopherols and tocotrienols)	Germ of all cereal grains.	HPLC	Induction of immune responses; lowering of cholesterol levels; defence against oxidative stress; antimutagenic and anticancer.	[50,51,52]
Phytosterols (Sitosterol, campesterol, stigmasterol, brassicasterol)	Aleurone, pericap and germ of rice, wheat, rye, oat and barley.	Gas chromatography analysis	Prevent CVDs.	[53,54,55]
Phenolics (Lignans, phenolic acids, alkylresorcinols, avenathramide, coumarins)	Bran layer of most cereals e.g. barley, sorghum, rice, rye, wheat, millet and oat.	HPLC, GC-MS	Believed to have anticancer activity; prevent oxidative stress, cholesterolemia, atherosclerosis and aging; anti-inflammatory and anti-irritant.	[56,57,52,58]
Carotenoids	Yellow endosperm of durum wheat.	UV/Vis spectrometry, HPLC and MS spectrometry	Prevent cataracts, age-related muscular degeneration, cancer and cardiovascular disease.	[59,52,60]
Flavonoids (anthocyanidins, flavonols, flavanones)	Yellow lemon sorghum, aleurone of blue and red coloured maize.	UV/Vis spectrometry, HPLC, mass spectrometry	Inhibitory effects on cancer, anti-inflammatory properties, reduce glycemia, combats complications of diabetes.	[61,52,62,63]
Phytate (Inositol hexaphosphate)	Aleurone layer and scutellum cells of germ of most cereals.	HPLC, HPIC	Gene regulation, anti-inflammatory, prevents complications of diabetes, antineoplastic in breast, colon and liver.	[64,65,66]

Table 4. Antioxidant compounds in cereals, human effects and methods of determination

According to [67], these antioxidant compounds may offer protection against heart disease, hormone-related breast and prostate cancers. Enterodiol and enterolactone inhibited colon cancer cell growth, induced cell cycle and apoptosis *in vitro* [68]. In a study conducted among post-menopausal women diagnosed with heart conditions, whole grains was associated with a slower build-up of artery-narrowing plaque among the post-menopausal women and in lowering the overall risk of mortality associated to CVDs [69,70]. Whole grains were also implicated in a 66% reduction in cancer in a study conducted in over 2000 people fed with a high-fibre whole grain diet [71]. Available epidemiological evidence suggests that sorghum consumption reduces the risk of certain types of cancer in humans compared to other cereals [19]. Positive effects of sorghum and/or millet consumption on cancer have been documented. Sorghum consumption consistently correlated with low incidence of oesophageal cancer [72] in various parts of the world (including several parts of Africa, Russia, India, China and Iran) whereas wheat and corn consumption correlated with elevated incidence [19]. Sorghum containing tannins are widely reported to reduce caloric availability and hence weight gain in animals. However, with obesity as a major and ever-increasing problem in the developed world (with more than 60% of Americans reported to be overweight), this attribute of sorghum tannins has the potential of mitigating the problem [19]. Although information on how sorghum phytochemicals affect human health is limited, overall epidemiological studies suggest that sorghum possesses anti-carcinogenic properties when consumed regularly in the diet.

Whole grains, oilseeds, nuts and legumes are rich in sterols and stanols. In humans, high intake of sterols or stanols is associated with lowering of serum and LDL cholesterol concentrations. Phytosterols compete with cholesterol for micelle formation in the intestinal lumen and inhibits cholesterol absorption [73],. Whole grains are good sources of health beneficial phytochemicals. These phytochemicals are in free soluble-conjugated and bound forms [74]. Most of them are bound to the cell wall materials and insoluble. This makes it difficult for these phytochemicals to be released during the upper gastrointestinal tract digestion. As a result of this, colonic digestion of such materials by microflora results in the release of the bulk of bound phytochemicals to exert their health benefits. Hence, the reduced risk of colon cancer associated with increased consumption of whole grain products. Higher beans consumption apart from being associated with reduced risk of diabetes and obesity, is inversely associated with prostate, breast and colon cancers [10]. This is due to the presence of elements which are able to retard the glycemic response, slowing the release of glucose into the blood [75]. This antioxidant and anticarcinogenic effect of beans has been attributed to the presence of phenolic and phytate acids, which were previously regarded as unwanted compounds with antinutritional factors.

Consuming whole grains and their products regularly is associated with risk reduction of developing chronic diseases such as CVDs, type 2 diabetes and some cancers. Therefore, dietary modification by increasing the consumption of wide variety of fruits, vegetables and whole grains daily is a practical strategy for consumers to optimize their health and reduce the risk of chronic diseases [76].

4. Fortified antioxidant grain-based products

Cereal extruded products are mainly composed of starches, and or vegetable proteins. The role of these constituents is mainly to impart structure, texture, bulk, mouth feel and other desired characteristics for finished products [77]. Infant cereals are one of the most common weaning foods. However, these foods in their natural form may lack some vital infant nutritional requirements for proper growth. The nutritional quality of raw cereal based infant products is low, hence they have to be processed (fortified) to improve their overall nutritional quality [78].

5. Novel antioxidant grain-based products

A novel way of consuming grain products is the consumption of functional foods. Functional here refers to foods that provide other health benefits to the body apart from those derived from its nutrients. Eating whole grain meals and functional food products will therefore enhance the nutritional intake derived from whole grain related diets [79].

6. Global policies affecting antioxidant-rich grain production

Recent dramatic increases in food prices are having severe consequences for poor countries and their populace. The Food and Agriculture Organization (FAO) of the United Nations, reports that food prices rose by nearly 40% in 2007 and made further large jumps in early 2008. Nearly all agricultural commodities including rice, maize, wheat, meat, dairy products, soybeans, palm oil, and cassava are affected. In response to the price hikes, food riots have occurred in many developing countries, including Burkina Faso, Cameroon, Côte d'Ivoire, Egypt, Haiti, Indonesia, Senegal, and Somalia. According to the FAO, 37 countries are now facing food crises [80].

7. Future research on natural antioxidant-rich grains

Many investigations continue to establish the protective cancer-preventive and healthful compounds in cereal grains [81-83,12]. In [84], it was reported that many epidemiological studies suggested that consumption of whole grain cereal is highly correlated to reduced incidences of chronic diseases. Experimental and epidemiological studies have shown that consumption of grains, lower the incidence of aging diseases, as well as other non-communicable diseases such as colorectal cancer, hypertension, stroke and heart diseases [85-87]. There is strong epidemiological evidence that whole-grain cereals protect the body against age-related diseases such as diabetes, CVDs and some cancers. This may be due to the fibre and micronutrients in the outer layer and germ fractions of the grain acting together to combat oxidative stress, inflammation, hyperglycaemia and carcinogenesis. It has been shown that the whole wheat flours of different wheat varieties contain significant amounts of phenolic antioxidants and dietary fibres). Cereal bran fibres, good for colon health, show good potential for high incorporation into extruded foods [88]. Sorghum phytochemicals have been shown to have potential impact on human [19]. There is now evidence that the consumption of whole grains and whole-grain products is implicated in the prevention of cancer and other chronic diseases [83]. Studies have shown that plant food material with polyphenolic constituents have more potent antioxidant

http://dx.doi.org/10.5772/57169

and anti-inflammatory activities. In many epidemiologic studies, an inverse association between high cereal intake and low cancer incidence has been observed [83,11].

Future research in antioxidant rich grains may address regional health issues. In Africa, future research on antioxidant- rich foods can also be directed to address nutritional issues. It was suggested that while corn starch provides all the features for production of highly acceptable extruded snack foods its nutritional value is far from satisfying the needs of health conscience consumers [78]. In the US, future prospective studies may address the question of whether whole grain intake is directly related to body weight and obesity and whether the associations are primarily driven by fiber, other dietary component of whole-grain foods, or some other related aspect of the diet [89].

Epidemiological studies have shown that the consumption of whole grain cereal foods reduces the risk of chronic diseases linked with metabolic syndrome, such as CVD and diabetes. Aggressive and consistent consumer education needs to be put in place by the government or relevant agencies to educate consumers on the health benefits of cereal foods especially in the developing countries where the level of ignorance is high and literacy is low. Furthermore, food scientists and engineers, nutritionists and consumer scientists should look into developing more varieties of appealing cereal based products from the already identified cereal grains rich in antioxidants and bioactive components. More clinical trials are required to strengthen the proposed link between the phenolic compounds found in rice and chronic disease prevention. Research is needed to evaluate the effects of both hydrophilic and lipophilic antioxidants on their antioxidant capacity. Clinical trials that ascertain the phytochemicals found in whole grains may be responsible for the health benefit derived from whole grain consumption.

8. Conclusion

The beneficial effects associated with whole grain consumption are in part due to the existence of the unique phytochemicals of whole grains [9]. Based on the epidemiological data, consumption of whole wheat grain has been recommended to improve insulin sensitivity and to lower serum insulin concentration [90,91].

Author details

Afam I.O. Jideani*, Henry Silungwe, Thakhani Takalani, Tonna A. Anyasi, Henry Udeh and Adewale Omolola

*Address all correspondence to: afam.jideani@univen.ac.za

Department of Food Science and Technology, School of Agriculture, University of Venda, Thohoyandou, South Africa

References

[1] Schmitz K, Marquart L. Labeling and regulatory issues related to functional cereal products. In: Hamaker BR. (ed.) Technology of functional cereal products. Cambridge: Woodhead publishing; 2008. p34.

[2] Espin JC, Garcia-Conesa MT, Tomas-Barberan FA. Nutraceuticals: Facts and fiction. Phytochemistry 2007;68, 2986-3008.

[3] Liu RH. Whole grain phytochemicals and health. Journal of Cereal Science 2007;46, 207-219.

[4] Slavin JL. Mechanisms for the impact of whole grain foods on cancer risk. Journal of the American College of Nutrition 2000;19, 300S-307S.

[5] Collar C. Novel high-fibre and whole grain breads. In: Hamaker BR. (ed.) Technology of functional cereal products. Cambridge: Woodhead publishing; 2008. p186.

[6] Rajasekaran A, Sivagnanam G, Xavier R. Nutraceuticals as therapeutic agents: a review. Research Journal in Pharmacy and Technology 2008;1(4) 328-340.

[7] Kasum CM, Jacobs DRJ, Nicodemus K, Folson AR. Dietary risk factors for upper aerodigestive tract cancers. International Journal of Cancer 2002;99, 267-272.

[8] Danish Food Composition Databank. http://www.foodcomp.dk/fcdb_search.asp. (accessed 1 August 2013).

[9] Ragaee S, Abdel-Aal EM, Noaman M. Antioxidant activity and nutrient composition of selected cereals for food use. Food Chemistry 2006;98, 32-38.

[10] Madhujith T, Shahidi F. Antioxidative and antiproliferative properties of selected barley (*Hordeum vulgare* L.) cultivars and their potential for inhibition of low-density lipoprotein (LDL) cholesterol oxidation. Journal of Agricultural and Food Chemistry 2007;55, 5018-5024.

[11] Shewry PR The health grain programme opens new opportunities for improving wheat for nutrition and health. Nutrition Bulletin 2009a;34, 225-231.

[12] Jideani IA. *Digitaria exilis* (acha/fonio), *Digitaria iburua* (iburu/fonio) and *Eluesine coracana* (tamba/finger millet) – Non-conventional cereal grains with potentials. Scientific Research and Essays 2012;7(45): 3834-3843. http://www.academicjournals.org/SRE DOI: 10.5897/SRE12.416 (accessed 20 June 2013).

[13] Aoe S. Nutritional and physiological effects of dietary fiber in oats and barley. Japanese Journal of Nutrition and Dietetics 2008;66, 311-319.

[14] Revanappa SB, Salimath PV. Phenolic acid profiles and antioxidant activities of different wheat (*Triticum aestivum* L.) varieties. Journal of Food Biochemistry 2010;35(3): 759-779.

[15] Sidhu JS, Kabir Y. Functional foods from cereal grains. International Journal of Food Properties 2007;10, 231-244.

[16] Sun T, Ho C. Total phenolic content and antioxidant activity of cereals. In: Shibamoto T, Kanazawa K, Ho C. (ed.) Functional food and healthy, ACS symposium series 993. Washington, DC: American Chemical Society; 2008. p143-150.

[17] Mazza G. Anthocyanins and heart health. Ann 1st Super Sanita 2007;43, 369-374.

[18] Kamran M, Saleem N, Umer ZN. Ready-to-eat (RTE) wheat bran breakfast cereal as a high-fibre diet. Journal of Food Processing and Preservation 2008;32, 853-867.

[19] Awika JM, Rooney LW. Sorghum phytochemicals and potential impact on human health. Phytochemistry 2004;65, 199-1221.

[20] Baublis AJ, Lu C, Clydesdale FM, Decker EA. Potential of wheat-based breakfast cereals as a source of dietary antioxidant. Journal of the American College of Nutrition 2000;19(3) 308S-311S.

[21] Dordevic TM, Siler-Marinkovic SS, Dimitrijevic-Brankovic SI. Effect of fermentation on antioxidant properties of some cereals and pseudo cereals. Food Chemistry 2010;119, 957-963.

[22] Sreeramulu D, Reedy CVK, Raghunath M Antioxidant activity of commonly consumed cereals, millets, pulses and legumes in India. Indian Journal of Biochemistry and Biophysics 2009;46, 112-115.

[23] Alvarez P, Alvarado C, Mathieu F, Jimenez L, De La Fuente M. Diet supplementation for five weeks with polyphenol-rich cereals improves several functions and the redox state of mouse leucocytes. British Journal of Nutrition 2006;45, 428-438.

[24] Hamid AA, Aiyelaagbe OO, Usman LA, Ameen OM, Lawal A. Antioxidants: Its medicinal and pharmacological applications – review. African Journal of Pure and Applied Chemistry 2010;4(8) 142-151.

[25] Graf E, Eaton JW. Antioxidant functions of phytic acid. Free Radical Biology and Medicine 1990;8, 61-69.

[26] Smith AP. Breakfast cereal consumption and subjective reports of health. International Journal of Food Sciences and Nutrition 1999c;50, 445-449.

[27] Dimitrios B. Sources of natural phenolic antioxidants – review. Trends in Food Science and Technology 2006;17, 505-512.

[28] Halvorsen BL, Holte K, Myhrstad MCW, Barikmo I, Hvattum E, Remberg SF, Anne-Brit Wold A-B, Haffner K, Baugerød H, Andersen LF, Moskaug JO, Jacobs DR Jr, Blomhoff R. A Systematic Screening of Total Antioxidants in Dietary Plants. The Journal of Nutrition 2002;132, 461-471

[29] Adom KK, Sorrels ME, Liu RH. Phytochemicals and antioxidant activity of milled fractions of different wheat varieties. Journal of Agricultural and Food Chemistry 2005;53, 2297-2306.

[30] Adom KK, Liu RH. Antioxidants activity of grains. Journal of Agricultural and Food Chemistry 2002;50, 6182-6187.

[31] Choi Y, Jeong HS, Lee JS. Antioxidant activity of methanolic extracts from some grains consumed in Korea. Food Chemistry 2007;103, 130-138.

[32] Zilica SC, Zita VH, Sukalovic S, Dodiga D, Maksimovi V, Maksimovi M, Basi Z. Antioxidant activity of small grain cereals caused by phenolics and lipid soluble antioxidants. Journal of Cereal Science 2011;54, 417-424.

[33] Gallardo C, Jimenez L, Garcıa-Conesa M-T. Hydroxycinnamic acid composition and in vitro antioxidant activity of selected grain fractions. Food Chemistry 2006;99, 455-463.

[34] Okarter N, Liu CS, Sorrells ME, Liu RH. Phytochemical content and antioxidant activity of six diverse varieties of whole wheat. Food Chemistry 2010;119, 249-257.

[35] Bramley PM, Elmadfa I, Kafatos A, Kelly FJ, Manios Y, Roxborough HE, Schuch W, Sheehy PJA, Wagner K-H. Vitamin E. Journal of the Science of Food and Agriculture 2000;80, 913-938.

[36] Panfili G, Fratianni A, Irano M. Normal phase high performance liquid chromatography method for the determination of tocopherols and tocotrienols in cereals. Journal of Agricultural and Food Chemistry 2003;51, 3940-3944.

[37] Ha T-Y, Ko S-N, Lee S-M, Kim H-R, Chung S-H, Kim S-R, Yoon H-H, Kim I-H. Changes in nutraceutical lipid components of rice at different degrees of milling. European Journal of Lipid Science and Technology 2006;108, 175-181.

[38] Cicero AFG, Gaddi A. Rice bran oil and γ-oryzanol in the treatment of hyperlipoproteinemias and other conditions. Phytotherapy Research 2001;15, 277-289.

[39] Quinde Z, Ullrich SE, Baik BK. Genotypic variation in colour and discolouration potential of barley-based food products. Cereal Chemistry 2004;81, 752-758.

[40] Baik B, Ullrich SE. Barley for food: Characteristics, improvement and renewed interest. Journal of Cereal Science 2008;48, 233-242.

[41] Stewart DC, Freeman G, Evans DE. Development and assessment of a small-scale wort filtration test for the prediction of beer filtration efficiency. Journal of the Institue of Brewing 2000;106, 361-366.

[42] Lusk LT, Duncombe GR, Kay SB, Navarro A, Ryder D. Barley-glucan and beer foam stability. Journal of the American Society of Brewing Chemists 2001;59, 183-186.

[43] Thompkinson DK, Bhavana V, Kanika P. Dietary approaches for management of cardiovascular health – a review. Journal of Food Science and Technology 2012; DOI 10.1007/s13197-012-0661-8.

[44] SEDRI. Dietary Reference intakes: proposed definition and plan for review of dietary antioxidants and related compounds. Standing Committee on the Scientific Evaluation of Dietary Reference Intakes Washington, DC: National Academic Press; 1998. p. 24.

[45] Petal RP, McAndrew J, Sellak H, White CR, Jo H, Freeman BA, Darley-Usmar VM. Biological aspects of reactive nitrogen species. Biochemical and Biophysical ACTA 1999;1411(2-3) 385-400.

[46] Castrol L, Freeman BA. Reactive oxygen species in human health and disease. Nutrition 2001;17(2) 161-165.

[47] Yao LH, Jiang YM, Shi J, Tomas,-Barneran FA, Datta N, Singanusong R, Chen SS. Flavonoids in food and their health benefits. Plant Foods Human Nutrition 2004;59, 113-122.

[48] Martinez DB, Ibanez GV, Rincon LF. Acido fitico: aspectos nutriocionales e implicaciones analiticas. Archivos Latinoamericanos de Nutricion 2002;52, 219-231.

[49] Food and Drug Administration. FDA allows barley productsto claim reduction in risk of coronary heart disease. FDA news release (December 23). http://origin.www.fda.gov/bbs/topics/news/2005/NEW01287.html (accessed June 28 2013).

[50] Nasaretnam K, Yew WW, Wahid MB. Tocotrienols and cancer: beyond antioxidant activity. European Journal of Lipid Science and Technology 2007;109, 445-452.

[51] Peterson DM, Jenson CM, Hoffman DL, Mannerstedt-Fogelfors B. Oat tocols: saponification vs. direct extraction and analysis in high oil genotypes. Cereal Chemistry 2007;84, 56-60.

[52] Serna-Saldivar SO. Cereal grains; properties, processing and nutritional attributes. Boca Raton, Florida: CRC Press; 2010. p607-609

[53] Lampi A, Piironen V, Toivo J. Analysis of phytosterols in foods. In: Dutta, P.C Phytosterols as Functional Food Components and Nutraceuticals. New York: Marcel Decker Inc; 2004. p33-73.

[54] Nurmi T, Nystrom L, Edelmann M, Lampi A, Piironen V. Phytosterols in wheat varieties in the HEALTHGRAIN diversity screen. Journal of Agricultural and Food Chemistry 2008;56, 9710-9715.

[55] Nystrom L, Paasonen A, Lampi A, Piironen V. Total plant sterols, steryl ferulates and steryl glycosides in milling fractions of wheat and rye. Journal of Cereal Science 2008;45, 106-115.

[56] Li L, Shewry PR, Ward JL. Phenolics acids in wheat varieties the HEALTHGRAIN diversity screen. Journal of Agricultural and Food Chemistry 2008;56, 9732-9739.

[57] Milder IE, Arts ICW, Venema DP, lasaroms JJP, Wahala K, Hollman PCH. Optimization of a liquid chromatography-tandem mass spectrometry method for quantification of plant lignans seciosolariciresinol, matairesinol, lariciresinol and pinoresinol in foods. Journal of Agricultural and Food Chemistry 2004;52, 4643-4651.

[58] Slanin A, Glatz Z. Separation procedures applicable to lignin analysis. Journal of Chromatography Biology 2004;812, 215-229.

[59] Olmedilla B, Granado F, Blanco I, Vaquero M, Cajigal C. Lutein in patients with cataracts and age related macular degeneration: a long term supplementary study. Journal of Science Food and Agriculture 2001;81, 904-909.

[60] Abdel-Aal E-SM, Akhtar MH. Recent advances in analyses of carotenoids and their role in human health. Current Pharmaceutical Analyses 2006;2, 195-204.

[61] Mazza G, Cacace JE, Kay CD. Methods of analysis for anthocyanins in plant and biological fluids. Journal of AOAC International 2004;87, 129-145.

[62] Yawadio R, Tanimori S, Morita N. Identification of phenolic compounds isolated from pigmented rices and their aldose reductase inhibitory activities. Food Chemistry 2007;101, 1616-1625.

[63] Tsuda T, Horio F, Uchida K, Aoki H,Osawa T. Dietary cyaniding 3-0-β-D-glucoside-rich purple corn colour prevents obesity and ameliorates hyperglycemia. Journal of Nutrition 2003;133, 2125-2130.

[64] Chen QC, Li BW. Separation of phytic acid and other related inositol phosphates by high perfomance ion chromatography and its application. Journal of Chromatography Analyses 2003;1018, 41-52.

[65] Claxon A, Morris C, Blake D, Siren M, Halliwell B, Gustaffson T, Lofkvist B, Bergelin I. The anti-inflammatory effects of D-myo-inositol-1,2,6-trisphosphate (PP56) on animal models of inflammation. Agents Actions 1990; 29, 68-70.

[66] York JD. Regulation of nuclear processes by inositol polyphosphates. Acta Molecular and Cell Biology of Lipids 2006;1761, 552-559.

[67] Johansen NF, Hausner H, Olsen A, Tetens I, Christensen J, Knudsen KE, Overvad K, Tjonneland A. Intake of whole grains and vegetables determines the plasma enterlactone concentration of Danish women. Journal of Nutrition 2004;134, 2691-2697.

[68] Qu H, Madl RL, Takemoto DJ, Baybutt RC, Wang W. Lignans are involved in the antitumor activity of wheat bran in colon cancer SW480 cells. Journal of Nutrition 2005;135, 598-602.

[69] Erkkila AT, Herrington DM, Mozaffarian D, Lichtenstein AH. Cereal fibre and whole-grain intake are associated with reduced progression of coronary-artery athe-

rosclerosis in postmenopausal women with coronary artery disease. American Heart Journal 2005;150(1) 94-101.

[70] Sahyoun NR, Jacques PF, Zhang XL, Juan W, McKeown NM. Whole-grain intake is inversely associated with the metabolic syndrome and mortality in older adults. American Journal of Clinical Nutrition 2006;83(1) 124-133.

[71] Slattery ML, Curtin KP, Edwards SL, Schaffer DM. Plant foods, fibre, and rectal cancer. American Journal of Clinical Nutrition 2004;79(2) 274-281.

[72] Van Rensburg SJ. Epidemiological and dietary evidence for a specific nutritional predisposition to esophageal cancer. Journal of the National Cancer Institute 1981;67, 243-251.

[73] Nissinen M, Gylling H, Vuoristo M, Miettinen TA. Micellar distribution of cholesterol and phytosterols after duodenal plant stanol ester infusion. American Journal of Physiology Gastrointestinal and Liver Physiology 2002;282, G1009-G1015.

[74] Adom KK, Sorrels ME, Liu RH. Phytochemical profiles and antioxidant activity of wheat varieties. Journal of agricultural and food Chemistry 2003;51, 7825-7834.

[75] Valdes ST, Coelho CMM, Michelluti DJ, Tramonte VLCG. Association of genotype and preparation methods on the antioxidant activity and antinutrients in common beans (*Phaseolus vulgaris* L.). Journal of Food Science and Technology 2011;44, 2104-2111.

[76] Rautenbach F, Venter I. Hydrophilic and lipophilic antioxidant capacity of commonly consumed South African fruits, vegetables, grains, legumes, fats/oils and beverages. Journal of Food Composition and Analysis 2010;23, 753-761.

[77] Anton AA, Fulcher RG, Arnfield SDPhysical and nutrition impact of fortification of corn starch-based extruded snacks with common bean (*Phaseoulus vulgaris* L.) flour: Effect of bean addition and extrusion cooking. Food chemistry 2009;113, 989-996.

[78] Li W, Friel J, Beta T. An evaluation of the antioxidant properties and aroma quality of infant cereals. Food chemistry 2010;121, 1095-1102.

[79] Dean M, Raats MM, Shepherd R. Consumers and functional cereal products. In: Hamaker BR. (ed.) Technology of functional cereal products. Cambridge, UK: Woodhead publishing; 2008. p9.

[80] Rosegrant MW. Biofuels and grain prices: Impact and policy responses. USA: International Food Policy Research Institute; 2008.

[81] Jenkins DJA, Kendall CWC, McKeown-Eyssen G, Josse RG, Silverberg J, Booth GL, Vidgen E, Josse AR, Nguyen TH, Corrigan S, Banach MS, Ares S, Mitchell S, Emam A, Augusin LSA, Parker TL, Leiter LA Effect of a low-gylcermic index or a high-cereal fiber diet on type 2 diabetes: A randomised trial. Journal of the American Medical Association 2008;300, 2742-2753.

[82] Kahlon TS Evaluating healthful properties of cereals and cereal fractions by their bile-acid-binding potential. Cereal Foods World 2009;54, 118-121.

[83] Poutanen K. Healthgrain: EU approach to use more grains for health maintenance. Cereal Foods World Supplement 2009;54, A9.

[84] Anderson JW. Whole grains protect against atherosclerotic cardiovascular disease. The Proceedings of the Nutrition Society 2003;62, 135-142.

[85] Miller HE, Rigelhof F, Marquart L, Prakash A, Kanter M. Antioxidant content of whole grain breakfast cereals, fruits and vegetables. Journal of American College of Nutrition 2000;19(3) 312S-319S.

[86] Schatzkin A, Mouw T, Park Y. Dietary fiber and whole-grain consumption in relation to colorectal cancer in the NIH-AARP diet and health study. American Journal Clinical Nutrition 2007;85, 1353-1360.

[87] Wang L, Gaziano JM, Liu S, Manson JAE, Buring JE, Sesso HD. Whole- and refined-grain intakes and the risk of hypertension in women. American Journal of Clinical Nutrition 2007;86, 472-479.

[88] Hamaker BR, Pai D, Campanella OH. High incorporation of cereal bran fibers into foods. Cereal Foods World Supplement 2009;54(4) A4 http://meeting.aaccnet.org. (accessed 20 June 2013).

[89] Koh-Banerjee P, Rimm EB. Whole grain consumption and weight gain: a review of the epidemiological evidence, potential mechanisms and opportunities for future research. Proceedings of nutritional Society 2003;62, 25-29.

[90] Anderson J, Hanna T. Whole grain and protection against coronary heart disease: what are the active components and mechanisms. American Journal of Clinical Nutrition 1999; 32, 346-363.

[91] Jacobs DR Jr, Meyer KA, Kushi LH, Folsom AR. Whole-grain intake may reduce the risk of ischemic heart diseases death in post-menopausal women: the Iowa women's health study. American Journal of Clinical Nutrition 1998;68, 248-257.

Chapter 8

Nutritional, Therapeutic, and Prophylactic Properties of *Vigna subterranea* and *Moringa oleifera*

Victoria Adaora Jideani and
Claudine Florett Diedericks

Additional information is available at the end of the chapter

http://dx.doi.org/10.5772/57338

1. Introduction

1.1. Bambara groundnut

Bambara groundnut (*Vigna subterranea* (L.) Verdc.) [BGN] is an easy-to-cultivate legume seed classified under the family Fabaceae, sub-family Faboidea and genus *Vigna* [1]. Two botanical varieties exist, namely *V. subterranea* var. *spontanea* (wild varieties) and *V. subterranea* var. *subterranea* (cultivated varieties). BGN originated in West Africa from the Bambara district near Timbuktu and is now widely grown throughout tropical Africa, Indonesia, Malaysia, Sri Lanka, Central and South America and some parts of Northern Australia [2-4]. BGN is known by many common names such as Madagascar groundnut, baffin pea, voandzou, indhlubu, underground bean, nzama [Malawi], Epa-Roro [Nigeria], jugo beans [South Africa] and Nyimo beans [Zimbabwe] [1, 5]. Considered as one of the main attributes of BGN, is its tolerance of poor soils and drought, as well as its ability to yield in conditions in which groundnut fails completely. BGN also has an extremely tough seed coat, which makes it resistant to weevil attack and allows for storage of the seeds for long periods without loss [6]. Favourable characteristics making BGN an ideal crop includes its ability to be intercropped with other crops (i.e. maize, babala and sorghum), therefore not taking up areas designated to crops seen as more lucrative/important, its abundance in nitrogen which improves soil fertility and makes it useful in crop rotation, and the possibility to be grown without the use of expensive chemicals and fertilisers which are usually difficult to obtain in isolated areas [4].

BGN is propagated by its seeds which can be bought at local markets or are retained from the previous harvest. The larger seeds are used for cultivation and to retain maximum viability the seeds are dehulled before sowing [5]. As a leguminous annual short-day plant, BGN is grown for its underground seeds. Similar to the peanut, the BGN plant grows close to the ground and pods and seeds are formed on or below the soil surface [5]. Depending on the cultivar and weather conditions, the BGN plant matures in three to six months. The flowers and pods have been identified as essential parts of the plant [7]. The onset of flowering is 30 – 35 days after sowing, followed by pod development 30 days after the fertilisation process and the seeds developing after the pods in ten days. Pods are approximately 1.5 cm long, they may be wrinkled and slightly oval or round shaped containing one to two seeds. Pod colour varies from yellowish-white for unripe pods to yellowish-brown or purple for mature pods [2, 6]. BGN seeds are usually round, hard and smooth and vary in size. The colour of the seeds vary from black, dark-brown, red, white, cream or a combination of these colours and it may also be speckled with or without hilum colouration [1,6]. Illustrations of the BGN plant and various seed varieties are shown in Figure 1.

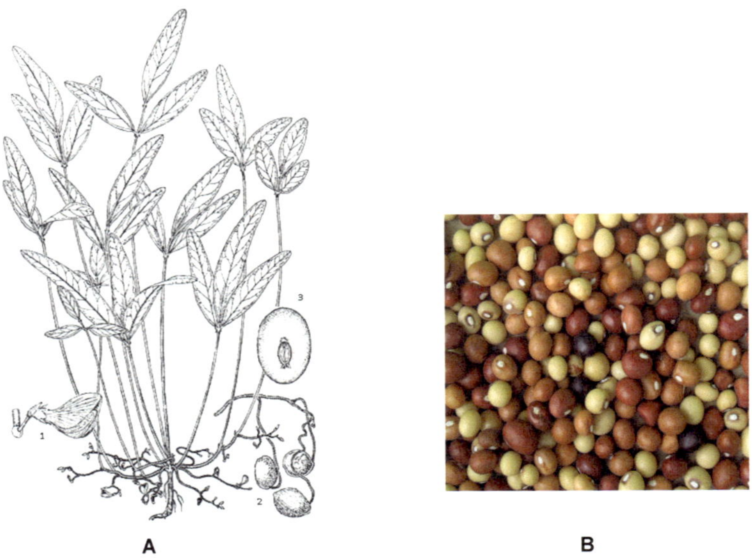

Figure 1. Bambara groundnut plant and seeds (A) Bambara groundnut flowering plant (1 – flower, 2 – fruits, 3 – seed); (B) Several varieties of Bambara groundnut seeds [8-9]

1.2. *Moringa oleifera*

The family of plants Moringaceae consists of 13 species outlined in Table 1. Out of the 13 species only *M. oleifera* has been accorded extensive research and development. They are important multipurpose crops in Africa and India. The species reported to have originated in India and Africa, are now grown around the world. Major production include Ghana, Senegal and Malawi, smaller production are in New Zealand and Fiji and more recent production in Nicaragua and Bolivia [10]. *Moringa* species are highly tolerant to arid conditions due to the formation of very large tuberous roots, and hence are often important famine foods [11]. Some common names for *M. oleifera* are detailed in Table 2. *Moringa* is a medium sized tree of 10 m

http://dx.doi.org/10.5772/57338

height, with a straight trunk (10-30 cm thick), whitish or gray, corky bark with longitudinal cracks. It has a tuberous taproot whose presence helps the species' tolerance to drought conditions. The tree is normally umbrella shaped with a lax crown of graceful, airy foliage, whose feathery effect is due to the finely tripinnnate division of the leaves (Figure 2). The leaves are densely crowded at the tops of the branchlets [12].

Species	Origin
Moringa oleifera	India
M. drouhardii	Madagascar
M. cocanensis	India
M. arborea	North Eastern Kenya
M. hildebrandtii	Madagascar
M. oleifera	India
M. borziana	Kenya and Somalia
M. ovalifolia	Namibia and extreme southwestern Angola
M. peregrina	Horn of Africa, Red sea, Arabia
M. longituba	Kenya, Ethiopia, Somalia
M. stenopetala	Kenya, Ethiopia
M. pygmaea	Northern Somalia
M. rivae	Kenya, Ethiopia
M. ruspoliana	Kenya

[1]Adapted from [12]

Table 1. *Moringa* species[1]

2. Food uses of the crops

2.1. Bambara groundnut

Primarily grown for human consumption, BGN seeds are consumed in various ways in both immature and fully matured form. Whilst immature, the BGN seeds may be consumed fresh (raw), grilled or it may be boiled before consumption. These seeds are also more palatable compared to the mature seeds which are hard. To soften the mature seeds and render them more pleasant tasting and sweet, the seeds are boiled or roasted [7, 5]. Immature seeds are frequently consumed as a snack by boiling the fresh seed with salt or roasting the seeds, and may also be pounded with or without hulls and boiled into a stiff porridge [8, 4, 13]. Mature seeds may be consumed as is by boiling in water, or it is often ground into flour and consumed as porridge by mixing the flour with butter or oil. The seeds may also be dried, boiled and consumed with plantains or maize [7-8]. Traditional uses of BGN inherent to certain areas in Africa are summarised in Table 3. Despite the many uses of BGN, the crop still remains underutilised due to several negative connotations such as being traditionally grown by women, an indigenous crop consumed by the poor in rural areas (from there the name "a poor man's food"), not being considered a lucrative cash crop and the difficulty in cooking and costs (including time, water and fuel) associated with cooking the seeds [4].

Language	Common name
English	*Moringa*, horseradish tree, drumstick tree, sujuna, ben tree, ben oil tree
French	Ben ailé, ben oléifère, benzolive, arbre radis du cheval
Spanish	Ben, árbol del ben, paraiso, morango, *Moringa*
Portuguese	acácia branca, marungo, muringa, moringuiero; cedro (Brazil)
Arabic	ruwag, alim, halim, shagara al ruwag (Sudan)
Swahili	mzunze, mlonge, mjungu moto, mboga chungu, shingo
German	Behenbaum, Behenussbaum, flügelsaniger Bennussbaum, Pferderettichbaum
Italian	Sàndalo ceruleo Fon: kpatima, yovokpatin,kpano,yovotin
Gun	èkwè kpatin, kpajima
Nigeria	
Yoruba & Nago	èwè igbale, èwè ile, èwè oyibo, agun oyibo, ayun manyieninu, ayèrè oyibo
Fulani	gawara, konamarade, rini maka, habiwal hausa
Hausa	zogall, zogalla-gandi, bagaruwar maka, bagaruwar masar, shipka hali, shuka halinka, barambo, koraukin zaila, rimin turawa
Ibo	Ikwe oyibo
Senegal	nebeday
Philippines	malunggay or malungai (Tagalog)
India	sujuna, sajina, lopa, horseradish or drumstick tree
Haiti	benzolive (Haitian Creole)

[1]Source: [12]

Table 2. *Moringa* common names[1]

Several research investigations are therefore aimed at highlighting the potential value of BGN as a sustainable food security crop. As in [14], milk was prepared from BGN by soaking the seeds in water, followed by homogenisation of the liquid and removal of the insoluble material. Acceptable BGN milk was obtained, and sensory analysis revealed panellists' preference for BGN milk in colour and taste compared to milk produced from soybean, cowpea and pigeon-pea. More recently, the functional properties of BGN flour and protein and starch fractions have also been investigated, as a means of better utilisation of this underutilised crop in food applications [15-19, 3].

2.2. *Moringa oleifera*

Moringa tree yields at least four different edibles namely pods, leaves, seeds and roots [12]. Figure 3 outlines some of the food uses of *Moringa*. The immature pods are the most valued and widely used of all the tree parts as it contains all the essential amino acids along with many vitamins and other nutrients. The tender pods have the general characteristics of a succulent string bean. It can be eaten raw or prepared like green peas or green beans. In India, they are usually added to curries and sometimes sliced, blanched and canned. The mature pods quickly turns tough as thick as a pencil and are too fibrous to eat like the string beans. In that form they are called drumsticks. However, they are cut into pieces to release the sweet frothy inside material which are well known ingredients in pickles in India.

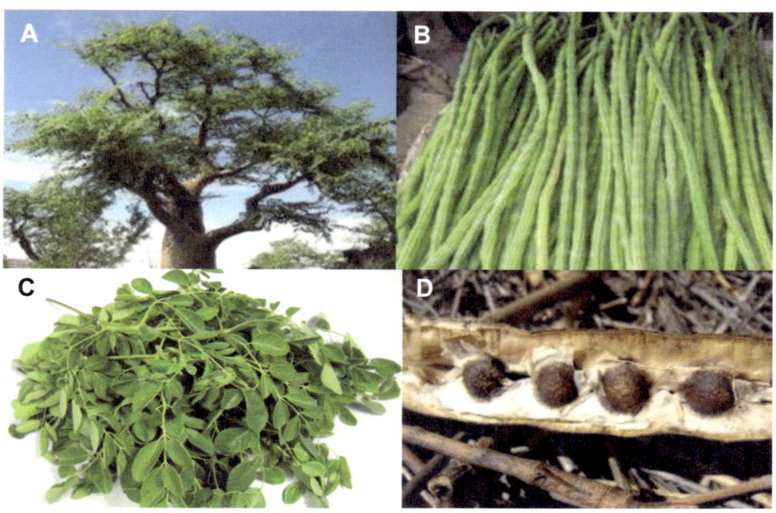

Figure 2. Part of *Moringa* tree (A) *Moringa* tree; (B) *Moringa* pods; (C) *Moringa* leaves and (D) *Moringa* pods with the seeds (www.ilove*Moringa*.com)

The fresh leaves are eaten as greens, in salads, in vegetable curries, as pickles and for seasoning. The dried leaves are crushed or pound and sifted into leaf powder which can then be added to sauces and foods as condiment. The flowers must be cooked and are eaten either mixed with other foods or fried in batter, and have been shown to be rich in potassium and calcium.

The seeds are often referred to as peas and can be used from the time they appear until they turn yellow and their shells begin to harden. They can be cooked like green peas. Hardened mature seeds are bitter and can be pressed yielding 38 – 40% of non-drying, edible oil which is clear, sweet and odourless and never becomes rancid and burns without smoke; its nutritional value resembles olive oil [20]. The seed powder can be used for water treatment where the powder coagulates solids and removes 90 – 99% bacteria.

The thickened root is used as substitute for horseradish although this is now discouraged as it contains alkaloids, especially moriginine, and a bacteriocide, spirochin, both of which can prove fatal following ingestion. Older roots and root bark are good sources of tanning agents.

Country	BGN food uses	Source
Cameroon	Testa-free fresh seeds – consumed as a complete meal by cooking with seasoning, or ground to prepare a traditional pudding sometimes with addition of taro leaves	[21]
Northern Ghana	Dry BGN seeds – boiled and crushed seeds used to form cakes/ balls followed by frying and adding to stews; BGN is also made into a paste and used in traditional dishes 'tubani' (steamed bean paste) and 'koose'/'akla' (fried bean paste)	[22-23]
Southern Ghana	'Aboboi' – prepared by soaking BGN seeds overnight followed by boiling (with/without capsicum pepper and salt) to produce a type of porridge/blancmange; served with 'gari' or plantain (ripe, fried or mashed)	
Kenya – Kambe & Giriama tribes	Dry BGN seeds are prepared by removal of the seed coat through pounding, winnowing and boiling the seeds until cooked; cooked seeds are pounded and mixed with coconut juice – this preparation is cooked and stirred until smooth, and served with 'ugali' or rice	[24]
Nigeria	Paste prepared from BGN flour used in preparation of 'moi moi' and 'akara' (bean balls); 'okpa' (steamed gel prepared by slurry of BGN)	[25-26]
South Africa	BGN (sometimes with peanuts) are added to millet or maize and the mixture boiled to form a stiff dough; this dough is salted and made into a ball known as 'tshidzimba' (Venda), 'sekome' (Sesotho) or 'tihove' (Shangaan)	[27]

Table 3. Some food uses of Bambara groundnut in parts of Africa

3. Nutritional characteristics

3.1. Bambara groundnut

BGN seeds contain on average 63% carbohydrate, 19% protein and 6.5% fat; amounts which are regarded as sufficient to make the seed a complete food [1]. Reference [4] compared the nutritional composition of BGN with more commonly utilised and commercialised grain legumes, and BGN compared favourably (see Table 4). The high carbohydrate content of BGN is mainly composed of starch and non-starch polysaccharides [1], fractions which are important in the human diet providing energy and imparting several physiological functions. BGN is also rich in calcium, potassium, iron and nitrogen [4, 6]. In [28] the proximate composition of seeds, flour and seed coats from different BGN varieties were compared. Results for BGN seeds and flour showed no big differences, concluding that the inherent nutrients would be provided in either raw or processed (milled) form. Nti [22] evaluated the chemical composition of five BGN varieties as well as the effects of different processing conditions on the chemical, mineral and anti-nutritional composition of BGN flour samples. The moisture content of all varieties (ranging from 8.8 ± 0.22 – 9.8 ± 0.23%) indicated good storage stability of BGN seeds. An increase in tannins content were observed in darker-coloured varieties, with black white-eye BGN having the highest tannin content (14.92 ± 0.85 mg CE/g).

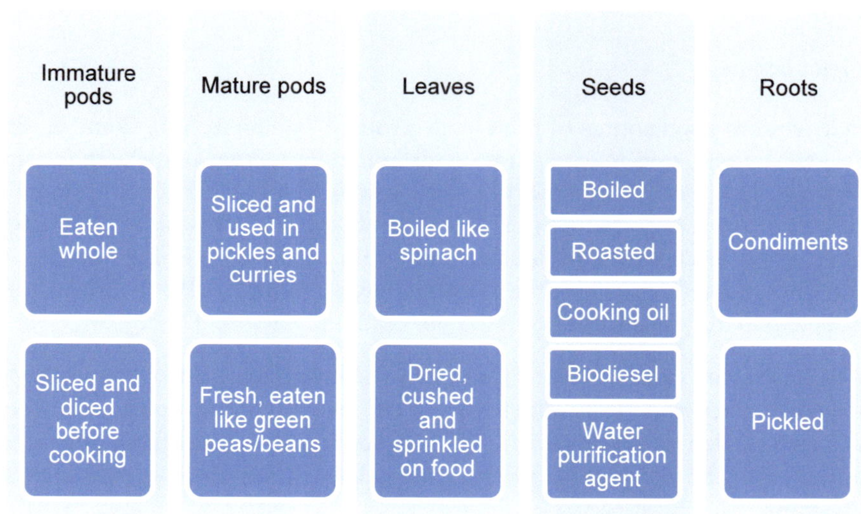

Figure 3. Some food uses of *Moringa* tree

These anti-nutritional components are mainly found in the seed coat and as in common beans, their concentration are correlated with the colour of the seeds [1]. Dehulling and boiling with dehulling having significant effects on the protein and tannins content of all varieties. Protein content which was highest in the undehulled (27.35 ± 0.27%) black white-eye variety as compared to the other varieties, increased significantly [$p < 0.05$] when dehulled (28.55 ± 0.26%) and boiled with dehulling (28.61 ± 0.51%). Tannins content in undehulled black white-eye BGN flour (15.40 ± 0.39 mg CE/g) decreased significantly [$p < 0.05$] when the sample was dehulled (1.16 ± 0.12 mg CE/g) and even more so when boiling and dehulling (0.09 ± 0.02 mg CE/g). These results demonstrate the positive effect of processing conditions on the nutritional properties of BGN, which could lead to increased utilisation in especially weaning products in which high-protein formulations are important.

The highly nutritious content of BGN and its unusually high content of the sulphur-containing essential amino acid methionine, makes BGN an important crop to consider for food security [4].

	Bambara groundnut	Soybean	Chickpea	Cowpea
Calories (kCal)	390.0	416.0	364.0	343.0
Protein (g)	20.8	36.5	19.3	23.8
Carbohydrates (g)	61.9	30.2	60.6	59.6
Fat (g)	6.6	19.9	6.0	2.1

[1] Adapted from [4]

Table 4. Nutritional composition of BGN and some commonly utilised legumes[1]

3.2. *Moringa oleifera*

M. oleifera leaves are good source of protein, β-carotene, vitamins, A, B, C and E, riboflavin, nicotinic acid, folic acid, pyridoxine, amino acids, minerals and various phenolic compounds [29-30]. *Moringa oleifera* leaf powder (25 g daily) is said to give a child the recommended daily allowance for protein (42%), calcium (125%), magnesium (61%), potassium (41%), iron (71%), vitamin A (272%), and vitamin C (22%). Gram for gram, *M. oleifera* leaves contain seven times the vitamin C in oranges, four times the calcium in milk, four times the β-carotene in carrots, twice the protein in milk and three times the potassium in bananas [31-33].

Leaves of *M. oleifera* are rich in palmitic (16:0) and linolenic (18:3) acids whereas the seeds are predominated by oleic acid (18:1). The roots are rich in palmitic and oleic acid whereas the stems and twigs are rich in palmitic acid [34]. It is becoming popular not only among the lower socio-economic class, but in the entire society irrespective of one's socio-economic background and health status.

4. Phytochemical properties of the crops

4.1. Bambara groundnut

Some phytochemistry studies have been done on species from the genus *Vigna*, with most focussing on *V. unguiculata* (cowpea) and limited information available on *V. subterreanea*. Pale et al. [35] investigated the anthocyanins present in bambara groundnut through column and preparative thin-layer chromatography. Three anthocyanins (delphinidin 3-*O*-β-glucoside, petunidin 3-*O*-β-glucoside and malvidin 3-*O*-β-glucoside) were identified. Anthocyanins have many beneficial effects on health, and further investigation into the health properties associated with BGN consumption is needed. In a study by [36], eleven species of *Vigna* were surveyed for canavanine, proanthocyanidin and flavonoid profiles. Canavanine, delphinidin

http://dx.doi.org/10.5772/57338

and cyanidin were absent in BGN seeds. The absence of canavanine is consistent in the species of *Vigna*. The flavonoid profiles revealed that the four BGN varieties studied accumulated four types of kaempferol glycosides. In all *Vigna* species, the prevalent flavonoid appears to be kaempferol. Kaempferol-3-*O*-glucoside-7-rhamnoside seemed to be restricted to BGN. As a polyphenol antioxidant, kaempferol imparts many health benefits and reduces the risk of many chronic illnesses such as cancer [37]. A recently published article by [38] also reveals the possible components in BGN which could have beneficial effects on health in their study on the effects of gas flaring on the African breadfruit and BGN. Valuable information on the phytochemical properties of BGN was found with high concentrations in the unpolluted samples for oxalate (0.38 ± 0.04%), saponin (0.24 ± 0.02%); vitamin E (3.18 ± 0.15 mg/100 g), vitamin C (1.17 ± 0.20 mg/100 g), vitamin A (26.05 ± 0.14 mg/100 g) and niacin (2.10 ± 0.06 mg/100 g). The concentrations of oxalate, saponin, alkaloid and flavonoid were increased by gas flaring, whilst the concentrations of vitamins were significantly [$p < 0.05$] reduced. Vitamin A which is important for maintaining good eye-sight and preventing eye diseases [39], were significantly higher [$p < 0.05$] in the BGN seeds as compared to the other vitamins detected. The information available on phytochemical components of BGN seeds is promising, and should be further investigated to determine and highlight their specific effects on human health, which could greatly influence the current underutilised status of this crop.

4.2. *Moringa oleifera*

Strickly speaking, phytochemicals are non-nutritive chemicals produced by plants which may have an impact on health, or on flavour, texture, smell or colour of the plants. Plants produce these chemicals to protect themselves but recent research demonstrates that they can also protect humans against diseases. The phytochemicals include the alkaloids, anthocyanins, carotenoids, coumestans, flavan-3-ols, flavonoids, hydroxycinnamic acids, isoflavones, lignans, monophenols, monoterpenes, organosulfides, phenolic acids, phytosterols and saponins. Each phytochemicals work differently. *M. oleifera* contains various phytochemicals namely, carotenoids, vitamins, minerals, amino acids, sterols, glycosides, alkaloids, flavonoids and phenolics [40, 29]. Table 5 details the phytochemicals found in *M. oleifera*. *Moringa* species are rich sources of various phytochemicals including uncommon sugar-modified glucosinolates, although there are only details on quantity and profiles for *M. oleifera*, *M. peregrine* and *M. stenopetala* [34, 41-42]. The predominant glucosinolate is 4-O-(α-L-rhamnopyranosyloxy)-benzylglucosinolate (glucomoringin) and depending on the tissues three mono-acetyl-rhamnose isomers of this glucosinolate have also been detected [41, 43]. Chlorogenic acids and flavonols have been reported in different tissues of *M. oleifera* and *M. stenopetala* but there is no information for other *Moringa* species [34, 40-41, 44-45]. The flavonoid profile was found to be quite complex and was predominated by flavonol glycosides (glucosides, rutinosides and malonylglucosides of quercetin, kaempferol and isorhamnetin). The predominant core aglycones are flavonols: quercetin > kaempferol > isorhamnetin. The leaves had the highest and most complex flavonoid contents, and no flavanoids were detected in roots or seeds. The antioxidant activity of leaves from *M. oleifera* was shown to be very high due to the high concentrations of polyphenolics [46-47]. Therefore *M. oleifera* tissues could be an important dietary source of antioxidant polyphenolics.

Guevara et al. [48] isolated eight compounds from the seeds of *M. oleifera* namely, O-ethyl-4-(α-L-rhamnosyloxy)-benzyl carbamate, 4-(α-L-rhamnosyloxy-benzyle isothiocyanate, niazimicin, niazirin, β-stiosterol, glycerol-1-(9-octadecanoate), 3-O-(6′-O-oleoyl-β-d-glucopyranosyl)-βsitosterol and β-sitosterol-3-O-β-d-glucopyranoside. 4-(α-L-rhamnosyloxy-benzyle isothiocyanate, niazimicin and β-sitosterol-3-O-β-d-glucopyranoside showed significant inhibitory activity against Epstein-Barr virus-early antigen (EBV-EA) and niazimicin in particular was found to have potent antitumor promoting acitivity in vivo in the two-stage carcinogenesis in mouse skin. They proposed that niazimicin could be a potent chemo-preventive agent in chemical carcinogenesis. Beta-sitosterol acts against some form of cancer and was found to reduce the growth of prostate and colon cancer cells. Other medical benefits of beta-sitosterol are boosting of immune defense, anti-inflammatory, normalising blood sugar, healing of ulcers and alleviating cramps.

Niaziridin and niazirin are present in leave and pods, respectively and are not detected in the bark of *M. oleifera*. Relatively higher amount of niazirin is present in leaves in comparison to the pods, while niaziridin content was about three times higher in the pods than the leaves [49]. Niaziridin rich fraction of *M. oleifera* pods enhances the bioactivity of commonly used antibiotics such as rifampicin, tetracycline and ampicillin against gram positive and negative bacteria and also facilitates the absorption of drugs, vitamins and nutrients through the gastro-intestinal membrane thus increasing their bio-availability [50]. Therefore, niaziridin can be used in combination therapy with drugs and nutrients resulting in reduced drug associated toxicity, reduced cost and duration of chemotherapy [49]. Hence, fruits of *M. oleifera* contain antitumor and anti-inflammatory compounds of the glycoside type (i.e. niazirin, niazimicin, niazicin A).

Phytochemical	Structure	Location	Ref.
Glucosinolates			
Benzylglucosinolate (Glucotropaeolin)	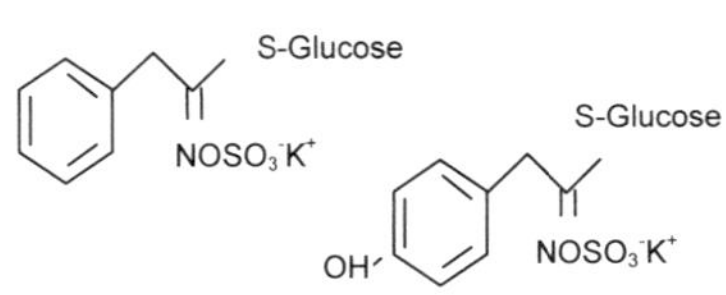		
4-Hydroxybenzylglucosinolate (Sinalbin)			
4-O-(α-L-Rhamnopyranosyloxy)-benzylglucosinolate (Glucomoringin) (G2) (R1, R2, R3 = H)	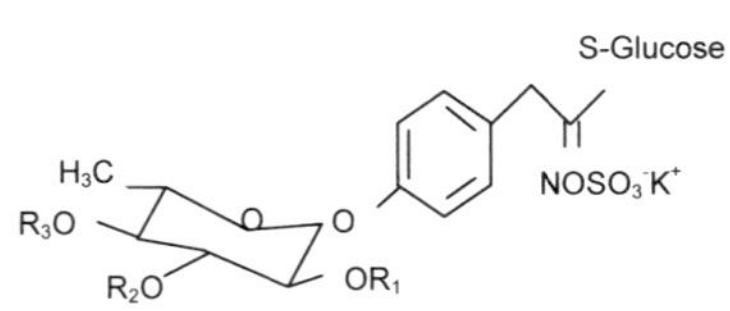	All tissues except the roots	
4-O-(α-L-Acetyl-rhamnopyranosyloxy)-benzylglucosinolate (G3-G5) (R1 & R2 = H, R3 = Ac; R1 & R3 = H, R2 = Ac; R1 = Ac; R2 & R3 = H)		Roots	
Hydrolysis Products & Related Derivatives			
4-O-(α-L-Rhamnopyranosyloxy)-benzylisothiocyanate (R1 = R2 = R3 = H, X = N = C = S)	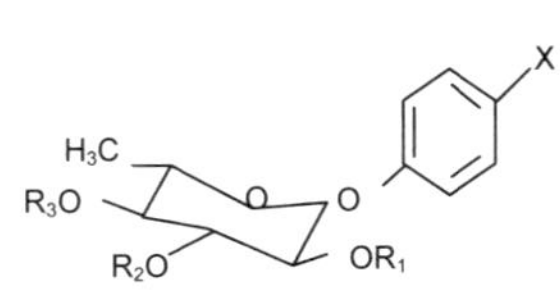	Leaves and pods	[48]
Niazirin (R1 = R2 = R3 = H, X = CN)		Roasted seeds	

http://dx.doi.org/10.5772/57338

Phytochemical	Structure	Location	Ref.
Niazirinin (R1 = R2 = H, R3 = Ac, X = CN			
Niazimin A/B (R1 = R2 = H, R3 = Ac, X = CH2-NH-CO-OEt)			
Niazinin A/B (R1 = R2 = R3 = H, X = CH2-NH-(C=S)-OMe)			
Niazicin A/B (R1 = R2 = H, R3 = Ac, X = CH2-NH-(C=S)-OMe)			
Niazimicin (R1 = R2 = R3 = H, X = CH2-NH-(C=S)-OEt)			
Niaziminin A/B (R1 = R2 = H, R3 = Ac, X = CH2-NH-(C=S)-OEt)			
Phenolics			
3-Caffeoylquinic acid (3-CQA) (Neochlorogenic acid)	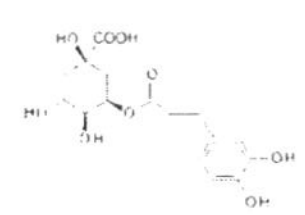 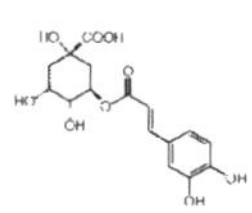	All tissues except the roots, pods and seeds	[41]
5-Caffeoylquinic acid (50CQA) (Chlorogenic acid)			
Major flavonoids (K = Kaempferol, Q = Quercetin)			
K 3-O-Rutinoside ((R3 =-GlcRha, R3′ = H & R4′ = OH) (F7)	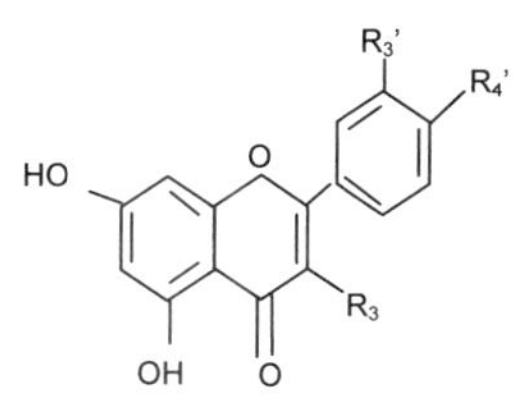		
K 3-O-Glucoside (R3 = -Glc, R3′ = H, R4′ = OH) (F9)			
K 3-O-(6″-Malonylglucoside) (R3 = -GlcMalm R3′ = H, R4′ = OH) (F13)			
Q 3-O-Rutinoside (R3 = -GlcRha, R3′ & R4′ = OH) (F4)			
Q 3-O-Glucoside (R3 = -Glc, R3′ & R4′ = OH) (F6)			
Q 3-O-(6″-Malonylglucoside) (R3 = -GlcMal, R3′ & R4′ = OH) (F8)			

[1]Source: [34]

Table 5. Phytochemicals found in *M. oleifera*[1]

Polyphenolic compounds exist widely in the plant kingdom and are used in humans to modulate lipid peroxidation involved in atherogenesis, thrombosis and carinogenesis due to their antioxidant activity and anti-inflammatory action [40, 51]. Both aqueous and acetone extracts of *M. oleifera* leaves have potent antioxidant activities; however, Moyo et al. [52] reported higher values of phenols, flavonoids, flavonol and proanthocyanidins in acetone extract of *M. oleifera* leaves than the aqueous extract. Similar observation was reported by other researchers [40, 46, 53-54]. The ability of the extracts to adsorb and neutralise free radicals or decompose peroxides are attributed to the synergistic effect of phenolic compounds in the *M. oleifera*. The redox properties, presence of conjugated ring structures and carboxylic group which can inhibit lipid peroxidation are responsible for its ability as free radical scavengers [55].

The aqueous extract of leaf (LE), fruit (FE) and seed (SE) of *M. oleifera* could significantly inhibit the OH-dependent damage of pUC18 plasmid DNA with an activity sequence of LE > FE > SE. Gallic acid, chlorogenic acid, ellagic acid, ferulic acid, kaempferol, quercetin and vanillin were present in the extracts. The leaf extract was comparatively higher in total phenolics [105.04 mg gallic acid equivalents (GAE/g)], total flavonoids [31.28 mg quercetin equivalents (QE/g)] and ascorbic acid (106.95 mg/100 g) with better antioxidant activity (85.8%), anti-radical power (74.3), reducing power [1.1 ascorbic acid equivalents (ASE/ml)], inhibition of lipid peroxidation, protein oxidation, OH-induced deoxyribose degradation and scavenging power of superoxide anion and nitric oxide radicals than did the FE, SE and standard α-tocopherol [56]. Many gram negative bacteria such as *Erwinia carotovora, Enterobacter agglomerans, Chromobacterium violaceum* and *Pseudomonas aeruginosa* use N-acyl homoserine lactones (AHLs) signal molecules to monitor their own population density. At a threshold population density, AHLs interact with cellular receptors and trigger the expression of a set of target genes including virulence, antibiotic production, biofilm formation, bioluminescence, mobility and warming, in a process called "quorum sensing" (QS) [57]. The discovery of the QS system and its critical role in bacteria virulence and survival has revealed a novel way to attack and attenuate bacterial pathogenicity. The major advantage of this novel strategy for anti-infective therapy is that it circumvents the problem of antibiotic resistance, which is intimately connected to the use of conventional antibacterial agents, as it specifically interferes with the expression of pathogenic traits rather than to impede growth of the bacteria. The efficacy and toxicity of previous reported QS blockers (halogenated furanones) have been important concerns. Hence, attention has been focused on identification of such QS blockers from natural and non-toxic sources for the development of novel non-antibiotic drugs for treating bacterial diseases in humans as well as in other animals. Singh et al. [56] reported that the leaf and the fruit extracts of *M. oleifera* inhibited violacein production, a QS-regulated behaviour in *Chromobacterium violaceum* 12472. This provides evidence on *M. oleifera* as natural antioxidant for its capacity to protect organism and cell from oxidative DNA associated with aging, cancer and denegerative diseases as well as inhibit lipid peroxidation and bacterial QS. Thus, *M. oleifera* may serve as an ideal ingredient for functional food, nutraceutical and bio-pharmaceutical industries.

The seeds of *Moringa oleifera* contain 4 (α-L-Rhamnosyloxy) benzyl isothiocyanate and benzyl isothiocyanate. These are antimicrobial agents effective against several bacteria and fungi. The minimal bactericidal concentration in vitro is 40 μmol/l for *Mycobacterium phlei* and 56 μmol/l for *Bacillus subtilis* [58]. Singh et al. [10] identified ten phenolic compounds (gallic acid, p-coumaric acid, ferulic acid, caffeic acid, protocatechuric acid, cinnamic acid, catechin, epicatechin, vanillin and quercetin) from defatted *M. oleifera* seed flour. These natural plant phenolics could be a good source of antioxidants and antimicrobials for food and pharmaceutical industries.

5. Therapeutic and prophylactic properties of the crops

5.1. Bambara groundnut

The medicinal role of BGN is mainly based on information obtained from communities in several parts of Africa, where this crop is reportedly responsible and useful for treatment of various ailments. As a treatment for diarrhoea, a mixture of BGN and water from boiled maize are consumed. Raw BGN seeds are chewed and swallowed by pregnant women to alleviate the nausea associated with pregnancy [7]. The medicinal value of the crop have also been highlighted and reviewed by [59]. The following uses of BGN as traditional medicine have been noted by the authors (i) In several countries in sub-Saharan Africa, BGN plays an important role in the diets of especially young rural children as it helps in overcoming the protein deficiency Kwashiorkor; (ii) The Igbos tribe in Nigeria use the seeds for treatment of venereal diseases; (iii) To treat polymenorrhea it is recommended that BGN seeds be roasted before consumption; (iv) The water in which BGN seeds are boiled is used as treatment for internal bruising, and a mixture of water and crushed seeds are prescribed for treatment of cataracts; (v) BGN seeds have the highest concentration of soluble fibre as compared to other beans; this could contribute to the reduction of heart disease incidence and prevention of colon cancer; (vi) Surveys amongst local communities in northern Côte d'Ivoire revealed that the BGN seeds are mainly used for medical treatments as opposed to other parts of the plant. The seeds are used to treat anemia, ulcers (black BGN variety mixed with an unidentified plant) and menorrhagia during pregnancy (hemostatic drink prepared by a mixture of BGN flour and *Pupalia lappacea* (L.) Amaranthaceae dissolved in water). The traditional uses of BGN to treat several ailments are noteworthy, and present a gap for detailed study on the pharmaceutical value of the crop. This would provide yet another means of highlighting the potential of BGN as an underutilised legume and tap into ways of encouraging more sustained production and use of BGN.

5.2. *Moringa oleifera*

Besides the rich nutritional value of *M. oleifera* it has curative and prophylactic properties [24]. Almost all the parts (root, bark, gum, leaf, pods, flowers, seed and seed oil) of M. oleifera have been used for various ailments including the treatment of inflammation and infectious diseases along with cardiovascular, gastrointestinal, haematological, hepatorenal disorders, diabetes mellitus, CNS depressant, and for antifertility effect [40]. The plant has been used for the treatment of ascites, rheumatism and for the enhancement of cardiac function. The seed extract have been reported to be administered nasally in diseases like rhinitis and the dried seeds used successfully as an 'anti-allergic' agent by the Ayurvedic practitioners [60]. Mahajan [61] reported an antiarthritic activity of ethanolic extract of seeds of *M. oleifera* against chemical induced rheumatoid arthritis as well as an antiasthmatic activity against immune-mediated inflammatory responses in rat [62]. *M. oleifera* seed extract can act against CCl4-induced liver injury and fibrosis in rats by a mechanism related to its antioxidant properties, anti-inflammatory effect and its ability to attenuate the hepatic stellate cells activation [63].

Siddhuraju and others [40] reported that leaf extracts (water, aqueous methanol, aqueous ethanol) were capable of scavenging peroxyl and superoxyl radicals. The major bioactive compounds of phenolics were found to be flavonoid groups such as quercetin and kaempferol. *Moringa* leaves are therefore potential source of natural antioxidants. The ethanol leaf extract of *Moringa oleifera* is used for hypertension [64-66]. The leaves are used as hypocholesterolemic and hypoglycemic agents [64, 67-68]. Additionally, the leaves have been reported for its antitumour [69], antioxidant [46, 54, 70], radio-protective [71-72], anti-inflammatory/diuretic properties [73], antihepatotoxic [74], antifertility [75], antiurolithiatic [76] and analgesic activities [77]. Choudhary and others [78] reported that ethanolic root-bark extract of *M. oleifera* possesses valuable antiulcer, antisecretory and cytoprotective activity in rats and thus can be used as source for an antiulcer drug.

An old report from Southeast Asia says a decoction of bark stimulates menses and is used for "morning after" birth control. In parts of West Africa, *Moringa* leaves or juice are taken for diabetes and high blood pressure [12]. Traditionally, leaves, fruits, roots and seeds of this plant are used for treating abdominal tumors, hysteria, scurvy, paralytic attacks, helminitic, bladder, prostate troubles, sores and skin infections [32].

Moringa oleifera possess genotoxicity at a high dose 3000 mg/kg b.wt of the powdered aqueous extract. However, intake is safe at levels ≤ 1000 mg/kg b.wt. [79].

6. Harnessing the rich nutritional and health properties of Bambara groundnut and *M. oleifera* for human nutrition

Bambara groundnut is a leguminous crop with great potential of sustaining the dietary needs of many people in both rural and urban communities. This indigenous African legume have been frowned upon as a 'poor man's food', but as more information emerges on the rich nutritional profile of BGN the importance of this crop to human nutrition is becoming more evident. In our laboratory we have demonstrated that Bambara groundnut could be used to produce a probiotic beverage as well as a rich source of soluble and insoluble fibre that can be used to enhance the nutrition and textural properties of white bread [80-81].

Moringa could be incorporated into programs on malnutrition. With four times the beta-carotene of carrot, *Moringa* has especial potential for programs dealing with avitaminosis, the vitamin A deficiency that causes 70 percent of childhood blindness. Consumption of diet supplemented with *M. oleifera* leaves could protect against diseases induced by oxidative stress. Many *Moringa* nutritional supplements exist in the market including *Moringa* dry leaf powder, capsules, nutrition shake and health booster. Perhaps using the multi mix approach of food product development more food products could be developed especially for programs on malnutrition.

Author details

Victoria Adaora Jideani* and Claudine Florett Diedericks

*Address all correspondence to: jideaniv@cput.ac.za

Department of Food Technology, Cape Peninsula University of Technology, Bellville, South Africa

References

[1] Bamishaiye, O.M., Adegbola, J.A. and Bamishaiye, E.I. Bambara groundnut: an under-utilized nut in Africa. Advances in Agricultural Biotechnology 2011; 1 60-72.

[2] Swanevelder, C.J. Bambara—Food for Africa (*Vigna subterranea* – bambara groundnut). Pp. 1-16. South Africa: National Department of Agriculture; 1998. p1-16.

[3] Eltayeb, A.R.S.M., Ali, A.O., Abou-Arab, A.A. & Abu-Salem, F.M. Chemical composition and functional properties of flour and protein isolate extracted from bambara groundnut (*Vigna subterranea* (L.) Verdc.). African Journal of Food Science 2011; 5(2) 82-90.

[4] De Kock, C. Bambara groundnut. http://www.underutilized-species.org/documents/Publications/bambara_groundnut_paper.pdf (accessed 03 September 2013)

[5] Stephens, J.M. Bambara Groundnut—*Voandzeia subterranea* (L.) Thouars. Gainesville, Florida: University of Florida; 2012. http://edis.ifas.ufl.edu/mv014 (accessed 11 June 2013).

[6] Mkandawire, C.H. Review of bambara groundnut (*Vigna subterranea* (L.) Verdc.) production in Sub-Sahara Africa. Agricultural Journal 2007; 2(4) 464-470.

[7] Directorate Plant Production (DPP). Production guidelines for Bambara groundnuts. Pretoria, South Africa: Department of Agriculture, Forestry and Fisheries; 2011. p1-10.

[8] Brink, M., Ramolemana, G.M. and Sibuga, K.P. *Vigna subterranea* (L.) Verdc. In: *Plant Resources of Tropical Africa/ Ressources végétales de l'Afrique tropicale* (edited by M. Brink & G. Belay). Wageningen, Netherlands: PROTA4U; 2006. http://www.prota4u.org/search.asp. (accessed 5 September 2013).

[9] Rulkens, T. Bambara groundnut (*Vigna subterranea*) from Buzi district in Mozambique. http://www.flickr.com/photos. (accessed 5 September 2013).

[10] Singh, R.S.G, Negi, P.S. and Radha, C. Phenolic composition, antioxidant and antimicrobial activities of free and bound phenolic extracts of *Moringa oleifera* seed flour. Journal of Functional Foods 2013 (Article in Press).

[11] Sena, L.P., VanderJagt, D.J., Rivera, C., Tin, A.C., Muhamadu, I., Mahamadou, O., Millton, M., Pastuszyn, A. And Glew, R.H. Analysis of nutritional components of eight famine foods of the Republic of Niger. Plant Foods for Human Nutrition 1998; 52 17-30.

[12] National Research Council (2006). Lost crops of Africa: Volume II: Vegetables. http://www.nap.edu/catalog/11763.html. (accessed 15 October 2013).

[13] Uebersax, M.A. and Occeña, L.G. Legumes in the diet. In: *Encyclopedia of Food Sciences and Nutrition*, 2nd Edition (edited by B. Caballero, L. Trugo & P.M. Finglas). New York: Elsevier Science Ltd; 2003. p3520-3528.

[14] Brough, S.H., Azam-Ali, S.N. and Taylor, A.J. The potential of bambara groundnut (*Vigna subterranea*) in vegetable milk production and basic protein functionality systems. Food Chemistry 1993; 47 277-283.

[15] Adebowale, K.O., Afolabi, T.A. and Lawal, O.S. Isolation, chemical modification and physicochemical characterisation of bambarra groundnut (*Voandzeia subterranean*) starch and flour. Food Chemistry 2002; 78 305-311.

[16] Adebowale, K.O. and Lawal, O.S. Comparative study of the functional properties of bambarra groundnut (*Voandzeia subterranean*), jack bean (*Canavalia ensiformis*) and mucuna bean (*Mucuna pruriens*) flours. Food Research International 2004; 37 355-365.

[17] Lawal, O.S., Adebowale, K.O. and Adebowale, Y.A. Functional properties of native and chemically modified protein concentrates from bambara groundnut. Food Research International 2007; 40 1003-1011.

[18] Sirivongpaisal, P. Structure and functional properties of starch and flour from bambara groundnut. Songklanakarin Journal of Science and Technology 2008; 30(1) 51-56.

[19] Yusuf, A.A., Ayedun, H. and Sanni, L.O. Chemical composition and functional properties of raw and roasted Nigerian benniseed (*Sesamum indicum*) and bambara groundnut (*Vigna subterranean*). Food Chemistry 2008; 111 277-282.

[20] Tsaknis, J., Lalas, S., Gergis, V., Douroglou, V. and Spiliotis. Characterisation of *Moringa oleifera* variety Mbololo seed oil of Kenya. Journal of Agricultural and Food Chemistry 1999; 47 4495-4499.

[21] Nguy-Ntamag, F.C. Country Reports: Cameroon. Bambara groundnut *Vigna subterranea* (L.) Verdc. Promoting the conservation and use of underutilized and neglected crops 9. In: Heller J, Begemann F, Mushonga J. (eds.). Proceedings of the workshop on Conservation and Improvement of Bambara Groundnut *(Vigna subterranea (L.) Verdc.)*. November 1995. Harare, Zimbabwe; 1997.

[22] Nti, C.A. Effects of bambara groundnut (*Vigna subterranea*) variety and processing on the quality and consumer appeal for its products. International Journal of Food Science and Technology 2009; 44 2234-2242.

[23] Doku, E.V. Country Reports: Ghana. Bambara groundnut *Vigna subterranea* (L.) Verdc. Promoting the conservation and use of underutilized and neglected crops 9. In: Heller J, Begemann F, Mushonga, J. (eds.). Proceedings of the workshop on Conservation and Improvement of Bambara Groundnut *(Vigna subterranea (L.) Verdc.)*. November 1995. Harare, Zimbabwe; 1997.

[24] Ngugi, G.W. Country Reports: Kenya. Bambara groundnut *Vigna subterranea* (L.) Verdc. Promoting the conservation and use of underutilized and neglected crops 9. In: Heller J, Begemann F, Mushonga J. (eds.). *Proceedings of the workshop on Conservation and Improvement of Bambara Groundnut (Vigna subterranea (L.) Verdc.)*. November 1995. Harare, Zimbabwe; 1997.

[25] Obizoba, I.C. Nutritive value of cowpea-bambara groundnut rice mixtures in adult rats. Nutrition Reports International 1983; 27 709-712.

[26] Uvere, P.O., Uwaegbute, A.C. and Adedji, E.M. Effects of malting on the milling performance and acceptability of bambara groundnut (*Voandzeia subterranea* Thouars) seeds and products. Plant Foods for Human Nutrition 1999; 54 49-57.

[27] Swanevelder, C.J. Country Reports: South Africa. Bambara groundnut *Vigna subterranea* (L.) Verdc. Promoting the conservation and use of underutilized and neglected crops 9. In: Heller J, Begemann F, Mushonga J. (eds.). *Proceedings of the workshop on Conservation and Improvement of Bambara Groundnut (Vigna subterranea (L.) Verdc.)* November 1995. Harare, Zimbabwe; 1997.

[28] Ojimelukwe, P.C. and Ayernor, G.S. Oligosaccharide composite and functional properties of flour and starch isolates from four cultivars of Bambara groundnut seeds. Journal of Food Science and Technology 1992; 29 319-321.

[29] Anwar, F., Latif, S., Ashraf, M. and Gilani, A.H. *Moringa oleifera*: A food plant with multiple medicinal uses. Phytotherapy Research 2007; 21 17–25.

[30] Khalafalla, M.M., Abdellatef, E., Dafalla, H.M., Nassrallah, A.A., Aboul-Enein, K.M. and Lightfoot, D.A. Active principle from *Moringa oleifera* Lam. leaves effective against two leukemias and a hepatocarcinoma. African Journal of Biotechnology 2010; 9 8467–8471.

[31] Ramachandran, C., Peter, K.V. and Gopalakrishnan, P.K. Drumstick (*Moringa oleifera*): a multipurpose Indian vegetable. Economic Botany 1980; 34, 276–283.

[32] Fuglie, L.J. Isolation and structure elucidation of new nitrile and mustard oil glycosides from *Moringa oleifera* and their effect on blood pressure. Journal of Natural Products (1999a); 57 1256–1261.

[33] Fuglie, L.J. The Miracle Tree. *Moringa oleifera*: Natural Nutrition for the Tropics. Dakar: Church World Service; (1999b). p. 68.

[34] Amaglo, N.K.; Bennett, R.N.; Lo Curto, R.B., Rosa, E.A.S., Turco, V.L, Giuffrida, A.; Curto, A.L., Crea, F. and Timpo, G.M. Profiling selected phytochemicals and nutrients in different tissue of the multipurpose tree *Moringa oleifera* L., grown in Ghana. Food Chemistry 2010; 122 1047-1054.

[35] Pale, E., Nacro, M., Vanhaelen, M. and Vanhaelen-Fastré. Anthocyanins from Bambara Groundnut (*Vigna subterranea*). Journal of Agricultural and Food Chemistry 1997; 45 3359-3361.

[36] Onyilagha, J.C., Islam, S. and Ntamatungiro, S. Comparative phytochemistry of eleven species of *Vigna* (Fabaceae). Biochemical Systematics and Ecology 2009; 37 16-19.

[37] Chen, A.Y. & Chen, Y.C. A review of the dietary flavonoid, kaempferol on human health and cancer chemoprevention. Food Chemistry 2013; 138(4) 2099-2107.

[38] Ujowundu, C.O., Nwagou, L.A., Ujowundu, F.N. & Belonwu, D.C. Effect of gas flaring on the phytochemical and nutritional composition of *Treculia Africana* and *Vigna subterranean*. British Biotechnology Journal 2013; 3(3) 293-304.

[39] Nwaogu, L.A. and Ujowundu, C.O. Effect of petroleum hydrocarbon pollution on the nutritional value of ripe guava (*Psidium guajava*) fruits grown in Imo State, Nigeria. International Journal of Biological and Chemical Sciences 2010; 4(2) 450-455.

[40] Siddhuraju, P. and Becker, K. Antioxidant properties of various solvent extracts of total phenolic constituents from three different agroclimatic origins of drumstick tree (*Moringa oleifera* Lam.) leaves. Journal of Agricultural and Food Chemistry 2003; 51(8) 2144-2155.

[41] Bennett, R.N., Mellon, F.A., Foidl, N., Pratt, J.H., DuPont, M.S., Perkins, L. and Kroon, P.A. Profiling glucosinolates and phenolics in vegetative and reproductive tissues of the multi-purpose trees *Moringa oleifera* L. (Horseradish tree) and *Moringa stenopetala* L. Journal of Agricultural and Food Chemistry 2003; 51 3546–3553.

[42] Fahey, J.W., Zalcmann, A.T. and Talalay, P. The chemical diversity and distribution of glucosinolates and isothiocyanates among plants. Phytochemistry 2001; 56 5–51.

[43] Kjaer, A., Malver, O., El-Menshawi, B. and Reischt, J. Isothiocyanates in myrosinase-treated seed extracts of *Moringa peregrina*. Phytochemistry 1979; 18 1485–1487.

[44] Lako, J., Trenerry, V.C., Wahlqvist, M., Wattanapenpaiboon, N., Sotheeswaran, S. and Premier, R. Phytochemical flavonols, carotenoids and antioxidant properties of a wide selection of Fijian fruit, vegetables and other readily available foods. Food Chemistry 2007; 101 1727–1741.

[45] Manguro, L.O.A. and Lemmen, P. Phenolics of *Moringa oleifera* leaves. Natural Products Research 2007, 21.

[46] Sreelatha, S. and Padma, P.R. Antioxidant activity and total phenolic content of *Moringa oleifera* leaves in two stages of maturity. Plant Foods for Human Nutrition 2009; 64 303–311.

[47] Verma, A.R., Vijayakumar, M., Mathela, C.S., & Rao, C.V. In vitro and in vivo antioxidant properties of different fractions of *Moringa oleifera* leaves. Food and Chemical Toxicology 2009; 47 2196–2201.

[48] Guevara, A.P., Vargas, C., Sakurai, H. Fujiwara, Y., Hashimoto, K. Maoka, T., Kozuka, M., Ito, Y., Tokuda, H. and Nishino, H. An antitumor promoter from *Moringa oleifera* Lam. Mutation Research 1999; 440 181-188.

[49] Shanker, K, Gupta, M.M., Srivastava, S.K.; Bawankule, D.U.; Pal, A. and Khanuja, S.P.S. Determination of bioactive nitrile glycoside(s) in drumstick (*Moringa oleifera*) by reverse phase HPLC. Food Chemistry 2007; 105 376-382.

[50] Khanuja, S.P.S., Arya, J.S., Tiruppadiripuliyur, R.S.K., Saikia, D., Kaur, H., Singh, M., Gupta, S. C., Shasany, A.K., Darokar, M.P., Srivastava, S.K., Gupta, M.M., Verma, S.C. and Pal, A. Nitrile glycoside useful as a bioenhancer of drugs and nutrients, process of its isolation from *Moringa oleifera*. (United States Patent 2005; 6,858,588 B2).

[51] Frankel, E.N., & Meyer, A.S. The problems of using one-dimensional methods to evaluate multifunctional food and biological antioxidants. Journal of the Science of Food and Agriculture 2000; 80 1925–1941.

[52] Moyo, B., Oyedemi, S., Masika, P.J. and Muchenje, V. Polyphenolic content and antioxidant properties of *Moringa oleifera* leaf extracts and enzymatic activity of liver from goats supplemented with *Moringa oleifera* leaves/sunflower seed cake. Meat Science 2012; 91, 441-447.

[53] Frum, Y., & Viljoen, A.M. In vitro 5-lipoxygenase and antioxidant activities of South African medicinal plants commonly used topically for skin diseases. Skin Pharmacology and Physiology 2006; 19 329–335.

[54] Atawodi, S.E., Atawodi, J.C., Idakwo, G.A., Pfundstein, B., Haubner, R., Wurtele, G., Bartsch, H. and Owen, R.W. Evaluation of the polyphenol content and antioxidant properties of methanol extracts of the leaves, stem, and root barks of *Moringa oleifera* Lam. Journal of Medicinal Food 2010; 13 710–716.

[55] Oyedemi, S.O., Bradley, G. and Afolayan, A. J. In-vitro and in-vivo antioxidant activities of aqueous extract of Strychnos henningsii Gilg. African Journal of Pharmacy and Pharmacology 2010; 4 70–78.

[56] Singh, B.N., Singh, B.R., Singh, R.L., Prakash, D., Dhakarey, R., Upadhyay, G. and Singh, H.B. Oxidative DNA damage protective activity, antioxidant and anti-quorum sensing potentials of *Moringa oleifera*. Food and Chemical Toxicology 2009; 47 1109-1116.

[57] Manefield, M., Rasmussen, T.B., Henzter, M., Steinberg, P., Kjelleberg, S. and Givsko, M. Halogenated furanones inhibit quorum sensing through accelerated LuxR turnover. Microbiology 2002; 148 1119–1127.

[58] Eilert, U., Wolters, B. and Nahrstedt, A. The antibiotic principle of seeds for *Moringa oleifera* and *Moringa stenopetala*. Planta Medica 1981; 42(5) 55-61.

[59] Koné. M., Paice, A.G. and Touré, Y. Bambara groundnut [*Vigna subterranea* (L.) Verdc. (Fabaceae)] usage in human health. In: *Nuts and Seeds in Health and Disease Prevention* (edited by V.R. Preedy, R.R. Watson & V.B. Patel). UK: Elsevier Inc.; 2011. p. 192-194.

[60] Chopra, R.N., Chopra, I.C., Handa, K.L., Kapur, I.D. (Eds.), 1938. Chopra's Indigenous Drugs of India. UN Dhur and Sons, Calcutta, India, 1938, p. 110.

[61] Mahajan, S.G., Mali, R.G. and Mehta, A.A. Protective effect of ethanolic extract of seeds of *Moringa oleifera* Lam. against inflammation associated with development of arthritis in rats. Journal of Immunotoxicology 2007a; 4 39–47.

[62] Mahajan, S.G., Mali, R.G. and Mehta, A.A. Effect of *Moringa oleifera* Lam. seed extract on Toluene Diisocyanate-induced immune-medicated inflammatory responses in rats. Journal of Immunotoxicology 2007b; 4 85–96.

[63] Hamza, A. A. Ameliorative effects of *Moringa oleifera* Lam seed extract on liver fibrosis in rats. Food and Chemical Toxicology 2010; 48 345-355.

[64] Siddiqui, S. and Khan, M.I. Pharmacological Study of *Moringa pterygosperma*. Central Laboratories. Pakistani Council of Science and Industrial Research 1968;p. 268–272.

[65] Kirtikar, K.R. and Basu, K. Indian Medicinal Plants. India: Lalit Mohan Basu MB, Allahabad; 1984. p.677–681.

[66] Nikkon, F., Saud, A., Rahman, M.H. and Haque, M.E. In vitro antimicrobial activity of the compound isolated from chloroform extract of *Moringa oleifera* Lam. Pakistani Journal of Biological Sciences 2006; 6 1888–1890.

[67] Ghasi, S., Nwobodo, E. and Ofili, J.O. Hypocholesterolemic effects of crude extract of leaf of *Moringa oleifera* Lam in high-fat diet fed wistar rats. Journal of Ethnopharmacology 2000; 69 21–25.

[68] Dangi, S.Y., Jolly, C.I. and Narayanan, S. Antihypertensive activity of the total alkaloids from the leaves of *Moringa oleifera*. Pharmaceutical Biology 2002; 40, 144–148.

[69] Aruna, K., Sivaramakrishnan, V.M. Plant products as protective agents against cancer. Indian Journal of Experimental Biology 1990; 28 1008–1011.

[70] Diallo, D., Marston, A., Terreaux, C., Toure, Y., Paulsen, B.S. and Hostettmann, K. Screening of Malian medicinal plants for antifungal, larvicidal, molluscidal, antioxidant and radical scavenging activities. Phytotherapy Research 2001; 15 401–406.

[71] Rao, V.A., Devi, P.U. and Kamath, R. In vivo radioprotective effect of *Moringa oleifera* leaves. Indian Journal of Experimental Biology 2001; 39 858–863.

[72] Arora, R., Gupta, D., Chawla, R., Sagar, R., Sharma, A., Kumar, R., Prasad, J., Singh, S., Samanta, N. and Sharma, R.K. Radioprotection by plant products: present status and future prospects. Phytotherapy Research 2005; 19, 1–22.

[73] Cáceres, A., Cabrera, O., Morales, O., Mollinedo, P. and Mendia, P. Pharmacological properties of *Moringa oleifera*. 1. Preliminary screening for antimicrobial activity. Journal of Ethnopharmacology 1991; 33 213–216.

[74] Ruckmani, K., Kavimani, S., Anandan, R. and Jaykar, B. Effect of *Moringa oleifera* Lam. on paracetamol-induced hepatoxicity. Indian Journal of Pharmaceutical Sciences 1998; 60 33–35.

[75] Prakash, A.O. Ovarian response to aqueous extract of *Moringa oleifera* during early pregnancy in rats. Fitoterapia 1988; 59 89–96.

[76] Karadi, R.V., Gadge, N.B., Alagawadi, K.R. and Savadi, R.V. Effect of *Moringa oleifera* Lam. root-wood on ethylene glycol induced urolithiasis in rats. Journal of Ethnopharmacology 2006; 105 306–311.

[77] Rao, C.V., Ojha, S.K. and Mehrotra, S. Analgesic effect of *Moringa oleifera* leaf extract on rats. In: Proceedings of the Second World Congress on Biotechnological Developments of Herbal Medicine, Lucknow, India; 2003. p. 42.

[78] Choudhary, M.K.; Bodakhe, S.H. and Gupta, S.K. Assessment of the antiulcer potential of *Moringa oleifera* root-bark extract in rats. Journal of Acupuncture and Meridian Studies 2013; 6(4) 214-220.

[79] Asare, G.A.; Gyan, B.; Bugyei, K., Adjei, S.A., Mahama, R.; Addo, P., Otu-Nyarko, L., Wiredu, E.K. and Nyarko, A. Toxicity potentials of the nutraceutical *Moringa oleifera* at supra-supplementation levels. Journal of Ethnopharmacology 2012; 139 265-272.

[80] Jideani, V. A. and Murevanhema, Y.Y. A Bambara groundnut milk beverage and probiotic yoghurt produced therefrom and a method for the production thereof. South Africa- Complete Patent 25 January 2013, 2013/00683.

[81] Jideani, V.A. & Diedericks, C.F. Dietary fibre from Bambara groundnuts (*Vigna subterranea*). South Africa Provisional Patent 14 June 2013, 2013/04395.

Chapter 9

Dietary Antioxidant Properties of Vegetable Oils and Nuts – The Race Against Cardiovascular Disease Progression

Wongama Given Pantsi, Dirk Jacobus Bester,
Adriaan Johannes Esterhuyse and
Guillaume Aboua

Additional information is available at the end of the chapter

http://dx.doi.org/10.5772/57184

1. Introduction

Cardiovascular disease (CVD) is a substantial and growing problem in most of the developing regions of the world. Evidence from experimental, clinical and epidemiological studies has unequivocally pointed to oxidative stress as the key culprit in the pathogenesis of CVD [1, 2]. CVD continues to remain a concern in developed countries and is a growing health concern worldwide. Although death rates from CVD have decreased in many countries due to advances in the field of medicine, the prevalence of CVD risk factors continues to increase. Diet is a centrally important, modifiable risk factor in the prevention of CVD [221-224].

The protection offered by foods is probably mediated through multiple beneficial nutrients contained in these foods, including mono- and polyunsaturated fatty acids, antioxidant vitamins, minerals, phytochemicals, fibre and plant protein. In dietary practice, healthy plant-based diets do not necessarily have to be low in fat. Instead, these diets may include unsaturated fats as the predominant form of dietary fat (e.g., fats from natural vegetable oils and nuts).

Consistent evidence suggests that diets rich in fruit and vegetables and other plant foods are associated with moderately lower overall mortality rates and lower death rates from chronic diseases including CVD [3- 6]. The 'antioxidant hypothesis' proposes that vitamin C, vitamin E, carotenoids and other antioxidant nutrients offer protection against CVD by decreasing oxidative damage [7-9]. As evidence began to mount from animal studies and human epidemiological studies on the potential protective effects of antioxidants, excitement in both the lay and medical communities also began to increase.

There has been a global increase in the use of medicinal plants that contain significant amounts of antioxidant-rich oils, offering multiple health benefits with fewer side effects compared to their synthetic counterparts. The idea is that natural compounds, if taken in supplement form, may offer a broad and inexpensive means of decreasing the risk for CVD. Natural products, such as vegetable oils and nuts, may be viewed as a cocktail of active ingredients that often have a synergistic effect on health. The (n-3) PUFAs have been shown in epidemiological and clinical trials to reduce the incidence of CVD. Large-scale epidemiological studies suggest that individuals at risk of coronary heart disease (CHD) benefit from the consumption of plant and marine derived (n-3) PUFAs, although the ideal intake is presently unclear. Overall, in view of the prevalence of CHD, consumption of (n-3) PUFA oils should be considered as a useful complementary option for the amelioration of CVD. Several researchers have shown encouraging findings on the protective effects of some vegetable oils and nuts. However, more research needs to be done with regards to the nutrients in these vegetable oils and nuts to elucidate the protective effects against CVD progression. This chapter focuses on the beneficial roles of antioxidant-rich vegetable oils and nuts in the management of CVD, their mechanisms of action and future prospects.

The term "cardiovascular disease (CVD)" encompasses the major clinical end-points related to the heart and vascular system, including ischaemic myocardium (heart failure and angina), myocardial infarction (heart attack), cerebrovascular disease (stroke), high blood pressure (hypertension), peripheral arterial disease (ischaemia of the limbs), arrhythmias, congenital heart disease and rheumatic heart disease. The facts are unequivocal and disturbing; CVD is the leading cause of death worldwide [10-12].

Chronic diseases are disorders with a long duration and generally slow progression. They comprise four major non-communicable diseases (NCDs) as listed by the World Health Organization (WHO), namely CVD, cancer, chronic respiratory disease and diabetes [13], which are now reaching epidemic proportions in low- and middle-income countries (LIMIC) of the world [14-18]. NCDs constitute the major global health burden of the 21st century [19-20] without discriminating among age groups [21]. Chronic diseases are implicated in 35 million deaths annually worldwide and a large portion of these deaths occurs due to CVD in LIMIC [22].

There is a rising epidemic of NCDs in sub-Saharan Africa (SSA). However, as in other LIMICs, individuals in SSA suffer from the dual burdens of infectious disease and NCDs [22, 23]. Walker and colleagues [24] reported that SSA continues to suffer under the weight of infectious diseases such as HIV and malaria, as well as high rates of undernutrition. Facing these issues in conjunction with the chronic diseases that accompany high rates of overnutrition is a daunting task [25] for the health burden in Africa. SSA has a disproportionate burden of both infectious and chronic diseases compared with other parts of the world [26]. South Africa (SA) is a country of great diversity extending from highly industrialized cities with an urban advanced-economy lifestyle to remote rural areas with more traditional lifestyles. SA, like many SSA countries, is not immune to the NCD epidemic accompanied by the continued burden of undernutrition. In SA, approximately 28% of deaths annually are attributed to

http://dx.doi.org/10.5772/57184

infectious diseases, while NCDs account for 25% of the lives lost [27]. The burden of diseases related to NCDs is predicted to rise substantially in SA over the next decade if necessary measures are not in place to combat the trend [28]. WHO estimates the burden from NCDs in SA to be two to three times higher than that in developed countries [13].

Approximately 35-65% of all deaths worldwide occur due to CVDs and death rates exceed these estimated figures owing to malnutrition and infections [29, 30]. CVDs and their risk factors are increasing in SSA [17, 31] with a high prevalence of ischaemic heart disease among men in their sixties followed by women of the same age group [17]. The common potential risk factors for NCDs are tobacco use, physical inactivity and an unhealthy diet, which all lead to CVD, diabetes and cancer [32, 33]. This burgeoning epidemic of NCDs has many root causes. Additional perpetuators of these epidemics are globalization and urbanization [34-37] with abdominal obesity contributing significantly to CVD in the SSA region [38]. Compelling evidence demonstrates a rise in mortality and morbidity from the NCDs in all strata of South African society. Leeder and colleagues [39] estimated that even without changes in the risk factor profile or the mortality rates from CVD, the demographic changes will result in a doubling of the number of cardiovascular deaths in SA by 2040. Chronic diseases such as CVD, obesity and diabetes have therefore become at least as important as infectious disease.

In summary, CVD is a substantial and growing problem in most of the developing regions of the world. The burden of NCD on the African continent and in SA in particular continues to demonstrate the potential for a sustained rise. A significant investment in the health care system and in particular the primary health care system is therefore justified. Further innovative strategies and plans are needed to address the determinants of this disease burden. However, indications still point to the paucity of community-based studies aimed at investigating NCD prevalence, incidence and risk factors. Consistent evidence suggests that diets rich in fruit and vegetables and other plant foods are associated with moderately lower overall mortality rates and lower death rates from chronic diseases including CVD [3-6]. The 'antioxidant hypothesis' proposes that carotenoids, polyphenols, vitamin C, vitamin E and other antioxidant nutrients afford protection against CVD by decreasing oxidative damage [7-9]. As the evidence began to mount from animal studies and human epidemiologic studies on potential protective effects of antioxidants, excitement in both the lay and medical communities also began to increase. The idea that natural compounds, if taken in supplement form, may offer a broad and inexpensive means of decreasing the risk for CVD and other age-related diseases is a very attractive hypothesis. Enthusiasm has grown to the point where people around the globe have become aware of the need to consume a diet with a high content of fruit and vegetables.

Indeed, evidence from experimental, clinical and epidemiologic studies has unequivocally pointed to oxidative stress as the key culprit in the pathogenesis of CVD [1, 2, 40, 41]. CVD continues to remain a significant problem in developed countries and is a growing health concern worldwide. Although death rates from CVD have decreased in many countries, due to advances in the field of medicine, the prevalence of CVD risk factors continues to increase. Diet is a centrally important, modifiable risk factor in the prevention of CVD [221-224].

2. Can vegetable oils and nuts be the natural solution for CVD?

Oxidative stress is common in many clinically important cardiac disorders, including ischaemia/reperfusion (I/R) injury, diabetes and hypertensive heart disease [42-46]. Several animal models suggest that when endogenous anti-oxidant systems are compromised, as is the case under oxidative stress conditions, exogenous antioxidant supplementation can be used for preventive and/or therapeutic intervention of CVD [42, 43, 47-49].

2.1. Composition and health benefits of vegetable oils

2.1.1. Dietary fats

Fats are the most concentrated form of energy for the body. They also aid in the absorption of fat-soluble vitamins (A, D, E and K) and other fat-soluble biologically active components [50]. Chemically, most of the fats in foods are triglycerides, made up of a unit of glycerol combined with free fatty acids, each of which may be the same or different. Other dietary fats include phospholipids, phytosterols and lipoproteins associated with cholesterol [50-52]. A balanced diet, including oils and fats that supply energy and essential fatty acids is needed for good health.

The different types of fatty acids are the most important characteristics of dietary fats. According to the degree of unsaturation (double bonds and hydrogen content), fatty acids are largely classified into three major types: saturated fatty acids, monounsaturated fatty acids (MUFA) and polyunsaturated fatty acids (PUFA). A fourth form, the trans fatty acids, are mainly produced by partial hydrogenation of polyunsaturated oils in food processing but also occur naturally in animal foods in small amounts [53].

Fatty acids consist of a hydrocarbon chain with a hydrophobic methyl group at one end and a hydrophilic carboxyl group at the other end. Greek letters (α, β, γ, ω) have been used to identify the location of the double bonds in fatty acids. The "alpha" carbon is the carbon closest to the carboxyl group. The methyl group of the molecule is also referred to as the omega end and the terminal carboxyl group is located at the delta end. Current chemical numerical terms number the carbon chain form one to "n", with n being the last carbon at the methyl end. The terms "n" and "omega" are synonymous [54].

2.1.2. Saturated fat

Saturated fatty acids contain no double bond; they are fully saturated with hydrogen. The main saturated fatty acids are lauric acid (C12:0), myristic acid (C14:0), palmitic acid (C16:0) and stearic acid (C18:0). Saturated fats are found in animal-based products, such as milk, cream, butter and cheese, meat from most land animals, palm oil and coconut oil, as well as manufactured products made from these, such as pies, biscuits, cakes and pastries [55].

2.1.3. Monounsaturated fat (MUFA)

MUFAs are predominant in vegetable oils, such as olive oil, canola oil and peanut oil and are also found in high proportions in animal fats [56]. Much of the interest in the role of MUFA in the prevention of coronary heart disease (CHD) stems from the observed beneficial effects of the Mediterranean diet [57], which includes high consumption of olive oil. MUFAs are less susceptible to oxidation when compared to PUFAs. This in turn leads to increased availability of antioxidants in the active form and better stability of olive oil [58-61]. Olive oil also contains some antioxidant micronutrients, namely polyphenols and squalene [58, 62-64]. The main MUFA in the human diet is oleic acid (C18:1n-9), which has one double bond. MUFA intake has been associated with a slight cardioprotective effect [65]. MUFAs are known to have a beneficial effect on the serum lipid profile and thus decrease the risk of CVD [66-68]. Furthermore, these fatty acids are stable in oxidative stress conditions and are less likely to react with reactive oxygen species (ROS) when compared with PUFA [58-59]. However, studies reporting associations between dietary intake of MUFAs and CHD risk have been inconclusive [69-71].

2.1.4. Polyunsaturated fat (PUFA)

PUFAs are naturally occurring endogenous substances, present in almost all tissues and are essential components of all mammalian cells. They are essential for survival and cannot be synthesized in the body. Hence, they have to be obtained in our diet and are therefore essential [54, 72]. There are two types of naturally occurring PUFAs in the body, the (n-6) PUFAs derived from linoleic acid (LA, C18:2) and the (n-3) PUFAs derived from α-linolenic acid (ALA, C18:3). They are categorized depending on the location of their first double bond: (n-3) PUFAs have their first double bond located at the third carbon molecule and (n-6) PUFAs at the sixth. Both of these two forms of PUFAs are metabolized by the same set of enzymes as their respective long-chain metabolites [73]. The differences between (n-3) and (n-6) PUFAs are shown in Table 1 below.

Vegetable oils are the predominant sources of alpha linolenic acid (ALA). ALA is found in legumes, flax seeds, walnuts, pinto beans, soybeans and spinach [74]. Dietary intake of ALA among Western adults is typically in the range of 0.5–2g/d [75]. The (n-6) PUFA is the main PUFA in most Western diets and is typically consumed in greater amounts than ALA [75, 76]. The evidence for a beneficial role of dietary (n-6) PUFAs is less convincing and for the purpose of this chapter we will focus on the (n-3) PUFA. The three main forms of (n-3) PUFAs are ALA, eicosapentaenoic acid (EPA, C20:5 n-3) and docosahexaenoic acid (DHA, C22:6 n-3) [77], with ALA being the simplest form. The (n-3) PUFAs are a family of biologically active fatty acids. The simplest member of this family, ALA, can be converted to the more biologically active and very long-chain (n-3) PUFAs; EPA and DHA. This process, as shown in Figure 1, occurs by a series of desaturation and elongation reactions, with stearidonic acid being an intermediate in the pathway [54, 75, 78].

Research has shown that long-chain (n-3) PUFAs protect against CVD [77, 79-82]. The cardioprotective effects of (n-3) PUFAs have long been recognized. Epidemiologic data suggest that (n-3) PUFAs derived from fish oil reduce CVD. Fish oil is a rich source of EPA (C20:5 n-3) and DHA (C22:6 n-3) (Table 1) [67, 83, 84]. The cardioprotective roles of these two forms of (n-3) PUFA are extensively reviewed by Bester and co-workers [48]. Fish oil may also reduce mortality after a cardiovascular incident, as it plays a role in reducing potentially fatal arrhythmias ([85-87]. There are several prospective studies relating the use of fish or the intake of long-chain (n-3) PUFAs to lower risk of CVD [88, 89]. Long chain (n-3) PUFAs have several beneficial cardiovascular properties, including antiatherothrombotic, antiarrhythmic, anti-inflammatory, antihypertensive and triglyceride lowering [81, 90, 91]. In summary, studies investigating the dietary roles of fatty acids demonstrate that dietary supplementation with (n-3) PUFAs decreases cardiac deaths, nonfatal cardiovascular events and all-cause mortality. These benefits are most apparent in high-risk patients. (n-3) PUFA supplementation appears to confer additional benefits in patients eating a Mediterranean diet.

The original observation is from almost 57 years ago, when Hugh M. Sinclair [92] published his observations on the negative effects of essential fatty acid deficiency on CVD. He strengthened his hypothesis by noting the low mortality rate from CHD (coronary heart disease) in Greenland Eskimos, a population consuming a high fat diet, but rich in (n-3) PUFAs [92]. Clinical studies suggest that (n-3) PUFAs reduce mortality from coronary heart disease and the rate of sudden cardiac death [92-95]. Significant antiarrhythmic effects of (n-3) PUFAs were observed in some but not all human studies on atrial fibrillation [96, 97]. In addition, animal studies show strong antiarrhythmic effects of (n-3) PUFAs [98-102].

	(n-3) PUFA	**(n-6) PUFA**
Molecular structure	First double-bond on the third carbon counting from the methyl end (the "nth" carbon)	First double-bond on the sixth carbon counting from the methyl end (the "nth" carbon)
Types	α-Linolenic acid (ALA) [C18:3] Eicosapentaenoic acid (EPA) [C20:5] Docosahexaenoic acid (DHA) [C22:6]	Linoleic acids (LA) [C18:2] Arachidonic acid (AA) [C20:4]
Food sources	Flaxseed oil (ALA) Canola oil (ALA) Soybean oil (ALA) Oily fish (EPA/DHA) Fish oil capsules (EPA/DHA)	Corn oil(LA) Soybean oil (LA) Sunflower oil (LA) Poultry (AA) Meats (AA)

Table 1. Molecular structure, types and food sources of (n-3) and (n-6) PUFAs.

Long-chain (n-3) PUFAs are important constituents of all cell membranes and confer on membranes properties of fluidity and thus, determine and influence the behaviour of membrane-bound enzymes and receptors [103-107]. These PUFAs are found in abundance in the myocardium, retina, brain and spermatozoa, and are essential for the proper functioning of these tissues and growth, being important modulators of many physiological processes. The fact that these tissues have developed the cellular machinery to preferentially incorporate these minor dietary components into their membranes suggests that these PUFAs play a role in the proper function of the cell [108-110].

The fatty acid composition of myocardial membrane phospholipids, in particular, is sensitive to the type of fatty acid consumed in the diet. Studies show that indeed the myocardium and

http://dx.doi.org/10.5772/57184

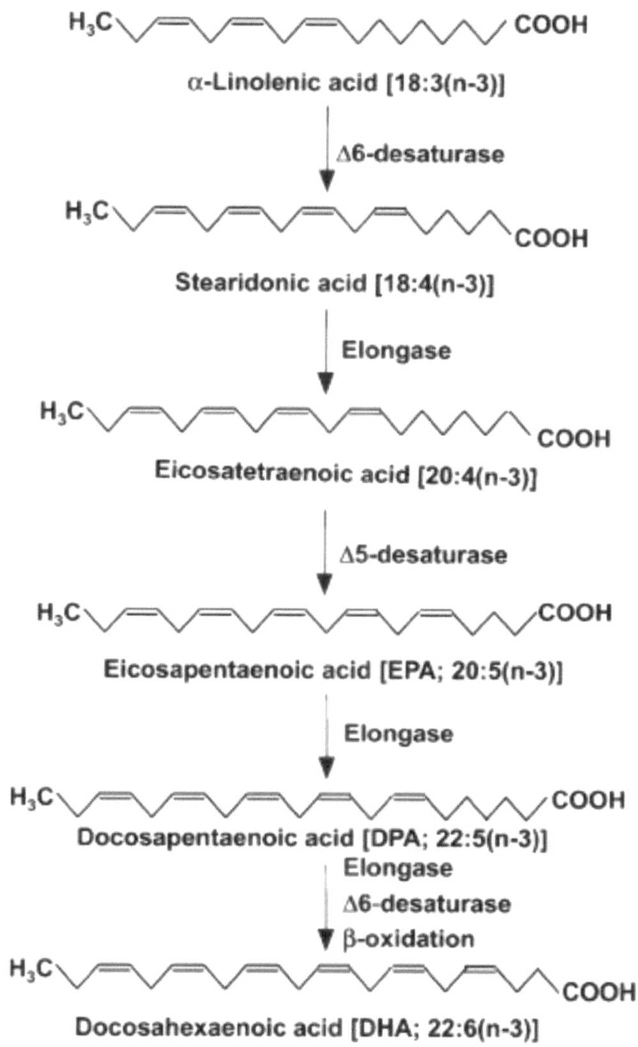

Figure 1. The biosynthesis of (n-3) PUFA.

myocardial membrane phospholipids are rich in (n-3) PUFAs after fish oil consumption [111, 112]. Diet-induced changes in the PUFA composition of a cell membrane have an impact on the cell's function, partly because these fatty acids represent a reservoir of molecules that perform important signalling roles within and between cells. In particular, dietary (n-3) PUFAs compete with dietary (n-6) PUFAs for incorporation into all cell membranes [113,114]. (n-3) PUFAs modulate the expression of adhesion proteins such as selectins [115] and exert an effect by modulating the intracellular signalling pathways associated with the control of transcription factors (e.g., nuclear factor-κB) and gene transcription [116,117]. Research has shown that enrichment of monocyte membranes with (n-3) PUFAs results in the synthesis and secretion of reduced quantities of cytokines (e.g., tumour necrosis factor-α, interleukin-1β) that are involved in the amplification of the inflammatory response [117,118]. Therefore, at a cellular level, (n-3) PUFAs from fish oils can directly or indirectly modulate a number of cellular activities associated with inflammation.

2.1.5. Polyphenols

Polyphenols constitute one of the most numerous and ubiquitously distributed groups of plant secondary metabolites, with more than 8000 phenolic structures currently known. Natural polyphenols can range from simple molecules (phenolic acids, phenylpropanoids, and flavonoids) to highly polymerised compounds (lignins, melanins, tannins), with flavonoids representing the most common and widely distributed sub-group [119]. These secondary plant metabolites are known to have potential antioxidant activity and radical scavenging capacity [120-124]. Polyphenols are gaining increased importance due to their beneficial effects on health. Flavonoids are the most abundant polyphenols in our diets. They can be divided into several classes according to the degree of oxidation of the oxygen heterocycle: flavones, flavonols, isoflavones, anthocyanins, flavanols, proanthocyanidins and flavanones [125]. A complication of the epidemiological observations regarding members of the flavonoid family is that subtle differences in their chemical structures can translate into marked differences in their absorption, metabolism and bioactivities [126]. South African herbal teas, rooibos (*Aspalathus linearis*) and honeybush (*Cyclopia ssp.*) are currently gaining popularity worldwide [127, 128], owing to their anti-oxidant, anti-cancer and anti-mutagenic properties [129-131]. Rooibos is a herbal tea made from the leaves and stems of the indigenous South African plant, *Aspalathus linearis* (*Brum.f*) *Dahlg.* (*family Fabaceae; tribe Crotalarieae*) [132,133]. Research has demonstrated that this herbal tea is rich in flavonoids [127, 134]. Animal studies that have investigated the cardioprotective effects of natural or synthetic flavonoids have focused mainly on the acute pharmacological activity of these compounds. For example, *in vivo* studies using animal models have reported acute cardioprotection obtained from intravenous injections of natural or synthetic flavonoids [135,136].

2.1.6. Vitamin E

Natural vitamin E is composed of eight chemical compounds: α-, β-, γ- and δ-tocopherols and their corresponding tocotrienols. α-Tocopherol is the most active form of vitamin E *in vitro*. The tocopherols are saturated forms of vitamin E, whereas the tocotrienols are unsaturated and have an isoprenoid side chain. Tocopherols possess a chromanol ring and a 15-carbon tail. The presence of three *trans* double bonds in the tail distinguishes tocopherols from tocotrienols [137-139]. This may account for the differences in their efficacy and potency *in vitro* and *in vivo* [140,141].

Red palm oil (RPO) is a rich source of vitamin E. It contains 560–1000 parts per million of vitamin E, of which approximately 18–22% are tocopherols and 78–82% tocotrienols [142-144]. RPO has been shown to offer protection against I/R injury [42, 43, 47, 48] leading to a reduction in oxidative stress [145]. It has also been suggested that palm oil may have some anti-arrhythmogenic effects, which may reduce sudden death after ischaemic incidents [146].

Of all the vegetable oils, RPO has the highest content of tocotrienols with γ-tocotrienol the most abundant. This form of vitamin E has been demonstrated to reduce cholesterol production and platelet aggregation [147-151]. RPO may also exert a neutral or positive effect on the serum lipid profile through the effects of its fatty acid composition and tocotrienols [152-155]. Investigations into vitamin E showed that tocotrienols are more potent than tocopherols as antioxidants. The tocotrienols present in palm oil have been shown to offer protection from myocardial I/R injury in an isolated perfused rat heart model [156, 157]. Animal studies with tocopherols and tocotrienols that investigate these compounds' potential against chronic diseases are extensively reviewed by Aggarwal and co-workers [158]. These authors argue that the evidence overwhelmingly suggests that tocotrienols may be superior in their biological properties than tocopherols and that their anti-inflammatory and antioxidant activities could prevent CVD among other chronic diseases.

2.1.7. Carotenoids

Carotenoids are nature's most widespread pigments, well known for their orange-red to yellow colours, which they impart to many fruits and vegetables. These fat-soluble phytochemicals have also received substantial attention because of their provitamin A and antioxidant roles [159]. Carotenoids are polyenoic terpenoids with conjugated trans double bonds. They include carotenes (β-carotene and lycopene), which are polyene hydrocarbons and xanthophylls (lutein, zeaxanthin, capsanthin, canthaxanthin, astaxanthin and violaxanthin) that have oxygen in the form of hydroxy, oxo, or epoxy groups [160]. The majority of the 600 carotenoids found in nature are 40 carbons in length and may be pure hydrocarbons, called carotenes, or possess oxygenated functional groups, in which case they are called xanthophylls [161]. The long-chain conjugated polyene structure accounts for the ability of these compounds to absorb visible light, but also makes them quite susceptible to oxidation. This latter property is closely related to their ability to act as antioxidants [162].

The properties and therefore functions of a carotenoid molecule are primarily dependent upon its structure and hence its chemistry [163]. In particular, the conjugated C = C double bond system is associated with energy transfer reactions, such as those found in photosynthesis [164]. In human plasma and tissues, several carotenoids have been well characterized including cyclic (such as β-carotene and α-carotene) and acyclic carotenes (such as lycopene and phytoene), together with a number of xanthophylls (such as zeaxanthin, lutein and beta-cryptoxanthin), all of which can be directly derived from dietary sources [165]. Carotenoids have generated considerable interest as several studies have suggested an inverse association between the dietary intake of carotenoids and the risk for CVD [166, 167]. Conversely prooxidant roles of these phytochemicals have also been reported [168-170].

2.1.8. Possible mechanism(s) of action

As mentioned earlier, RPO supplementation does offer protection against myocardial I/R injury via several suggested mechanisms. Amongst the proposed mechanisms are the NO–cyclic GMP pathway, phosphorylation of mitogen-activated protein kinases and scavenging of deleterious reactive oxygen species by RPO [42, 43, 47, 48].

Investigations concerning (n-3) PUFAs show that these forms of essential fatty acids reduce the risk of sudden cardiac death as well as fatal and nonfatal myocardial infarction [171-173]. A number of mechanisms have been implicated in the protective effects of (n-3) PUFAs [174, 175]. The (n-3) PUFAs have been demonstrated as altering the transcription of specific genes. These effects are mediated by a variety of mechanisms that involve indirect (i.e., by eicosanoids, hormones) and direct nuclear effects on genes. The PUFAs (i.e., both (n-3) and (n-6) PUFAs) modulate the expression of genes involved in lipogenesis, glycolysis, production of glucose transporters, inflammatory mediators, early response genes and genes for cell adhesion molecules [176, 177].

The primary source of MUFA that lowers cholesterol levels is olive oil [178, 179]. It is evident that olive oil, due to its micronutrient content and fatty acid composition, can play a vital role in maintaining beneficial serum lipid profiles. Together with its ability to reduce systemic oxidative stress, blood pressure and inflammation, it has become an appropriate dietary supplement for lowering the risk of CHD.

2.2. Composition and health benefits of nuts

Nuts are highly nutritious and of prime importance for people in several regions in Asia and Africa. Most nuts contain a great deal of fat (e.g., pecan 70%, macadamia nut 66%, Brazil nut 65%, walnut 60%, almonds 55% and peanut butter 55%). Most have a good protein content (in the 10–30% range) and only a few have a very high starch content [180]. Many nuts have also been identified as especially rich in antioxidants [181, 182]. Nuts therefore constitute one of the most nutritionally concentrated kinds of food available. Most nuts, left in their shell, have a remarkably long shelf life and can conveniently be stored for winter use [183]. Nuts are foods rich in fat, ranging from 46% in cashews and pistachios to 76% in macadamia nuts and provide 20–30 kJ/g per nut. Despite their high fat content, they are not harmful because they contain a low proportion (4–16%) of saturated fatty acids. Nearly one half of the fat content of nuts consists of unsaturated fatty acids, including both mono- (oleic acid) and poly- (linoleic and α-linolenic acid) unsaturated fatty acids (MUFA and PUFA respectively). The fatty fraction of nuts also contains plant sterols with anti-oxidants [184] and cholesterol-lowering effects [185]. Nuts are also rich sources of other bioactive macronutrients, such as protein (25% of energy) and dietary fibre, which ranges from 4 to 11g/100 g and in standard servings provide 5–10% of daily fibre requirements. They also contain significant micronutrients (Table 2), among them folate [185] antioxidant vitamins (e.g., tocopherols) and phenolic compounds [183].

By virtue of their unique composition, nuts are likely to benefit modern cardiovascular risk biomarkers, such as LDL oxidizability, soluble inflammatory molecules and endothelial dysfunction. The complex pathophysiology of atherosclerotic disease has evolved beyond the accumulation of cholesterol in the arterial wall. A series of circulating, functional, structural and genomic biological markers that reflect arterial vulnerability have been proposed as potential novel risk factors for the development of CVD (Vasan, 2006). Among them, biomarkers for oxidation [186], inflammation [187] and endothelial dysfunction [188] have received increasing attention.

http://dx.doi.org/10.5772/57184

Average nutrient composition of nuts (per 100 g)[1]

Nuts	Energy	Total fat	SFA	MUFA	PUFA	Plant sterols	Total protein	Arginine	Fiber	Folate	α-Tocopherol	Calcium	Magnesium	Potassium
	kJ	*g*	*g*	*g*	*g*	*mg*	*g*	*g*	*g*	*μg*	*mg*	*mg*	*mg*	*mg*
Almonds	2418	50.6	3.9	32.2	12.2	120	21.3	2.47	8.8	29	25.9	248	275	728
Brazil nuts	2743	66.4	15.1	24.5	20.6	NR	14.3	2.15	8.5	22	5.7	160	376	659
Cashews	2314	46.4	9.2	27.3	7.8	158	18.2	2.12	5.9	25	0.9	37	292	660
Hazelnuts	2629	60.8	4.5	45.7	7.9	96	15.0	2.21	10.4	113	15.0	114	163	680
Macadamias	3004	75.8	12.1	58.9	1.5	116	7.9	1.40	6.0	11	0.5	85	130	368
Peanuts (dry roasted)	2448	49.7	6.9	24.6	15.7	NR	23.7	3.1	8.0	145	6.9	54	176	658
Pecans	2889	72.0	6.2	40.8	21.6	102	9.2	1.18	8.4	22	1.4	70	121	410
Pine nuts (dried)	2816	68.4	4.9	18.8	34.1	141	13.7	2.41	3.7	34	9.3	16	251	597
Pistachios	2332	44.4	5.4	23.3	13.5	214	20.6	2.03	9.0	51	2.3	107	121	1025
Walnuts	2738	65.2	6.1	8.9	47.2	72	15.2	2.28	6.4	98	0.7	98	158	441

Table 2. Composition of Nuts (data from the US department of agriculture nutrient database)

Studies had shown that whole, unprocessed and unpeeled nuts have a unique composition that consists of important macro- and micronutrients, which give nuts their multiple beneficial effects on cardiovascular outcomes [189-192]. Most nut constituents have shown beneficial effects when clinically tested, in isolation or as part of enriched foods, for effects on diverse cardiovascular outcomes, including novel risk markers [189-192].

2.2.1. *Antioxidant effects*

Nuts are important sources of tocopherols and phenolic antioxidants, which protect against LDL oxidation [183]. Walnuts have been shown to contain substantial amounts of melatonin, which contributed to a significant antioxidant effect in an experimental rat model [193]. In addition, a substantial fraction of nut fat comes from MUFAs, which are not susceptible to oxidation. The PUFAs are contained mainly in walnuts and are more susceptible to oxidation. However, nuts are a rich source of many antioxidants, which protect the PUFA *in vivo* against oxidative modification [194].

2.2.2. *Anti-inflammatory effects*

Plasma high-sensitivity CRP, an accepted measure for systemic low-grade inflammation, was a secondary outcome in several controlled nut feeding trials conducted in hypercholesterolemic subjects with almonds [195-198] or walnuts [197, 199]. Some of them have demonstrated a CRP-lowering effect [196, 197, 198]. Zhao et al., who used walnuts and walnut oil to enrich the diet in PUFA and especially ALA, showed a decrease in inflammatory markers [197] and proinflammatory cytokine production by mononuclear cells [197].

2.2.3. *Effects on endothelial function*

Endothelial dysfunction is a critical event in atherogenesis and is implicated both in early disease and in advanced atherosclerosis [201]. Short-term feeding studies have shown consistently that diets rich in saturated fatty acids impair endothelial function [181, 202, 203] and that even a single fatty meal rich in saturated fatty acids is followed by transient endothelial dysfunction [204, 205]. These detrimental effects can be counteracted by the administration of PUFA and other nutrients contained in nuts, such as antioxidant vitamins and arginine [179]. Another feeding trial showed that, compared with an isoenergetic Mediterranean diet with similar saturated fatty acid content, a walnut diet attenuated the endothelial dysfunction associated with hypercholesterolemia [199]. Moreover, changes in circulating levels of cellular adhesion molecules critical to leukocyte recruitment on the arterial wall also reflect endothelial dysfunction [201]. Several studies have shown that diets enriched with ALA from walnuts [197, 199, 206] reduce endothelial activation as assessed by decreased plasma cellular adhesion molecules. Walnut feeding also reduced the expression of endothelin-1, a potent endothelial activator in an animal model of accelerated atherosclerosis [207].

2.2.4. Effects on body weight changes

As the interest in incorporating nuts into the diet grows, it is important that consumers understand how to include them in a healthy diet without promoting weight gain. They are high-fat, energy dense foods and are therefore a potential threat for contributing to positive energy balance. Numerous epidemiological and clinical studies have shown that nuts are not associated with higher body weight [208, 209] or weight gain [210-215]. This could be attributed along with other potential mechanisms for the high satiety properties of nuts [216]. The enhanced satiety, which is also achieved via other mechanisms such as the decreased eating rate [217], leads to reduced energy consumption and therefore a decreased risk of weight gain and obesity.

Blomhoff et al. [190] argued that the inverse association between nut intake and cardiovascular and coronary heart diseases in epidemiological studies may, or may not, be associated with antioxidants. According to these authors, epidemiologic studies are not ideally suited for studying the role of specific nuts or biological mechanisms. Nevertheless, they are in agreement with findings supporting the theory that a complex and rich mix of nut constituents is able to offer protection against CVD and perhaps other chronic diseases [183].

2.2.5. Possible mechanism(s) of action

Epidemiologic and clinical trial evidence has demonstrated the beneficial effect of nut consumption on coronary heart disease and its associated risk factors. The cardioprotective properties of nuts, due partially to their favourable lipid fatty acid profile (rich in unsaturated fatty acids), exceed the LDL-C lowering. Nuts, especially walnuts, contain (n-3) PUFAs, which have been shown to have a favourable impact on multiple factors related to CVD, such as inflammation, platelet function, arrhythmias, hypertriglyceridemia and nitric oxide-induced endothelial relaxation [218]. Nuts are also excellent sources of other bioactive compounds such as vegetable protein, dietary fibre, potassium, calcium, magnesium, tocopherols, phytosterols, phenolic compounds, resveratrol and arginine [179]. This unique nutrient composition explains the benefits of nut consumption for the prevention of CVD through mechanisms of oxidation, inflammation and vascular reactivity.

3. Conclusions and future directions

Investigation of the mechanisms underlying CVD showed that the disease has a complex cause beyond the accumulation of cholesterol on the arterial wall, with enhanced oxidative stress and a prominent inflammatory response. Diet has been shown to be associated with cardiovascular events. PUFAs are essential in our diet because we cannot synthesize them. They are also essential nutrients for optimal health of the cardiovascular, nervous and undoubtedly other organ systems. Dietary (n-3) PUFAs are incorporated into the cellular membranes of all tissues. The extent of incorporation into tissue membranes is dependent on dietary intake. The enrichment of membranes with (n-3) PUFAs can modulate cellular signalling events, membrane protein function and gene expression.

Interest in the possible health benefits of flavonoids has increased owing to their potent antioxidant and free-radical scavenging activities observed *in vitro*. There is growing evidence from human feeding studies that the absorption and bioavailability of specific flavonoids is much higher than originally believed. However, epidemiologic studies exploring the role of flavonoids in human health have been inconclusive. Some studies support a protective effect of flavonoid consumption in CVD and cancer; other studies demonstrate no effect and a few studies suggest potential harm. More recently, results from human studies provide evidence that rooibos can offer protection against oxidative stress conditions such as CVD [131,219]. In a study by Pantsi et al., the beneficial effects of dietary rooibos flavonoids were observed *ex vivo* in isolated perfused rat hearts. Epidemiological studies suggest that the beneficial cardiovascular health effects of diets rich in fruit and vegetables are in part mediated by their flavonoid content, with particular benefits provided by one member of this family, the flavonols [49].

Polyphenols are abundant micronutrients in our diet and evidence for their role in the prevention of degenerative diseases is emerging. Bioavailability differs greatly from one polyphenol to another, so the most abundant polyphenols in our diet are not necessarily those leading to the highest concentrations of active metabolites in target tissues. Because there are many biological activities attributed to the flavonoids, some of which could be beneficial or detrimental depending on specific circumstances, further studies in both the laboratory and with populations are warranted.

However, the fatty acid components of nuts may differently influence oxidation processes and this needs to be considered for the synergy or opposition to the effects of constituent antioxidants. There is growing evidence that dietary polyphenols in nuts, tea and wine may have anti-inflammatory effects, mediated by both their antioxidant action and modulation of signal transduction pathways, such as the nuclear transcription factor kB, with ensuing down-regulation of inflammatory genes in endothelial cells and macrophages [220]. The increased diversity and availability of sources of dietary fatty acids will likely allow the continued expansion of food products fortified with these fatty acids, a trend that may result in the attainment of the recommended dietary intake of these nutrients.

Future studies in oils should be carried out in order to elucidate the effects of oils in various models in which effects remain unknown. Little is known about the effects of nuts on a diseased heart. Studies should be performed to test whether nuts may offer protection against the severity or progression of various models of CVD.

Author details

Wongama Given Pantsi, Dirk Jacobus Bester, Adriaan Johannes Esterhuyse and Guillaume Aboua

Department of Biomedical Sciences, Faculty of Health and Wellness, Cape Peninsula University of Technology, Bellville, South Africa

References

[1] Ceconi C, Boraso A, Cargnoni A, Ferrari R. Oxidative stress in cardiovascular disease: myth or fact? *Biochemistry and Biophysics* 2003; 420: 217-221.

[2] Dalle-Donne I, Rossi R, Colombo R, Giustarini D, Milzani A. Biomarkers of oxidative damage in human disease. *Clin Chem* 2006; 52: 601–623.

[3] He FJ, Nowson CA, Lucas M, MacGregor GA. Increased consumption of fruit and vegetables is related to a reduced risk of coronary heart disease: meta-analysis of cohort studies. *J Hum Hypertens* 2007; 21: 717–728.

[4] Dembitsky VM, Poovarodom S, Leontowicz H, Leontowicz M, Vearasilp S, Traktenberg S. The multiple nutrition properties of some exotic fruits: Biological activity and active metabolites. *Food Research International* 2011; 44: 1671–1701.

[5] Devalaraja S, Jain S, Yadav H. Exotic fruits as therapeutic complements for diabetes, obesity and metabolic syndrome. *Food Research International* 2011; 44: 1856–1865.

[6] Sant'Ana AS. Special issue on exotic fruits. *Food Research International* 2011; 44: 1657.

[7] Rufino MSM, Ricardo E, Alves RE, Brito ES, Jiménez JP, Calixto FS et al. Bioactive compounds and antioxidant capacities of 18 non-traditional tropical fruits from Brazil. *Food Chemistry* 2010; 121: 996–1002.

[8] Borges GSC, Vieira FGK, Copetti C, Valdemiro GL, Zambiazi RC, Mancini Filho J. Chemical characterization, bioactive compounds, and antioxidant capacity of Jussara (Euterpe edulis) fruit from the Atlantic Forest in southern Brazil. *Food Research International* 2011; 44: 2128–2133.

[9] Coimbra MC, Jorge N. Proximate composition of guariroba (Syagrus oleracea), jerivá (Syagrus romanzoffiana) and macaúba (Acrocomia aculeata) palm fruits. *Food Research International* 2011; 44: 2139–2142.

[10] Yach D, Hawkes C, Gould CL, Hofman KJ. The global burden of chronic diseases: overcoming impediments to prevention and control. *JAMA* 2004; 291: 2616 –2622.

[11] Fuster V, Voute J. MDGs: chronic diseases are not on the agenda. *Lancet* 2005; 366: 1512-1514.

[12] Goyal A, Yusuf S. The burden of cardiovascular disease in the Indian subcontinent. *Indian J Med Res* 2006; 124: 235-244.

[13] World Health Organization. The Global Burden of Disease: 2004 Update. *Geneva: WHO*, 2008.

[14] Ezzati M, Vander Hoorn S, Lawes CM et al. Rethinking the 'diseases of affluence' paradigm: global patterns of nutritional risks in relation to economic development. *PLoS Med* 2005; 2: e133.

[15] Connor MD, Walker R, Modi G, Warlow CP. Burden of stroke in black populations in sub-Saharan Africa. *Lancet Neurol* 2007; 6: 269–278.

[16] Daar AS, Singer PA, Persad, et al. Grand challenges in chronic non-communicable diseases. *Nature* 2007; 450: 494-496.

[17] Mensah GA. Ischaemic heart disease in Africa. *Heart* 2008; 94: 836–843.

[18] Parkin DM, Sitas F, Chirenje M et al. Cancer in indigenous Africans—burden, distribution and trends. *Lancet Oncol* 2008; 9: 683–692.

[19] Alwan A, Maclean DR, Riley LM, d'Espaignet ET, Mathers CD, Stevens GA, Bettcher D, Narayan KM, Ali MK, Koplan JP. Global noncommunicable disease - where worlds meet. *N Engl J Med* 2010; 363: 1196-1198.

[20] Beaglehole R, Horton R. Chronic diseases: global action must match global evidence. *Lancet* 2010; 376: 1619-1621.

[21] Narayan KM, Ali MK, Koplan JP. Global noncommunicable diseases - where worlds meet. *N Engl J Med* 2010;363:1196-1198.

[22] Lopez AD, Mathers CD, Ezzati M, Jamison DT, Murray CJ. Global and regional burden of disease and risk factors, 2011: systematic analysis of population health data. *Lancet* 2006; 367: 1747-1757.

[23] Mathers CD, Loncar D. Projections of global mortality and burden of disease from 2002 to 2030. *PLoS Med* 2006; 3: e442.

[24] Walker A, Walker B, Segal I. Some puzzling situations in the onset, occurrence and future of coronary heart disease in developed and developing populations, particularly such in sub-Saharan Africa. *Journal of the Royal Society for the Promotion of Health* 2004; 124: 40–46.

[25] Salman Z, Kirk G, DeBoer M. High rate of obesity-associated hypertension among primary schoolchildren in Sudan. *International Journal of Hypertension, Volume* 2011, Article ID 629492, 5 pp.

[26] Dalal S, Beunza JJ, Volmink J, Adebamowo C, Bajunirwe F, Njelekela M, Mozaffarian D, Fawzi W, Willet W, Adami H, Holmes MD. Non-communicable disease in sub-Saharan Africa: what we know. *International Journal of Epidemiology* 2011; 40: 885-901.

[27] Steyn K, Bradshaw D, Norman R, Laubscher R. Determinants and Treatment of Hypertension in South Africa/Determinants of Hypertension and Its Treatment in South Africa During 1998: The First Demographic and Health Survey. *Tygerburg, South Africa: South Africa Medical Research Council*; 2003.

[28] Abegunde DO, Mathers CD, Adam T, Ortegon M, Strong K. The burden and costs of chronic diseases in low-income and middle-income countries. *Lancet* 2007; 370: 1929–1938.

[29] Critchley J, Liu J, Zhao D, Wei W, Capewell S. Explaining the increase in coronary heart disease mortality in Beijing between 1984 and 1999. *Circulation* 2004; 110: 1236–1244.

[30] Gaziano T. Global burden of cardiovascular disease. Braunwald's Heart Disease: A Textbook of Cardiovascular Medicine, 8th ed. Saunders; 2008: 1–22.

[31] Vorster HH. The emergence of cardiovascular disease during urbanisation of Africans. *Public Health Nutr* 2002; 5: 239–243.

[32] Medical Research Council. South Africa Demographic and Health Survey 2003. Pretoria: Department of Health, 2007.

[33] Norman R, Bradshaw D, Schneider M, et al. and the SA CRA Collaborating Group. A Comparative risk assessment for South Africa in 2000: towards promoting health and preventing disease. *S Afr Med J* 2007; 97: 637–641.

[34] Misra A, Khurana L. Obesity and the metabolic syndrome in developing countries. *Journal of Clinical Endocrinology and Metabolism* 2008; 93: S9–S30.

[35] Abdulai A. Socio-economic characteristics and obesity in underdeveloped economies: does income really matter? *Applied Economics* 2010; 42: 157–169.

[36] Maher D, Smeeth L, Sekajugo J. Health transition in Africa: practical policy proposals for primary care. *Bulletin of the World Health Organization* 2010; 88: 943–948.

[37] Greenberg H, Raymond S, Leeder S. The prevention of global chronic disease: academic health's new frontier. *American Journal of Public Health* 2011; 101: 1386–1391.

[38] Steyn K, Sliwa K, Hawken S et al. Risk factors associated with myocardial infarction in Africa: the INTERHEART Africa study. *Circulation* 2005; 112: 3554–3561.

[39] Leeder SR, Raymond SU, Greenberg H. A race against time: the challenge of cardiovascular diseases in developing economies. *New York: Columbia University*, 2004.

[40] Manikandan P, Sumitra M, Aishwarya S, Manohar BM, Lokanadam B, Puvanakrishnan R. Curcumin modulates free radical quenching in myocardial ischaemia in rats. *Int J Biochem Cell Biol* 2004; 36: 1967–1980.

[41] Ungvari Z, Gupte SA, Recchia FA, Batkai S, Pacher P. Role of oxidative-nitrosative stress and downstream pathways in various forms of cardiomyopathy and heart failure. *Curr Vasc Pharmacol* 2005; 3: 221–229.

[42] Esterhuyse AJ, du Toit EF, Benade AJS, van Rooyen J. Dietary red palm oil improves reperfusion cardiac function in the isolated perfused rat heart of animals fed a high cholesterol diet. *Prostaglandins, Leukotrienes and Essential Fatty Acids* 2005; 72: 153 161.

[43] Engelbrecht AM, Esterhuyse J, du Toit EF, Lochner A, van Rooyen J. p38-MAPK and PKB/Akt, possible role players in red palm oil-induced protection of the isolated perfused rat heart? *Journal of Nutritional Biochemistry* 2006; 17: 265-271.

[44] Qin CX, Williams SJ, Woodman OL. Antioxidant activity contributes to flavonol cardioprotection during reperfusion of rat hearts. *Free Radical Biology and Medicine* 2011; 51: 7-1437.

[45] Yu E, Mercer J, Bennett M. Mitochondria in vascular disease, *Cardiovascular Research* 2012; 95: 2-173.

[46] Morsy MD, Bashir SO. Alpha-tocopherol ameliorates oxidative renal insult associated with spinal cord reperfusion injury. *Journal of Physiology and Biochemistry* 2013; 69, 3-487.

[47] Kruger M, Engelbrecht AM, Esterhuyse J, du Toit EF, van Rooyen J. Dietary Red Palm Oil (RPO) reduces ischaemia/reperfusion injury in a hypercholesterolemic diet. *Br J Nutr* 2007; 97: 653-660.

[48] Bester D, Esterhuyse AJ, Truter EJ, van Rooyen J. Cardiovascular effects of edible oils: a comparison between four popular edible oils. *Nutrition Research Reviews* 2010; 23: 334–348.

[49] Pantsi WG, van Rooyen J, Marnewick JL, Esterhuyse AJ, Rautenbach F. Rooibos (Aspalathus linearis) offers cardiac protection against ischaemia/reperfusion in the isolated perfused rat heart. *Phytomedicine* 2011; 18: 1220–1228.

[50] Fahy E, Subramaniam S, Murphy RC, et al. Update of the LIPID MAPS comprehensive classification system for lipids. *J Lipid Res* 2009; 50(suppl): S9–S14.

[51] Quehenberger O, Armando AM, Brown AH, et al. Lipidomics reveals a remarkable diversity of lipids in human plasma. *J Lipid Res*. 2010; 51: 3299-3305.

[52] Quehenberger O, Dennis EA. The human plasma lipidome. *N Engl J Med*. 2011; 365: 1812-1823.

[53] Innis SM. Dietary triacylglycerol structure and its role in infant nutrition. *Adv Nutr.* 2011; 2: 275-283.

[54] Das UN. Essential fatty acids: Biochemistry, physiology, and pathology. *Biotechnology J* 2006; 1: 420-439.

[55] Hu FB, Stampfer MJ, Manson JE, Ascherio A, Colditz GA, Speizer FE, et al. Dietary saturated fats and their food sources in relation to the risk of coronary heart disease in women. *Am J Clin Nutr* 1999; 70: 1001–1008.

[56] Guthrie HA, Pcciano MF. Human nutrition. Boston, MA7 WCB/ McGraw Hill; 1995, pp. 419.

[57] Keys A. Mediterranean diet and public health: personal reflections. *Am J Clin Nutr* 1995; 61: 1321S–1323S.

[58] Owen RW, Mier W, Giacosa A, et al. Phenolic compounds and squalene in olive oils: the concentration and antioxidant potential of total phenols, simple phenols, secoiridoids, lignans and squalene. *Food Chem Toxicol* 2000; 38: 647–659.

[59] Diniz YSA, Cicogna AC, Padovani CR, et al. Diets rich in saturated and polyunsaturated fatty acids: metabolic shifting and cardiac health. *Nutrition* 2004; 20: 230–234.

[60] Wahle KW, Caruso D, Ochoa JJ, et al. Olive oil and modulation of cell signaling in disease prevention. *Lipids* 2004; 39: 1223–1231.

[61] Eder E, Wacker M, Lutz U, et al. Oxidative stress related DNA adducts in the liver of female rats fed with sunflower-, rapeseed-, olive- or coconut oil supplemented diets. *Chem Biol Interact* 2006; 159: 81–89.

[62] Newmark HL. Squalene, olive oil, and cancer risk: a review and hypothesis. *Cancer Epidemiol Biomarkers Prev* 1997; 6: 1101–1103.

[63] Quiles JL, Ochoa JJ, Ramirez-Tortosa C, et al. Dietary fat type (virgin olive vs. sunflower oils) affects age-related changes in DNA double-strand-breaks, antioxidant capacity and blood lipids in rats. *Exp Gerontol* 2004; 39: 1189–1198.

[64] Caravaca AMG, Pancorbo AC, Diaz BC, et al. Electrophoretic identification and quantitation of compounds in the polyphenolic fraction of extra-virgin olive oil. *Electrophoresis* 2005; 26: 3538–3551.

[65] Hu FB, Stampfer MJ, Manson JE, Rimm E, Colditz GA, Rosner BA, et al. Dietary fat intake and the risk of coronary heart disease in women. *New Engl J Med* 1997; 337: 1491–149.

[66] Heyden S. Polyunsaturated and monounsaturated fatty acids in the diet to prevent coronary heart disease via cholesterol reduction. *Ann Nutr Metab* 1994; 38: 117–122.

[67] Demonty I, Chan YM, Pelled D, et al. Fish-oil esters of plant sterols improve the lipid profile of dyslipidemic subjects more than do fish-oil or sunflower oil esters of plant sterols. *Am J Clin Nutr* 2006; 84: 1534–1542.

[68] Metcalf RG, James MJ, Gibson RA, et al. Effects of fish-oil supplementation on myocardial fatty acids in humans. *Am J Clin Nutr* 2007; 85: 1222–1228.

[69] McGee DL, Reed DM, Yano K, Kagan A, Tillotson J. Ten-year incidence of coronary heart disease in the Honolulu Heart Program. Relationship to nutrient intake. *Am J Epidemiol* 1984; 119: 667–676.

[70] Pietinen P, Ascherio A, Korhonen P, Hartman AM, Willett WC, Albanes D, et al. Intake of fatty acids and risk of coronary heart disease in a cohort of Finnish men. The Alpha-Tocopherol, Beta-Carotene Cancer Prevention Study. *Am J Epidemiol* 1997; 145: 876–87.

[71] Jakobsen MU, Overvad K, Dyerberg J, Schroll M, Heitmann BL. Dietary fat and risk of coronary heart disease: possible effect modification by gender and age. *Am J Epidemiol* 2004; 160: 141–149.

[72] Lerman RH. Essential fatty acids. *Altern Ther Health Med* 2006;12: 20-29.

[73] Das UN. Essential fatty acids and their metabolites could function as endogenous HMG-CoA reductase and ACE enzyme inhibitors, anti-arrhythmic, anti-hypertensive, antiatherosclerotic, anti-inflammatory, cytoprotective, and cardioprotective molecules. *Lipids Health Dis* 2008; 7: 37.

[74] Simopoulos AP. Summary of the NATO advanced research workshop on {omega} 3 and {omega} 6 fatty acids: Biological effects and nutritional essentiality. *J Nutr* 1989; 119: 521-528.

[75] Burdge GC, Calder PC. Dietary α-linolenic acid and health-related outcomes: a metabolic perspective. *Nutr Res Rev* 2006; 19: 26–52.

[76] Blasbalg TL, Hibbeln JR, Ramsden CE, Majchrzak SF, Rawlings RR. Changes in consumption of omega-3 and omega-6 fatty acids in the United States during the 20th century. *Am J Clin Nutr.* 2011; 93: 950–962.

[77] De Caterina R, Massaro M. Omega-3 fatty acids and the regulation of expression of endothelial pro-atherogenic and pro-inflammatory genes. *J Membr Biol* 2005; 206: 103 -116.

[78] Calder PC. Mechanisms of Action of (n-3) Fatty Acids. *J. Nutr* 2012; 142: 592S–599S.

[79] Kris-Etherton PM, Harris WS, Appel LJ. Fish consumption, fish oil, omega-3 fatty acids, and cardiovascular disease. *Circulation* 2002; 106: 2747–2757.

[80] Lands WE. Dietary fat and health: the evidence and the politics of prevention: careful use of dietary fats can improve life and prevent disease. *Ann N Y Acad Sci* 2005; 1055: 179–192.

[81] Lee JH, O'Keefe JH, Lavie CJ, Marchioli R, Harris WS. Omega-3 fatty acids for cardioprotection. *Mayo Clin Proc* 2008; 83: 324–332.

[82] Lavie CJ, Milani RV, Mehra MR, Ventura HO. Omega-3 polyunsaturated fatty acids and cardiovascular diseases. *J Am Coll Cardiol* 2009; 54: 585–594.

[83] Dahl L, Bjorkkjaer T, Graff IE, et al. Fish – more than just omega 3. Tidsskr *Nor Laegeforen* 2006; 126: 309–311.

[84] Conde CMS, Cyrino FZGA, Bottino DA, et al. Longchain n-3 polyunsaturated fatty acids and microvascular reactivity: observation in the hamster cheek pouch. *Microvasc Res* 2007; 3: 237–247.

[85] McLennan PL. Relative effects of dietary saturated, monounsaturated, and polyunsaturated fatty acids on cardiac arrhythmias in rats. *Am J Clin Nutr* 1993; 57: 207-212.

[86] Mclennan PL, Abeywardena MY. Membrane basis for fish oil effects on the heart: linking natural hibernators to prevention of human sudden cardiac death. *Membrane Biol* 2005; 206: 85–102.

[87] Hlavackova M, Neckar J, Jezkova J, et al. Dietary polyunsaturated fatty acids alter myocardial protein kinase-C expression and affect cardioprotection induced by chronic hypoxia. *Exp Biol Med* 2007; 232: 823–832.

[88] Mozaffarian D, Lemaitre RN, Kuller LH, Burke GL, Tracy RP, Siscovick DS. Cardiac benefits of fish consumption may depend on the type of fish meal consumed: the cardiovascular health study. *Circulation* 2003; 107: 1372–1377.

[89] He K, Song Y, Daviglus ML, Liu K, Van Horn L, Dyer AR, et al. Accumulated evidence on fish consumption and coronary heart disease mortality: a meta-analysis of cohort studies. *Circulation* 2004; 109: 2705–11.

[90] Anand RG, Alkadri M, Lavie CJ, et al. The role of fish oil in arrhythmia prevention. *J Cardiopulm Rehabil Preven*. 2008; 28: 92–98.

[91] Jung UJ, Torrejon C, Tighe AP, et al. n-3 Fatty acids and cardiovascular disease: mechanisms underlying beneficial effects. *Am J Clin Nutr*. 2008; 87: S2003–2009.

[92] Sinclair HM. Deficiency of essential fatty acids and atherosclerosis, etcetera. *Lancet* 1956; 270: 381–383.

[93] Leaf A, Kang JX, Xiao YF, Billman GE. Clinical prevention of sudden cardiac death by n-3 polyunsaturated fatty acids and mechanism of prevention of arrhythmias by n-3 fish oils. *Circulation* 2003; 107: 2646–2652.

[94] Mozaffarian D. Fish and n-3 fatty acids for the prevention of fatal coronary heart disease and sudden cardiac death. *Am J Clin Nutr* 2008; 87: 1991S–1996S.

[95] Mozaffarian D, Wu JH. Omega-3 fatty acids and cardiovascular disease: effects on risk factors, molecular pathways, and clinical events. *J Am Coll Cardiol.* 2011; 58: 2047-2067.

[96] Calo L, Bianconi L, Colivicchi F, et al. N-3 fatty acids for the prevention of atrial fibrillation after coronary artery bypass surgery: a randomized, controlled trial. *J Am Coll Cardiol* 2005; 45: 1723–1728.

[97] Virtanen JK, Mursu J, Voutilainen S, Tuomainen TP. Serum long-chain n-3 polyunsaturated fatty acids and risk of hospital diagnosis of atrial fibrillation in men. *Circulation* 2009; 120: 2315–2321.

[98] Matthan NR, Jordan H, Chung M, Lichtenstein AH, Lathrop DA, Lau J. Asystematic review and meta-analysis of the impact of omega-3 fatty acids on selected arrhythmia outcomes in animal models. *Metabolism* 2005; 54: 1557–1565.

[99] Sarrazin JF, Comeau G, Daleau P, et al. Reduced incidence of vagally induced atrial fibrillation and expression levels of connexins by n-3 polyunsaturated fatty acids in dogs. *J Am Coll Cardiol* 2007; 50: 1505–1512.

[100] Fischer R, Dechend R, Qadri F, et al. Dietary n-3 polyunsaturated fatty acids and direct renin inhibition improve electrical remodeling in a model of high human renin hypertension. *Hypertension* 2008; 51: 540–546.

[101] Gao JY, Yasuda S, Tsuburaya R, et al. Long-term treatment with eicosapentaenoic acid ameliorates myocardial ischemia–reperfusion injury in pigs in vivo. *Circ J* 2011; 75: 1843–1851.

[102] Kitamura K, Shibata R, Tsuji Y, Shimano M, Inden Y, Murohara T. Eicosapentaenoic acid prevents atrial fibrillation associated with heart failure in a rabbit model. *Am J Physiol Heart Circ Physiol* 2011; 300: H1814–H1821.

[103] Stubbs CD, Smith AD. The modification of mammalian membrane polyunsaturated fatty acid composition in relation to membrane fluidity and function. *Biochim Biophys Acta*. 1984; 779: 89–137.

[104] Murphy MG. Dietary fatty acids and membrane protein function. *J Nutr Biochem.* 1990; 1: 68–79.

[105] Yaqoob P. The nutritional significance of lipid rafts. *Annu Rev Nutr.* 2009; 29: 257–282.

[106] Das UN. Metabolic Syndrome Pathophysiology: The Role of essential fatty acids and their metabolites. *Ames, IA, USA: Wiley-Blackwell Publishers*; 2010.

[107] Das UN. Molecular Basis of Health and Disease. *New York: Springer*; 2011.

[108] Zuijdgeest-van Leeuwen SD, Dagnelie PC, Rietveld T, et al. Incorporation and washout of orally administered n-3 fatty acid ethyl esters in different plasma lipid fractions. *Br J Nutr* 1999; 82: 481-488.

[109] Connor WE. Importance of n-3 fatty acids in health and disease. *Am J Clin Nutr* 2000; 71: 171–175S.

[110] Surette ME, Koumenis IL, Edens MB, et al. Inhibition of leukotriene synthesis, pharmacokinetics, and tolerability of a novel dietary fatty acid formulation in healthy adult subjects. *Clin Ther* 2003; 25: 948-971.

[111] Nair SS, Leitch J, Falconer J, Garg ML. Cardiac (n-3) nonesterified fatty acids are selectively increased in fish oil-fed pigs following myocardial ischemia. *J Nutr* 1999; 129: 1518–1523.

[112] McLennan PL. Myocardial membrane fatty acids and the antiarrhythmic actions of dietary fish oil in animal models. *Lipids* 2001; 36: S111–114S.

[113] Healy DA, Wallace FA, Miles EA, et al. Effect of low-to-moderate amounts of dietary fish oil on neutrophil lipid composition and function. *Lipids* 2000; 35: 763-768.

[114] Calder PC. n-3 polyunsaturated fatty acids, inflammation and inflammatory diseases. *Am J Clin Nutr* 2006; 83: 1505S-1519S.

[115] De Caterina R, Massaro M. Omega-3 fatty acids and the regulation of expression of endothelial pro-atherogenic and pro-inflammatory genes. *J Membr Biol* 2005; 206: 103 -116.

[116] Weber C, Erl W, Pietsch A, et al. Docosahexaenoic acid selectively attenuates induction of vascular cell adhesion molecule-1 and subsequent monocytic cell adhesion to human endothelial cells stimulated by tumor necrosis factor-alpha. *Arterioscler Thromb Vasc Biol* 1995; 15: 622-628.

[117] Novak TE, Babcock TA, Jho DH, et al. NF-kappa B inhibition by omega-3 fatty acids modulates LPS-stimulated macrophage TNF-alpha transcription. *Am J Physiol Lung Cell Mol Physiol* 2003; 284: L84-L89.

[118] Caughey GE, Mantzioris E, Gibson RA, et al. The effect on human tumor necrosis factor alpha and interleukin 1 beta production of diets enriched in n-3 fatty acids from vegetable oil or fish oil. *Am J Clin Nutr* 1996; 63: 116-122.

[119] Bravo L. Polyphenols: chemistry, dietary sources, metabolism, and nutritional significance, *Nutr. Rev.* 1998; 56: 317–333.

[120] Higdon JV, Frei B. Tea catechins and polyphenols: health effects, metabolism, and antioxidant functions. *Critical Reviews in Food Science and Nutrition* 2003; 43: 89–143.

[121] Yilmaz Y. Novel uses of catechins in foods. *Trends in Food Science and Technology* 2006; 17: 64–71.

[122] Lobo V, Patil A, Phatak A, Chandra N. Free radicals, antioxidants and functional foods: impact on human health. *Pharmacognosy Review* 2010; 4: 118–126.

[123] Wootton-Beard PC, Ryan L. Improving public health? The role of antioxidant-rich fruit and vegetable beverages. *Food Research and Technology* 2011; 44: 3135–3148.

[124] Ignat I, Volf I, Popa VI. A critical review of methods for characterisation of polyphenolic compounds in fruits and vegetables. *Food Chemistry* 2012; 126: 1821–1835.

[125] Heiss C, Keen CL, Kelm M. Flavanols and cardiovascular disease prevention. *European Heart Journal* 2010; 31: 2583–2592.

[126] Erdman JW Jr, Balentine D, Arab L, Beecher G, Dwyer JT, Folts J, Harnly J, Hollman P, Keen CL, Mazza G, Messina M, Scalbert A, Vita J, Williamson G, Burrowes J. Flavonoids and heart health: proceedings of the ILSI North America Flavonoids Workshop, May 31–June 1, 2005, Washington, DC. *J Nutr* 2007; 137: 718S–737S.

[127] Joubert E, Joubert ME, Bester C, De Beer D, De Lange JH. Honeybush(Cyclopia spp.): From local cottage industry to global markets – the catalytic and supporting role of research. *South African Journal of Botany* 2011; 77: 887–907.

[128] Joubert E, De Beer D. Rooibos (Aspalathus linearis) beyond farm gate: from herbal tea to potential phytopharmaceutical. *South African Journal of Botany* 2011; 77: 869–886.

[129] Joubert E,Gelderblom WC, Louw A, De Beer D. South African herbal teas: Aspalathus linearis, Cyclopia spp. and Athrixia phylicoides–a review. *Journal of Ethnopharmacology* 2008a; 119: 376–412.

[130] Joubert E, Gelderblom WC, De Beer D. Phenolic contribution of South African herbal teas to a healthy diet. *Natural Product Communications* 2009; 4: 701–718.

[131] Marnewick JL, Rautenbach F, Venter I, Neethling H, Blackhurst DM, Wolmarans P, Macharia M. Effects of rooibos (Aspalathus linearis) on oxidative stress and biochemical parameters in adults at risk for cardiovascular disease. *J. Ethnopharmacol.* 2011; 133: 46–52.

[132] McKay DL, Bloemberg JB. A review of the bioactivity of South African herbal teas: Rooibos (Aspaluthus Linearis) and Honeybush (Cyclopia intermedia). *Physiother. Res* 2007; 21: 1–16.

[133] Marnewick JL. Rooibos and honeybush: recent advances in chemistry, biological activity and pharmacological activity and pharmacogynosy. In: Juliana HR, Simon JE, Ho CT. (Eds.), African Natural Plant Products: New Discoveries and Challenges in Chemistry and Quality. ACS Symposium Series, 1021. *Oxford University Press*, 2009; pp. 277–294.

[134] Bramati L, Minoggio M, Gardana C, Simonetti P, Mauri P, Pietta P. Quantitative characterization of flavonoid compounds in rooibos tea (Aspalathus linearis) by LC–UV/DAD. J. *Agric. Food Chem.* 2002; 50: 5513–5519.

[135] Ji ES, Yue H, Wu YM, He RR. Effects of phytooestrogen genistein on myocardial ischaemia reperfusion and apoptosis in rabbits. *Acta Pharmacol. Sin* 2004; 25; 306–312.

[136] Wang S, Dusting GJ, May CN, Woodman OL. 3_,4_-Dihydroxyflavonol reduces infarct size and injury associated with myocardial ischaemia and reperfusion in sheep. *Br. J. Pharmacol.* 2004; 42: 352–443.

[137] Qureshi AA, Sami SA, Salser WA, Khan FA. Synergistic effect of tocotrienol-rich fraction (TRF(25)) of rice bran and lovastatin on lipid parameters in hypercholesterolemic humans. *J Nutr Biochem* 2001; 12: 318–329.

[138] Qureshi AA, Sami SA, Salser WA, Khan FA. Dose-dependent suppression of serum cholesterol by tocotrienol-rich fraction (TRF25) of rice bran in hypercholesterolemic humans. Atherosclerosis 2002; 161: 199–207.

[139] Sen CK, Khanna S, Rink C, Roy S. Tocotrienols: the emerging face of natural vitamin E. *Vitam Horm* 2007; 76: 203–261.

[140] Serbinova E, Kagan V, Han D, Packer L. Free radical recycling and intramembrane mobility in the antioxidant properties of alpha-tocopherol and alpha-tocotrienol. *Free Radic Biol Med* 1991; 10: 263–275.

[141] Yoshida Y, Niki E, Noguchi N. Comparative study on the action of tocopherols and tocotrienols as antioxidant: chemical and physical effects. *Chem Phys Lipids* 2003; 123: 63–75.

[142] Nagendran B, Unnithan UR, Choo YM. Characteristics of red palm oil, a-carotene- and vitamin E-rich refined oil for food uses. *Food Nutr Bull* 2000; 2: 189–194.

[143] Sundram K, Sambanthamurthi R, Tan YA. Palm fruit chemistry. *Asia Pac J Clin Nutr* 2003; 12: 355–362.

[144] Schroeder MT, Becker EM, Skibsted LH. Molecular mechanism of antioxidant synergism of tocotrienols and carotenoids in palm oil. *J Agric Food Chem* 2006; 54: 3445–3453.

[145] Narang D, Sood S, Thomas MK, et al. Effect of dietary palm oil on oxidative stress associated with ischaemic–reperfusion injury in isolated rat heart. *BMC Pharmacol* 2004; 4: 29.

[146] Charnock JS, Sundram K, Abeywardena MY et al. Dietary fats and oils in cardiac arrhythmia in rats. *Am J Clin Nutr* 1991; 53: 1047S–1049S.

[147] Steiner M, Anatasi J. Vitamin E and platelet aggregation. *J Clin Invest* 1975; 57: 732–737.

http://dx.doi.org/10.5772/57184

[148] Chan AC, Leith MK. Decreased prostacyclin synthesis in vitamin E deficient rabbit aorta. *Am J Clin Nutr* 1981; 34: 2341–2347.

[149] Helub BJ, Sicilia I, Mahadevappa VG. Effect of tocotrienol derivatives on collagen and ADP-induced plasma platelet aggregation. Abstracts, PORUM International Palm Oil Development Conference, 1989; 5–9 September, Kuala Lumpur, N 9.

[150] Qureshi AA, Qureshi N, Weight JJK, et al. Lowering of serum cholesterol in hypercholesterolaemic humans by tocotrienols (palmvitee). *Am J Clin Nutr* 1991; 53: 1021S–1026S.

[151] Pearce BC, Parker RA, Deason ME, et al. Hypocholesterolaemic activity of synthetic and natural tocotrienols. *J Med Chem* 1992; 35: 3595–3606.

[152] Hornstra G. Dietary lipids and cardiovascular disease: effects of palm oil. *Oleagineux* 1988; 43: 75–81.

[153] Qureshi AA, Bradlow BA, Brace L, et al. Response of hypercholesterolaemic subjects to administration of tocotrienols. *Lipids* 1995; 30: 1171–1177.

[154] Sundram K, Anisah I, Hayes KC, et al. Trans (elaidic) fatty acids adversely impact lipoprotein profiles relative to specific saturated fatty acids in humans. *J Nutr* 1997; 127: 514S–520S.

[155] Kritchevsky D. Impact of red palm oil on human nutrition and health. *Food Nutr Bull* 2000; 2: 182–188.

[156] Simopoulos AP. Omega-3 fatty acids in health and disease and in growth and development. *Am J Clin Nutr* 1991; 54: 438–463.

[157] Serbinova E, Khavaja S, Catudioc J, et al. Palm oil vitamin E protects against ischaemia/reperfusion injury in the isolated perfused Langendorff heart. *Nutr Res* 1992; 12: 989S–1009S.

[158] Aggarwal BB, Sundaram C, Prasad S, Kannappan R. Tocotrienols, the vitamin E of the 21st century: Its potential against cancer and other chronic diseases. *Biochemical Pharmacology* 2010; 80: 1613-1631.

[159] Ribayamercado JD, Solon SF, Tang G, Cabal-Borza M, Perfecto SC, Russel RM. Bionconversion of plant carotenoids to vit-A in Filipino school-aged children varies inversely with vit-A status. *Am J Clin Nutr* 2000; 72: 455–465.

[160] Choe E, Min DB. Mechanisms of antioxidants in the oxidation of foods. Comp Rev Food Sci Food Safe 2009; 8: 345–358.

[161] Krinsky NI. The antioxidant and biological properties of carotenoids. *Ann NY Acad Sci* 1998; 854: 443–447.

[162] Reboul E, Thap S, Tourniaire F, Andre M, Juhel C, Morange S, Amiot MJ, Lairon D, Borel P. Differential effect of dietary antioxidant classes (carotenoids, polyphenols, vitamins C and E) on lutein absorption. *Br J Nutr* 2007; 97: 440–446.

[163] Young AJ, Lowe GM. Antioxidant and prooxidant properties of carotenoids. *Arch Biochem Biophys* 2001; 385: 20–27.

[164] Christensen RL. The photochemistry of carotenoids. In: Frank HA, Young AJ, Britton G, Cogdell RJ, (Eds.), *Dordrecht, The Netherlands: Kluwer Academic* 1999; 137–157.

[165] Khachik F, Spangler CJ, Smith, JC, Canfield LM, Steck A, Pfander H. Identification, quantification, and relative concentrations of carotenoids, and their metabolites in human milk and serum. *Anal Chem* 1997; 69: 1873–1881.

[166] Chen J, Jarvi M, Lo PC, Stefflova K, Wilson BC, Zheng G. Using the singlet oxygen scavenging property of carotenoid in photodynamic molecular beacons to minimize photodamage to non-targeted cells. *Photochem Photobiol Sci* 2007; 6: 1311–1317.

[167] McNulty H, Jacob RF, Mason RP. Biologic activity of carotenoids related to distinct membrane physicochemical interactions. *Am J Cardiol* 2008; 101: 20–29.

[168] Burton GW, Ingold KU. beta-Carotene: an unusual type of lipid antioxidant. *Science*. 1984; 224: 569–73.

[169] Sies H, Stahl W. Vitamins E and C, β-carotene, and other carotenoids as antioxidants. *Am J Clin Nutr* 1995; 62: 1315S–1321S.

[170] Amengual J, Lobo GP, Golczak M, Li HN, Klimova T, Hoppel CL, Wyss A, Palczewski K, von Lintig J. A mitochondrial enzyme degrades carotenoids and protects against oxidative stress. *FASEB J* 2011; 25: 948–959.

[171] Daviglus ML, Stamler J, Orencia AJ, et al. Fish consumption and the 30-year risk of fatal myocardial infarction. *N Engl J Med*.1997; 336: 1046–1053.

[172] Albert CM, Hennekens CH, O'Donnell CJ, et al. Fish consumption and risk of sudden cardiac death. *JAMA*. 1998; 279: 23–28.

[173] Leaf A, Albert CM, Josephson M, et al. Prevention of fatal arrhythmias in high-risk subjects by fish oil n-3 fatty acid intake. *Circulation*. 2005; 112: 2762–2768.

[174] Zaloga GP. Dietary lipids: ancestral ligands and regulators of cell signaling pathways. *Crit Care Med*. 1999; 27: 1646–1648.

[175] Siddiqui RA, Shaikh SR, Sech LA, et al. Omega 3-fatty acids: health benefits and cellular mechanisms of action. *Mini Rev Med Chem*.2004; 4: 859–871.

[176] Clarke SD, Jump DB. Regulation of gene transcription by polyunsaturated fatty acids. *Prog Lipid Res*. 1993; 32: 139–149.

[177] Abia R, Perona JS, Pacheco YM, Montero E, Muriana FJ, Ruiz-Gutierrez V. Postprandial triacylglycerols from dietary virgin olive oil are selectively cleared in humans. *J Nutr* 1999; 129: 2184–2191.

[178] Kris-Etherton PM, Yu-Poth S, Sabaté J, Ratcliffe HE, Zhao G, Etherton TD. Nuts and their bioactive constituents: effects on serum lipids and other factors that affect disease risk. *Am J Clin Nutr* 1999; 70: 504–511.

[179] Davidson A. The Oxford Companion to Food. Oxford, UK: *Oxford University Press* 1999.

[180] Halvorsen BL, Holte K, Myhrstad MC, et al. A systematic screening of total antioxidants in dietary plants. *J Nutr* 2002; 132: 461–471.

[181] Wu X, Beecher GR, Holden JM, Haytowitz DB, Gebhardt SE, Prior RL. Lipophilic and hydrophilic antioxidant capacities of common foods in the United States. *J Agric Food Chem* 2004; 52: 4026–4037.

[182] Blomhoff R, Carlsen MH, Andersen LF, Jacobs DR J. Health benefits of nuts: potential role of antioxidants. *Br J Nutr* 2006; 96: 52–60.

[183] Vivancos M, Moreno JJ. beta-Sitosterol modulates antioxidant enzyme response in RAW 264.7 macrophages. *Free Radic Biol Med* 2005; 39: 91–97.

[184] Segura R, Javierre C, Lizarraga MA, Ros E. Other relevant components of nuts: phytosterols, folate and minerals. *Br J Nutr* 2006; 96: 36–44.

[185] Fraley AE, Tsimikas S. Clinical applications of circulating oxidized low-density lipoprotein biomarkers in cardiovascular disease. *Curr Opin Lipidol* 2006; 17: 502–509.

[186] Ferri N, Paoletti R, Corsini A. Biomarkers for atherosclerosis: pathophysiological role and pharmacological modulation. *Curr Opin Lipidol* 2006; 17: 495–501.

[187] Deanfield JE, Halcox JP, Rabelink TJ. Endothelial function and dysfunction. Testing and clinical relevance. *Circulation* 2007; 115: 1285–95.

[188] Brown AA, Hu FB. Dietary modulation of endothelial function: implications for cardiovascular disease. *Am J Clin Nutr* 2001; 73: 673–686.

[189] Blomhoff R. Dietary antioxidants and cardiovascular disease. *Curr Opin Lipidol* 2005; 16: 47–54.

[190] Basu A, Devaraj S, Jialal I. Dietary factors that promote or retard inflammation. *Arterioscler Thromb Vasc Biol* 2006; 26: 995–1001.

[191] Kay CD, Kris-Etherton PM, West SG. Effects of antioxidant-rich foods on vascular reactivity: review of the clinical evidence. *Curr Atheroscler Rep* 2006; 8: 510–522.

[192] Reiter RJ, Manchester LC, Tan DX. Melatonin in walnuts: influence on levels of melatonin and total antioxidant capacity of blood. Nutrition 2005; 21: 920–924.

[193] Alexiadou K, Katsilambros N. Nuts: Anti-atherogenic food? *European Journal of Internal Medicine* 2011; 22: 141–146.

[194] Abbey M, Noakes M, Belling GB, Nestel PJ. Partial replacement of saturated fatty acids with almonds or walnuts lowers total plasma cholesterol and low-densitylipoprotein cholesterol. *Am J Clin Nutr* 1994; 59: 995–999.

[195] Jenkins DJ, Kendall CW, Marchie A, Faulkner DA, Wong JM, de Souza R, et al. Effects of a dietary portfolio of cholesterol-lowering foods vs lovastatin on serum lipids and C-reactive protein. *JAMA* 2003; 290: 502–510.

[196] Zhao G, Etherton TD, Martin KR, West SG, Gillies PJ, Kris-Etherton PM. Dietary alpha-linolenic acid reduces inflammatory and lipid cardiovascular risk factors in hypercholesterolemic men and women. *J Nutr* 2004; 134: 2991–2997.

[197] Jenkins DJ, Kendall CW, Marchie A, Faulkner DA, Josse AR, Wong JM, et al. Direct comparison of dietary portfolio vs statin on C-reactive protein. *Eur J Clin Nutr* 2005; 59: 851–860.

[198] Ros E, Núñez I, Pérez-Heras A, Serra M, Gilabert R, Casals E, et al. A walnut diet improves endothelial function in hypercholesterolemic subjects: a randomized crossover trial. *Circulation* 2004; 109: 1609–1614.

[199] Zhao G, Etherton TD, Martin KR, Gillies PJ, West SG, Kris-Etherton PM. Dietary alpha-linolenic acid inhibits proinflammatory cytokine production by peripheral blood mononuclear cells in hypercholesterolemic subjects. *Am J Clin Nutr* 2007; 85: 385–391.

[200] Bonetti PO, Lerman LO, Lerman A. Endothelial dysfunction: a marker of atherosclerotic risk. *Arterioscler Thromb Vasc Biol* 2003; 23: 168–175.

[201] West SG. Effect of diet on vascular reactivity: an emerging marker for vascular risk. *Curr Atheroscler Rep* 2001; 3: 446–455.

[202] Sanderson P, Sattar N, Olthof M, Grimble RF, Calder PC, Griffin BA, et al. Dietary lipids and vascular function: UK Food Standards Agency workshop report. *Br J Nutr* 2004; 91: 491–500.

[203] de Koning EJ, Rabelink TJ. Endothelial function in the post-prandial state. *Atheroscler* 2002; 3: 11–16.

[204] Tentolouris N, Arapostathi C, Perrea D, Kyriaki D, Revenas C, Katsilambros N. Differential effects of two isoenergetic meals rich in saturated or monounsaturated fat on endothelial function in subjects with type 2 diabetes. *Diab Care* 2008; 31: 2276–2278.

[205] Estruch R, Martínez-González MA, Corella D, Salas-Salvadó J, Ruiz-Gutiérrez V, Covas MI, et al. PREDIMED study investigators. Effects of a Mediterranean-style diet on cardiovascular risk factors: a randomized trial. *Ann Intern Med* 2006; 145: 1–11.

[206] Davis P, Valacchi G, Pagnin E, Shao Q, Gross HB, Calo L, et al. Walnuts reduce aortic ET-1 mRNA levels in hamsters fed a high-fat, atherogenic diet. *J Nutr* 2006; 136: 428-432.

[207] Sabaté J. Nut consumption and body weight. *Am J Clin Nutr* 2003; 78: 647–650.

[208] Griel AE, Eissenstat B, Juturu V, Hsieh G, Kris-Etherton PMJ. Improved diet quality with peanut consumption. *Am Coll Nutr* 2004; 23: 660–668.

[209] Alper CM, Mattes RD. Effects of chronic peanut consumption on energy balance and hedonics. *Int J Obes Relat Metab Disord* 2002; 26: 1129–1137.

[210] Fraser GE, Bennett HW, Jaceldo KB, Sabaté J. Effect on body weight of a free 76 kilojoule (320 calorie) daily supplement of almonds for six months. *J Am Coll Nutr* 2002; 21: 275–83.

[211] Sabaté J, Cordero-Macintyre Z, Siapco G, Torabian S, Haddad E. Does regular walnut consumption lead to weight gain? *Br J Nutr* 2005; 94: 859–64.

[212] Rajaram S, Sabaté J. Nuts, body weight and insulin resistance. *Br J Nutr* 2006; 96: 79-86.

[213] Hollis J, Mattes R. Effect of chronic consumption of almonds on body weight in healthy humans. *Br J Nutr* 2007; 98: 651–656.

[214] Bes-Rastrollo M, Wedick NM, Martinez-Gonzalez MA, Li TY, Sampson L, Hu FB. Prospective study of nut consumption, long-term weight change, and obesity risk in women. *Am J Clin Nutr* 2009; 89: 1913–1919.

[215] Mattes RD, Kris-Etherton PM, Foster GD. Impact of peanuts and tree nuts on body weight and healthy weight loss in adults. *J Nutr* 2008; 138: 1741–1745.

[216] Kokkinos A, le Roux CW, Alexiadou K, Tentolouris N, Vincent RP, Kyriaki D, et al. Eating slowly increases the postprandial response of the anorexigenic gut hormones, peptide YY and glucagon-like peptide-1. *J Clin Endocrinol Metab* 2010; 95: 333.

[217] Defilippis AP, Blaha MJ, Jacobson TA. Omega-3 Fatty acids for cardiovascular disease prevention. *Curr Treat Options Cardiovasc Med* 2010; 12: 365–380.

[218] Villano D, Pecorari M, Testa MF, Raguzzini A, Stalmach A, Crozier A, Tubili C, Serafini M. Unfermented and fermented rooibos teas (*Aspalathus linearis*) increase plasma total antioxidant capacity in healthy humans. *Food Chem.* 2010; 123: 679–683.

[219] Rahman I, Biswas SK, Kirkham PA. Regulation of inflammation and redox signaling by dietary polyphenols. *Biochem Pharmacol* 2006; 72: 1439–1452.

[220] Stephens NG, Parsons A, Schofield PM, Kelly F, Cheeseman K, Mitchinson MJ. Randomised controlled trial of Vitamin E in patients with coronary disease: Cambridge Heart Antioxidant Study (CHAOS). Lancet1996; 347: 781–786.

[221] Pryor WA. Vitamin E and heart disease: basic science to clinical intervention trials. Free Radic Biol Med 2000; 28: 141–164.

[222] Guidelines for the prevention of hypertension and associated cardiovascular disease. Joint World Health Organization/International Society of Hypertension Meeting. J Hypertens 1992; 10: 97-99.

[223] Goyal A, Yusuf S. The burden of cardiovascular disease in the Indian subcontinent. Indian J Med Res 2006; 124: 235-244.

Section 3

Plants with Hypolipidaemic Properties

Chapter 10

Plants with Hypolipidaemic Effects from Nigerian Flora

Ngozi Justina Nwodo, Charles Okeke Nnadi,
Akachukwu Ibezim and Chika John Mbah

Additional information is available at the end of the chapter

http://dx.doi.org/10.5772/57181

1. Introduction

Definition: Hyperlipidemia is a heterogeneous group of disorders characterized by high level of lipids (fats) in the bloodstream. These lipids include cholesterol, cholesterol esters, phospholipids, and triglycerides. Lipids are transported in the blood as large 'lipoproteins'. Alternatively, the disease refers to elevated levels of lipids and cholesterol in the blood, or the manifestations of different disorders of lipoprotein metabolism (dyslipidemia).

Causes: Hyperlipidemia could be caused by: (i) Familial combined hypercholesterolemia (ii) Familial hypertriglyceridemia (iii) other disease states such as *insulin and non-insulin dependent diabetes mellitus, hypothyroidism, Cushing's syndrome*, dysproteinemias, *nephrotic syndrome* and *renal failure*, cholestatic disorders and low thyroid (iv) drugs such as anabolic steroids, beta-blockers, birth control pills and estrogens, corticosteroids, protease inhibitors, retinoids, thiazide diuretics (v) diets like cholesterol intake greater than 300 mg per day, fat intake per total calories greater than 40 %, saturated fat intake per total calories greater than 10 % (vi) life style involving habitual excessive alcohol use, lack of exercise, smoking (vii) risk factors such as advancing age, sex (male), stress and postmenopause.

Classification: Lipoproteins are divided into five major classes, based on density and they include: (i) chylomicrons (ii) very low-density lipoproteins (VLDL) (iii) intermediate-density lipoproteins (IDL) (iv) low-density lipoproteins (LDL) and (v) high-density lipoproteins (HDL). Most triglyceride is transported in chylomicrons or VLDL, while most cholesterol is carried in LDL and HDL. Hyperlipidemia, a major, modifiable risk factor for atherosclerosis and cardiovascular disease, including coronary heart disease (CHD) is classified under (1) Primary hyperlipidemias - are probably genetically based, but the genetic defects are known for only a minority of patients. Examples are (i) primary chylomicronemia- recessive traits of deficiency of lipoprotein lipase or its cofactor (ii) familial hypercholesterolemia- an autosomal dominant trait, although levels of LDL tend to increase with normal VLDL; familial combined (mixed) hyperlipoproteinemia- elevated levels of VLDL, LDL (iii) familial dysbetalipoproteinemia-increased LDL with increased TG and cholesterol levels (iv) familial hypertriglyceridemia-increased VLDL production with normal or decreased LDL (v) familial mixed hypertriglyceridemia-serum VLDL and chylomicrons are increased. (2) Secondary hyperlipidemia- results from disease states such as Cushing's syndrome, diabetes, liver disorders, renal disorders, thyroid disease, obesity, as well as alcohol consumption, estrogen administration, and other drug-associated changes in lipid metabolism.

Symptoms: Hyperlipidemia usually does not cause symptoms. Very high levels of lipids or triglycerides can cause yellowish nodules of fat in the skin beneath eyes, elbows and knees, and in tendons (xanthomas). Sometimes pain, swelling of organs such as the liver, spleen or pancreas (pancreatitis) or whitish rings around the eye's iris occur. **Diagnosis**: Diagnosis is typically based on medical history, physical examination and most importantly blood test done after overnight fasting. The blood test, measure the levels of lipids in the blood and consist of, a fasting blood test for total cholesterol (TC), LDL (bad cholesterol), HDL (good cholesterol), triglycerides (TG). American Cholesterol Education Program advises that lipids be checked at least once every five years, starting at age 20. However, more frequent or earlier testing is recommended if family history of hyperlipidemia; risk factor or disease that may cause hyperlipidemia; complication that may result from hyperlipidemia exist. Also, the American Academy of Pediatrics recommends lipid screening for children at risk (example, a family history of hyperlipidemia and/or diabetes). Table 1 provides specifications for making a determination.

Cholesterol level	Acceptable	Borderline	High
Total Cholesterol (mg/dl)	<170	170 – 199	≥ 200
LDL Cholesterol (mg/dl)	<110	110 – 129	≥ 130
HDL Cholesterol (mg/dl)	<40	40-59	≥ 60
Total glycerides (mg/dl)	<150	150-200	≥ 200

Table 1. Classification of cholesterol level

Prevalence: (i) A significant percentage of world population has an increased plasma lipid level, resulting in increased risk of coronary heart disease (ii) Ethnic groups adopting a 'western' lifestyle tend to have higher levels of plasma lipids (iii) Men >30 years and women >55 years (in the U.S.) have10 % rise in fasting triglyceride level >200 mg/dl (iv) Severe hypertriglyceridemia (>2000 mg/dl) higher in diabetic patients or patients suffering alcoholism (iv) Lipoprotein lipase deficiency prevalence is much higher in Quebec, Canada. (v) total C and LDL-C rise steadily about 20% in men aged 20 to 50 years, 30% in women aged 20 to 60 years and younger women have lower levels than men while homozygous familial hypercholesterolemia manifests itself from birth (vii) hyperlipidermia is higher among men than women (gender factor) (viii) total cholesterol and LDL-C levels are similar in whites and blacks, triglycerides are lower and HDL-C levels tend to be higher in the African-American population. Asian-Indians have the highest risk, Europeans have an intermediate risk while Chinese have the lowest risk (race factor) (ix) familial combined hyperlipidemia inheritance is autosomal dominant and likely to involve one of multiple enetic defects, familial hypertriglyceridemia is most likely inherited as an autosomal dominant defect, lipoprotein lipase deficiency and hepatic lipase deficiency are very rare autosomal recessive conditions hypercholesterolemia in the majority of the general public is attributed to high-fat diets and poorly understood susceptibility and modifier genes (genetics factor). Published data on the prevalence of lipid abnormalities in Nigeria are scanty. This could be attributed to low prevalence of hyperlipidemia in Nigeria prior to occidental lifestyle. Osuji et al, 2012, reported that the current state of dyslipidemia in Nigeria clearly contradicts the previous perceptions. In their report, dsylipidemia was found to be highly prevalent in Nigeria with consistent low HDL-cholesterol and high LDL-c especially amongst the upper social class and people with other risk factors. Other studies reported low HDL-c, with TC/HDL-c to be prevalent in the Northern part of the country while high prevalence of TC, TG and low HDL were observed in the Southern part of the country amongst people of upper social class.

2. Treatment

Dietary intervention: is the primary treatment strategy, but drug therapy may often be added later to augment treatment. The main component of a "heart-healthy" diet is a food pattern that is low in saturated fat and dietary cholesterol and provides adequate energy to support growth and maintain an appropriate weight. Specific dietary recommendations include: (i) decreased intakes of saturated fat- most effective in lowering LDL. Sources include stick margarine, partially hydrogenated oils and fats, hydrogenated peanut butters, commercial bakery products, commercial fried food (e.g., French fries) and high fat animal products (ii) decreased intakes of trans-fatty acids- trans-fatty acids are thought to increase LDL levels nearly as much as saturated fat and appear to lower HDL. (iii) decreased intakes of dietary cholesterol- lead to LDL reduction. Diabetic patients tend to be more sensitive to dietary cholesterol intake, which is only found in animal products (iv) balance the fatty acid composition of diet- polyunsaturated and monounsaturated fatty acids can lower LDL and could be good substitutes for saturated fats (v) increased fiber intakes- soluble fiber can contribute to LDL reduction and is now a formal part of hyperlipidemia dietary recommendations. Common sources of fiber include oats, psyllium, guar gum, pectin, barley, dried beans, fruits, vegetables, cereals, whole grains, and legumes are good sources of soluble fiber (vi) encourage antioxidant food sources such as carotenoids, vitamins C and E and antioxidant-rich foods such as whole grains, citrus fruits, melons, berries and leafy green vegetables rather than supplements (vii) reduce serum homocysteine levels- adequate intakes of folate and vitamins B_6 and B_{12} as well as total fat restriction may keep homocysteine levels low. Food sources of these nutrients include fruits, dark green and leafy vegetables, fortified cereals, whole grains, lean meats and poultry.

Drug Therapy: Currently, there are many classes of medications that may be utilized in the pharmacologic management of hyperlipidemia. They are (1) HMG-CoA (3-hydroxy-3-methylglutaryl-coenzyme A) reductase inhibitors (statins). The cornerstone of the lipid-lowering therapy in adults has rested with the HMG CoA reductase inhibitors or statins. The use of these drugs has resulted in important reductions in overall cardiovascular morbidity and mortality. Mechanism of action- reduction of cholesterol synthesis in liver; inhibiting the rate-limiting step in endogenous cholesterol synthesis; compensatory increase in synthesis of LDL receptors on hepatic and extra hepatic tissues; increase in hepatic uptake of circulating LDL which decreases plasma LDL cholesterol; increase in HDL, decrease in TGs and vasodilatation and decrease in atherosclerosis. Pharmacological indication: Clinically used in the treatment of all types of hyperlipidemia except those who are homozygous for familial hypercholesterolemia (lack of LDL receptors). Table 2 summarizes the statins and their clinically applications.

Drug	Starting Dose (mg)	FDA-Approved Maximum (mg)	Half-life (hours)	Average Decrease in LDL-C Per Dose (mg:%)
Atorvastatin (lipitor)	10-20	80	14 or 20-30	10:39 20:43 80:60
Fluvastatin (Lescol)	20	80	3	20:22 80:35
Lovastatin (Mevacor)	20	80	2	20:28
Pitavastatin (Livalo)	2	4	12	2:36 4:43
Pravastatin (Pravachol)	40	80	2	40:34 80:37
Rosuvastatin (Crestor)	5-10	40	19	5:45 10:52 40:63
Simvastatin (Zocor)	20	80	4	20:38 80:36-47
Simvastatin/Ezetimibe (Vytorin)	10/10	10/40	22	10/10:45 10/40:55

Table 2. HMG-CoA INHIBITORS

(2) Fibrates (activators of lipoprotein lipase): Mechanism of action- agonists at peroxisome proliferator-activated receptor (PPAR); hydrolysis of VLDL and chylomicrons; decrease in serum TGs; increase clearance of LDL by liver and increase in HDL and expression of genes responsible for increased activity of plasma lipoprotein lipase enzyme. Pharmacological indication: most effective in reduction TGs (hypertriglyceridemia); combined hyperlipidemia (type III) if statins are contraindicated. Typical examples are fenofibrate(prodrug) and gemfibrozil (lopid) (3) Ezetimibe: Mechanism of action- inhibits intestinal cholesterol and

related phytosterol absorption; decrease in concentration of intrahepatic cholesterol; increase in uptake of circulating LDL; decrease in serum LDL cholesterol levels and compensatory increase in LDL receptors. Pharmacological indication: Effective in hypercholesterolemia together with statins and diet regulation; utilization of ezetimibe along with a statin allows for lower doses of the statin to be used, therefore reducing the likelihood of dose-related side effects of the statin. (4) Nicotinic acid; Niacin (Inhibitor of lipolysis): Mechanism of action- a potent inhibitor of lipolysis in adipose tissues; decreases mobilization of FFAs (major precursor of TGs) to the liver; increases HDL levels; decreases LDL, decreases endothelial dysfunction and thrombosis. Pharmacological indication- Used in the treatment of familial hyperlipidemias (type IIB) (increase in VLDL and LDL); combined with fibrates or cholestyramine in the treatment of hypercholesterolemia (5) Bile acids- Sequestrants(resins): The bile acid binding resins have been felt to be preferred in the pediatric age group as they are not systemically absorbed. Mechanism of action- are anion exchange resins; bind bile acids in the intestine forming complex that leads to loss of bile acids in the stools; increase the conversion of cholesterol into bile acids in the liver; compensatory increase in LDL receptors leading to decreased concentration of intrahepatic cholesterol; increase hepatic uptake of circulating LDL and decrease serum LDL cholesterol levels. Pharmacological indication: Effective in the treatment of type IIA and IIB hyperlipidemias (along with statins when response to statins is inadequate or they are contraindicated); treatment of pruritus in biliary obstruction (as rising from increase in bile acids). Typical examples are cholestyramine, colestipol and colesevelam. (6) Lovaza (Omega-3-acid ethyl ester): Mechanism of action: is unclear; however, proposed mechanisms include decreasing lipogenesis in the liver, increasing plasma lipoprotein lipase activity, and increasing mitochondrial and perixosomal lipase activity. The drug may increase aspartate aminotransferase (AST) and alanine aminotransferase (ALT) levels and has also been known to prolong bleeding time. Pharmacological indication: is indicated as adjunct therapy to diet in patients with triglyceride levels greater than or equal to 500 mg/dl (hypertriglyceridemia). It provides significant reduction in triglycerides, of approximately 44.9%, making it an ideal drug choice in patients with high triglycerides (7) Fish oil is another common over-the-counter (OTC) product that provides an alternative to the prescription product Lovaza (8) OTC herbal product: (i) Red yeast rice (RYR)- herbal supplements used for lipid-lowering effects. RYR is obtained by fermenting *Monascus purpureus*, a form of yeast, on rice, which is then dried, pulverized, and encapsulated. This process leads to the formation of 14 monacolins, which are compounds that inhibit HMG-CoA reductase. One of the mona-colins, monacolin K (lovastatin or mev-inolin) was the first synthesized HMG-CoA reductase inhibitor. RYR is commercially available in 600-mg capsules (ii) Plant sterols and stanols also assist in the reduction of LDL-C. Plant sterols reduce cholesterol absorption by competing with cholesterol for space within bile salt micelles in the intestinal lumen. The plant stanols, which are the result of the hydrogenation of sterols, are not absorbed as well as sterols. Ingestion of about 2 g per day of plant sterols or stanols, produces LDL-C reduction of 6% to 15%. Prevention: Cardiovascular disease (CVD) is the leading cause of mortality in advance countries, with hyperlipidemia a common risk factor for CVD, in adults having abnormal cholesterol values and elevated low-density lipoprotein (LDL) cholesterol levels. Prevention could be subdivided into: Primary prevention- (i) initial treatment is diet/exercise and should be given three to six months on dietary therapy prior to beginning medication and longer if lipids are improving and nearing LDL thresholds (ii) obtain cholesterol tests starting at the age of 20 (iii) eat a diet low in total fat, saturated fat, and cholesterol namely eat poultry without the skin, fish, vegetables, most fruits, whole grains, and skim milk (iv) reduce sugar intake (v) eat foods high in soluble fiber (vi) eat more cold water fish and soy products (vii) avoid cigarette smoking (viii) drink alcohol in moderation (two drinks per day for men, one drink per day for women) (ix) avoid overweight (x) exercise regularly and control blood sugar if diabetes is implicated (xi) increase physical activity (xii) consume a diet that contains adequate potassium, calcium, and magnesium to facilitate blood pressure control. Secondary prevention: Measuring lipids in adolescents that have strong family history of two or more coronary heart disease risk factors. In summary, US National Cholesterol Education Program (NCEP) Adult Treatment Panel III (ATP III in its guidelines has communicated the importance of early identification of risk, lifestyle modification, and pharmacologic treatment as the mainstay of therapy for hyperlipidemia and in the prevention of cardiovascular-related death.

The Promise of Nigeria Natural Products: Since the recognition of hyperlipiermia, a large number of plant species have been identified as having antihyperlipidermic properties and natural products are part of the current therapy for hyperlipidermia. Numerous natural products with antihyperlipidemic effect have been described in the literature. The objective of this chapter is to summarize the role of Nigeria natural products in the treatment and prevention of hyperlipidermia to date and to highlight specific classes of compounds that possess a requisite level of activity that would be considered worthy of further investigation as potential drug candidate.

3. Discussion

3.1. Antilipidemic agents from Nigeria flora

In Nigeria, traditional medicine has been the most popular means of healthcare from the olden days, before the emergence of alternative medicine in the form of synthetic agents. Traditional medicine can be said to be indigenous and a culture handed over to us by our anscestors as a means of surviving from various ailment obvious in every society. Due to high cost of synthetic drugs and side effects, natural products have become the best alternative strategy for the development of safe antilipidemic drugs. Various natural products both crude and isolated components found from plants are effective remedies for hyperlipidemia cases. Several proves are available in nature, indicating the positive effects of many natural product components that can be employed for the treatment of hyperlipidemia. Ibrahim *et al*, 2013 stated that polyphenols as apigenin, genistein and catechins as well as saponins, sterols, stanols polyunsaturated fatty acids, mucilage and carbohydrates are good examples of agents found to exhibit potent hypocholesterolemic activities. Table3 summarizes the continuous investigations of Nigerian plants used as antihyperlipidemia from ethnopharmacological approach based on the folkloric claims.

http://dx.doi.org/10.5772/57181

Sources	Morphological parts	Comments	References
PerseaAmerican (Avocado pea)	Leaves, methanolic extract	Hypolipidemic activity at 40 mg/kg	Kolawole *et al.*, 2012
Garciniakola	Root and seed, normal saline extracts	Hypolipidemic activity at 300-900 mg/kg	Udenze *et al.*, 2012
Viscumalbum	Plant parts, methanolic extract	Hypolipidemic activity at 50-100 mg/kg	Oluwatosin *et al.*, 2012
Caricapapaya	Seed, aqueous extract	Hypolipidemic activity at 100-400 mg/kg	Nwangwa and Ekhoye 2013
Emilapraetermissa	Leaves, aqueous extract	Hypolipidemic activity	Anaka *et al.*, 2013
Cleistopholis patens	Leaves, aqueous extract	Hypolipidemic activity at 400-600 mg/kg	Udem *et al.*, 2011
Solanumanguivi, *S. macrocarpum*	Fruit, aqueous extract	Hypolipidemic activity at 20-100 mg/kg	Elekofehiniti *et al.* 2012; Sodipo *et al.*, 2011
Annonamuricata	Plant parts, methanolic extract	Hypolipidemic activity	Adeyemi *et al.*, 2009
Nauclealatifolia	Root and stem bark, ethanolic extract	Hypolipidemic activity at 100-150 mg/kg	Odey *et al.*, 2013
Acalypha torta A. capitata	Leaves, aqueous extract	Hypolipidemic activity at 100-200 mg/kg	Nnodim *et al*, 2011
Scopariadulcis	Plant (herb) parts, methanolic extract	Hypolipidemic activity	Orhue and Nwanze, 2006
Alchorneacordifolia	Leaves, butanolic extract	Hypolipidemic activity at 800 mg/kg	Mohammed *et al.*, 2012
Vernonia amygdalina Vernonia amygdalina	Plant parts, methanolic extract; Leaves, ethanolic extract; root, normal saline extract	Hypolipidemic activity Hypolipidemic activity at 100-200 mg/kg	Oluwatosin *et al.*, 2008 Igbakin 2009, Owen *et al.*, 2011
Moringa oleifera	Leaves, aqueous extract	Hypolipidemic activity at 1 mg/g	Ghasi *et al.*, 2000
Clerodendrumcapitalum	Leaves, aqueous extract	Hypolipidemic activity at 100-800 mg/kg	Adenaya *et al.*, 2008
Parkiabiglobosa	Plant parts, methanolic extract	Hypolipidemic activity at 30-60 mg/kg	Odetola *et al.*, 2006
Citrusparadisi	Seed, methanolic extract	Hypolipidemic activity at 100-600 mg/kg	Adeneye, 2008
Cymbopogoncitrates	Leaves, aqueous extract	Hypolipidemic activity at 125-500 mg/kg	Adeneye & Agbaje, 2007
Catharanthusroseus	Leaves, aqueous extract	Hypolipidemic activity at1 ml/kg	Antia & Okokon, 2005
Albizziachevalieri	Root, aqueous extract	Hypolipidemic activity at 100-300 mg/kg	Saidu *et al.*, 2010
Stachytarphelaaugustifolia	Aerial part, methanolic extract	Hypolipidemic activity	Garba *et al.*, 2013
Vitexdoniana	Leaves, ethanolic extract	Hypolipidemic activity	Oche *et al.*, 2012

Sources	Morphological parts	Comments	References
Morindamorindoides	Root bark, methanolic extract	Hypolipidemic activity	Olukunle *et al.*, 2012
Arachishypogaea	Plant parts, aqueous extract	Hypolipidemic activity at 175 mg/kg	Bilbis *et al.*, 2002
"Ata-Ofa' (polyherbal tea)	Leaves, methanolic extract	Hypolipidemic activity at 50 mg/kg	Atawodi, 2001
Xylopiaaethiopica	Seed, methanolic extract	Hypolipidemic activity at 250 mg/kg	Nwozo *et al.*, 2011
Parinaripolyandra	Fruit, ethanolic extract	Hypolipidemic activity at 50-250 mg/kg	Abolaji *et al.*, 2007
Telfairia occidentalis	Plant parts, methanolic extract	Hypolipidemic activity	Adaramoye *et al.*, 2007
Curcuma longa	methanol extract of the rhizomes	hypoglycemic and hypolipidemic acitivity 100 mg/kg	Nwozo *et al*, 2009.
Spondiamombia	Aqueous leave extract	Lipid lowering effect at the doses of 250, 500and 750 mg/kg	Igwe *et al*, 2008
Crotonzambesicus	Ethanolic leaf extract	Lipid lowering effect	Ofusori *et al*, 2012.
Momordicacharantia Linn	Methanolic extract of the fruits	Anti-Diabetic and Hypolipidemic Effects at the doses of 200, 400 and 600 mg/kg	Kolawole and Ayankunle, 2012.
Bauhiniathoningii	Aqueous crude extract	Hypoglycemic and lipidemic effecte	Ojezele and Abatan, 2011.
Cajanuscajan	Methanolic leaf extract	Antioxidant and hypolipidemic activity at the dose of 200 mg/kg	Akinloye and Solanke 2011.
Jatrophatanjorensis	Methanolic leaf extract	Serum lipid profile and phytochemical composition at 100, 200 and 500mg/kg dose ranges	Oluwole *et al*, 2011.
Melantherascandens	Ethanolic leaf extract	Antidiabetic and hypolipidemic activities at the doses of 37, 74 &111 mg/kg	Akpan *et al*, 2012.
Ricinuscommunis	Aqueous root extract	Hypoglycaemic potential, lipid profile effects At a dose of 500mg/kg	Matthew *et al*, 2012.

Table 3. Medicinal plants investigated in Nigeria for use as Antihypolipidemic agent

These plants have been identified, authenticated and investigated from Nigeria flora against hyperlipidemia, using pharmacological validated animal models. They all have levels and with some levels of increase in LDL, TC, TG and decrease in HDL. Furthermore, there has been recent interest on the research towards hyperlipidemia due to its obvious relationship with

http://dx.doi.org/10.5772/57181

diabetes and other ailments like cushing's syndrome, renal disorder, pregnancy, polycystic ovary syndrome, underactive thyroid gland etc. Hyperlipidemia arising from high serum triglyceride or total cholesterol concentration or both has been reported in diabetic and hypertensive patients. Diabetics have been reported to be more prone to cardiovascular diseases including hypertension than non-diabetics (Bilbis et al, 2002). An overview of 40 medicinal plant species from Nigerian indigenous plants reported to have hypolipidemic effects are presented. Most of the reported hypolipidemic effects were on crude extracts and active constituents. Above 30 % of the investigated plant parts had effects on both lipid profile and glyceamic index. However, much still needs to be done on several phytoconstituents of these plants, as well as conduct clinical research on active constituents derived from them, especially in the determination of their levels of toxicity. Other Nigerian plants claimed to have positive effects on lipid profile but found to act as soup thickeners are yet to be investigated. The reported Nigerian plants in Table 3 are rich in soluble and dietary fibres (examples, legumes, fruits and vegetables) and if found to have minimal toxicities, can be incorporated into dietary supplements. According to Ibrahim *et al*, (2013), the major advantage of natural hypolipidemic drugs over synthetic drugs is that many natural drugs exhibit their hypolipidemic activity by different mechanisms. Plants are known to have a striking potential in the management of lipid metabolism and providing better therapeutic effects as an alternative medicine.

4. Conclusion

The use of herbal or natural medicines for the treatment of various disorders has a long and extensive history. The reported plants have the potential to act as lipid-lowering agents with minimal side effects (advantage over currently synthetic drugs) and thus could find their way onto the world market as alternatives to prescribed drugs currently available to treat hyperlipidermia. Most of the studies were carried out with crude extract and administered orally. The principal families in which such activity has been reported are Acanthaceae, Apiaceae, Asteraceae, Azoaceae, Combretaceae, Cucurbitaceae, Euphorbiaceae, Fabaceae, Lamiaceae, Liliaceae, Malvaceae, Myrtaceae, Rubiaceae, Rutaceae and Zingiberaceae, Finally, all the plant species appear to be promising as hypolipidemic agents with activity mediated through various mechanisms.

Author details

Ngozi Justina Nwodo*, Charles Okeke Nnadi, Akachukwu Ibezim and Chika John Mbah

*Address all correspondence to: ngozi.nwodo@unn.edu.ng

Department of Pharmaceutical and Medicinal Chemistry, Faculty of Pharmaceutical Sciences, University of Nigeria, Nsukka Enugu State, Nigeria

References

[1] Abolaji, A. O, Adebayo, A. H, & Odesanmi, O. S. (2007). Effects of Parinari polyandra (Rosaceae) on serum lipid profile and some electrolytes in pregnant rabbits. Res. J. of Med.Plant , 1(4), 121-127.

[2] Adaramoye, O. A, Achem, J, Akintayo, O. O, & Fafunso, M. A. (2007). Hypolipidemic effect of Telfairia occidentalis (fluted pumpkin) in rats fed a cholesterol-rich diet. J Med Food. , 10(2), 330-6.

[3] Adeneye, A. A, Adeleke, T. I, & Adeneye, A. K. (2008). Hypoglycemic and hypolipidemic effects of the aqueous fresh leaves extract of *Clerodendrum* capitatum in Wistar rats. J. Ethnopharmacol , 116(1), 7-10.

[4] Adeneye, A. A. (2008). Hypoglycemic and hypolipidemic effects of methanol seed extract of *Citrus paradisi* Macfad (Rutaceae) in alloxan-induced diabetic Wistar rats. *Nig Q J Hosp Med.;* , 18(4), 211-5.

[5] Adeneye, A. A, & Agbaje, E. O. (2007). Hypoglycemic and hypolipidemic effects of fresh leaf aqueous extract of *Cymbopogon citratus* Stapf. in rats. J. Ethnopharmacol. 25;, 112(3), 440-4.

[6] Adeneye, A. A, & Olagunju, A. J. (2009). Preliminary hypoglycemic and hypolipidemic activities of the aqueous seed extract of *Carica papaya*. Biology and Medicine , 1

[7] Aderamoye, O, Amanlou, M, Habibi-rezaei, M, Pasalar, P, & Ali, M. M. (2012). Methanolic extract of African mistletoes (*Viscum album*) improves carbohydrate metabolism and hyperlipidemia in streptozotocin-induced diabetic rats. Asian Pac J. Trop. Med. , 5(6), 427-33.

[8] Adeyemi, D. O, Komolafe, O. A, Adewole, S. O, & Obuotor, E. M. (2009). Anti-hyperlipidemic activities of *Annona muricata* (Linn). Int. J.Altern. Med. DOI:b, 7

[9] Akinloye, O. A, & Solanke, O. O. (2011). Evaluation of hypolipidemic and potential antioxidant effects of Pigeon pea (*Cajanus cajan* (l) mill sp.) leaves in alloxan-induced hyperglycemic rats. J. of Med. Plants Res. , 5, 2521-2524.

[10] Akpan, E. J, Okokon, J. E, & Offong, E. (2012). Antidiabetic and hypolipidemic activities of ethanolic leaf extract and fractions of *Melanthera scandens*. Asian Pacific J. of Tropical Biomedicine, , 523-527.

[11] Akuyam, S. A, Anya, P. O, Isah, H. S, Aliyu, I. S, & Yusuf, R. (2010). Lipid abnormalities: "A Case Study of Ahadu Gello University Hospital, Zaria, Nigeria". Ann. Nig. Med. , 4, 10-13.

[12] Alli Smith YRAdenlawo IG, (2013). Tissue lipid profile of rats administered saponin extract from the root of *bitter kola*. Adv, in Biochem., , 1(1), 1-4.

[13] American Diabetes Association(2001). Nutrition recommendations and principles for people with diabetes mellitus. Diabetes Care. 24:SS47., 44.

[14] Anaka Ogochukwu NgoziOwolabi Omonkhelin Josephine, EmenikeChinwendu, (2013). Anti-hyperlipidemic effect of aqueous leaf extracts *Emilia praetermissa* nilineredh (Asteraceae) in rats. Inter J, of Biosciences. , 3(5), 68-77.

[15] Antia, B. S, & Okokon, J. E. (2005). Effect of leaf juice of *Catharanthus roseus* Linn on cholesterol, triglyceride and lipoproteins levels in normal rats. Indian J Pharmacol. , 37, 401-2.

[16] Atawodi, S. E. (2011). Evaluation of the hypoglycemic, hypolipidemic and antioxidant effects of methanolic extract of *"Ata-Ofa" Polyherbal* Tea (*A-Polyherbal)* in Alloxan-induced diabetic rats. Drug Invention Today. , 3(11), 270-276.

[17] Bilbis, L. S, Shehu, R. A, & Abubakar, M. G. (2002). Hypoglycemic and hypolipidemic effects of aqueous extract of *Arachis hypogaea* in normal and alloxan-induced diabetic rats. Phytomedicin*e* , 9(6), 553-5.

[18] Burkill, H. M. (1997). The useful plants of west tropical Africa. 2. Roya Botanic Gardens, kew., 4

[19] Chait, A, & Brunzell, J. D. (1990). Acquired hyperlipidemia (secondary dyslipoprotein-emias). Endocrinol Metab Clin North Am. , 19, 259-278.

[20] Dixon, L. B, & Ernst, N. D. (2001). Choose a diet that is low in saturated fat and cholesterol and moderate in total fat:subtle changes to a familiar message. J. Nutr. 131(2S-1):510S-526S

[21] Duplaga, B. A. (1999). Treatment of childhood hypercholesterolemia with HMG-CoA reductase inhibitors. Ann. Pharmacother; , 33(11), 1224-1227.

[22] Elekofehinti, O. O, Adanlawo, I. G, Salin, J. A, & Sodehinde, S. A. (2012). Saponins from *Solanum anguivi* fruits extracts hypolipidemic potential in Rattusnovergicus. Der Pharmacia Lettre. , 4(3), 811-814.

[23] Executive Summary of The Third Report of The National Cholesterol Education Program (NCEP) Expert Panel on DetectionEvaluation, and Treatment of High Blood Cholesterol in Adults (Adult Treatment Panel III). Jama (2001). , 285(19), 2486-2497.

[24] Ezekwesili, C. N, & Obidoa, O. Nwodo OFC, (2008). Effect of ethanol extract of Acalypha torta leaves on the lipid profile and serum electrolytes of rabbits. Nig. J. of Biochem. Mol. Bio., , 23(1), 15-21.

[25] Fletcher, B, Berra, K, Ades, P, et al. (2005). Managing blood lipids: a collaborative approach. Circulation., 112, 3184-3209.

[26] Garba, **A**, Mada, S. B, & Ibrahim, G. Dauran IA Hamza AB, (2013). Studies on hypoglycemic and hypolipidemic effects of methanolic extract of *Stachytarpheta angustifolia*(mill) in streptozotoin induced diabetic rats. Asian J. Bio. Sci. Doi:10.3923/ajbs.2013

[27] Ghasi, S, Nwobodo, E, & Ofili, J. O. (2000). Hypocholesterolemic effects of crude extract of leaf of *Moringa oleifera* Lam in high-fat diet fed wistar rats. J. Ethnopharmacol. , 69, 21-25.

[28] Gordon, T, Castelli, W. P, Hjortland, M. C, et al. (1977). High density lipoprotein as a protective factor against coronary artery disease: the Framingham Study. Am J Med. , 62, 707-14.

[29] Grundy, S. M. (1998). Hypertriglyceridemia, atherogenic dyslipidemia and the metabolic syndrome. Am. J. Cardiol. 81:18B-25B.

[30] Hepper, F. N. (1963). Emilia in: Hutchinso JJ. and Dalziel JM. (eds) Flora of West Tropical Africa, 2nd ed. Crown Agents for Overseas Governments and Administrations, London, Uk. , 2, 244-245.

[31] Igbakin, A. P. (2009). Comparative studies on hypoglycaemic, hypoproteinaemic, hypocholesterolaemic and hypolipidaemic properties of ethanolic and normal saline extracts of the root of *V. amygdalina* in diabetic rats. Adv. Enviro. Bio. , 3(1), 33-38.

[32] Igwe, C. U, Ojiako, O. A, & Nwaogu, L. A. Onyeze, GOC, (2008). Lipid Lowering Effect of Aqueous Leaf Extract Of Spondias Mombin Linn J. of Pharmacol. 6 (1) , 10.

[33] Insull, W. (2006). Clinical utility of bile acid sequestrants in the treatment of dyslipidemia: a scientific review. South Med J.; , 99(3), 257-73.

[34] Knopp, R. H. (1999). Drug treatment of lipid disorders. N. Engl. J. Med. , 341, 498-511.

[35] Kolawole, O. T, Kolawole, S. O, Ayankunle, A. A, & Olaniran, I. O. (2012). Methanolic leaf extract of *Persea americana* protects rats against cholesterol-induced hyperlipidemia. *British J. of Med. Medical Res.*, , 2(2), 235-42.

[36] Kolawole, O. T, & Ayankunle, A. A. (2012). Seasonal Variation in the Anti-Diabetic and Hypolipidemic Effects of *Momordica charantia* Fruit Extract in Rats *European Journal of Medicinal Plants* , 2(2), 177-185.

[37] Krauss, R. M. (1982). Regulation of high density lipoprotein levels. Med. Clin. North. Am. , 66, 403-30.

[38] Krauss, R. M, Eckel, R. H, Howard, B, Appel, L. J, Daniels, S. R, Deckelbaum, R. J, et al. (2003). AHA Dietary guidelines: Revision 2000: A statement for healthcare professionals from the Nutrition Committee of the American Heart Association. Circulation 2000:102(18):2284-99.

[39] Lipka, L. Ezetimibe: a first-in-class, novel cholesterol absorption inhibitor. Cardiovasc Drug Rev. , 21(4), 293-312.

[40] Mckenney, J. (2003). Niacin for dyslipidemia: considerations in product selection. Am J Health Syst Pharm., 60(10), 995-1005.

[41] Mohammed, R. K, Ibrahim, S, Atawodi, S. E, Eze, E. D, Suleiman, J. B, & Malgwi, I. S. (2012). The study of the effects of n-butanol fraction of *Alchornea cordifolia* leaf extract on lipid profile and liver enzymes in streptozotocin-induced diabetic rats. Global Journal of medicinal Plant Research. , 1(1), 1-7.

[42] Moutzouri, E, Kei, A, Elisaf, M. S, & Milionis, H. J. (2010). Management of dyslipidemias with fibrates, alone and in combination with statins: role of delayed-release fenofibric acid. Vasc Health Risk Manag. , 6, 525-539.

[43] Nwangwa, E. K, & Ekhoye, E. I. (2013). Anti-hyperlipidemic Activity of aqueous extracts of *Carica papaya* seeds in albino rats fed with high fat diet. Current Trends in Technology and Science, Vol.II, 2279.

[44] Nwozo, S, Adaramoye, O, & Ajaiyeoba, E. (2009). Oral Administration of Extract from *Curcuma longa* Lowers Blood Glucose and Attenuates Alloxan-Induced Hyperlipidemia in Diabetic Rabbits, Pakistan Journal of Nutrition , 8(5), 625-628.

[45] Nwozo, S. O. Orojobi BF Adaramoye OA, (2011). Hypolipidemic and antioxidant potentials of Xylopia aethiopica seed extract in hypercholesterolemic rats. J. Med.Food 14(1-2) 114-19.

[46] Odetola, A. A, Akinloye, O, Egunjobi, C, Adekunle, W. A, & Ayoola, A. O. (2006). Possible antidiabetic and antihyperlipidaemic effect of fermented *Parkia biglobosa* (JACQ) extract in alloxan-induced diabetic rats. Clin. Exp. Pharmacol. Physiol. , 33(9), 808-12.

[47] Odey, M. O, Johnson, J. T, Iwara, I. A, Gauje, B, Akpan, N. S, Luke, U. O, Robert, A. E, & Ukpong, K. M. (2012). Effect of anti-hypertensive treatment with root and stem bark extracts on *Nauclea latifolia* on serum lipid profile. G.J.P. and A. Sc. and Tech., , 0214, 78-84.

[48] Ofusori, D. A, Komolafe, O. A, Adewole, O. S, Obuofor, E. M, Fakunle, J. B, & Ayoka, A. O. (2012). Effect of ethanolic leaf extract of *Croton zambesicus* (Mull arg.) on lipid profile in streptozotocin-induced diabetic rat. Diabetologia croatica. , 41-2.

[49] Oguejiofor, O. C, Onwukwe, C. H, & Odenigbo, C. U. (2012). Dyslipidemia in Nigeria: "Prevalence and pattern", (Review). Ann. African Med. 11(4), 197-202.

[50] Ojezele, M. O, & Abatan, O. M. (2011). Hypoglycaemic and coronary risk index lowering effects of *Bauhinia thoningii* in alloxan induced diabetic rats. Afr. Health Sci. , 11(1), 85-9.

[51] Okpe OcheAbdullahi Salman A, Nkeonye Ogechi L, Ilechukwu Chijioke C, Nweke Ogechi, Ihuoma Onyeyirichi, (2012). Hypoglycemic and hypolipidemic Effects of aqueous and ethanolic leaf extracts of *Vitex doniana* (Verbenaceae) in normoglycemic albino rats. Global Advanced Research Journal of Microbiology , 1, 173-179.

[52] Olukunle, J. O, Abatan, M. O, Adenubi, O. T, & Amusan, T. A. (2012). Hypoglycaemic and hypolipidaemic effects of crude extracts and chromatographic fractions of *Morinda morindoides* root bark in diabetic rats. Acta Vet. Brno. , 81, 269-74.

[53] Oluwatosin, A. Adaramoye, Olajumoke Akintayo, Jonah Achem, Michael A, Fafunso, (2008). Lipid-lowering effects of methanolic extracts of *V. amygdalina* leaves in rats fed on high cholesterol diet. J. Am. Med. Assoc. , 251, 351-64.

[54] Oluwole, I. Oyewole1 and Peter F. Akingbala, (2011). Phytochemical Analysis and Hypolipidemic Properties of *Jatropha tanjorensis* Leaf Extract Eur. J.l of Med. Plants1(4): 180-185,

[55] OrhueNEJ and Nwanze, EAC, (2006). *Scoparia dulcis* reduces the severity of trypanosome brucei-induced hyperlipidaemia in the rabbit. Afr. J. of Biotech. , 5, 883-887.

[56] Osuji, C. U, Nzerem, B. A, Meludu, S, Dioka, C. E, Nwobodo, E, & Amilo, G. I. (2010). The prevalence of over weight/obesity and dyslipidemia amongst a group of women attending "August" meeting. Nig. Med. J. 51(4), 155-159.

[57] Out, C, Groen, A. K, & Brufau, G. (2012). Bile acid sequestrants: more than simple resins. Curr Opin. Lipidol. , 23(1), 43-55.

[58] Owen, O. J. Amakiri AOA, Karibi-Botoye TA, (2011). Lipid-lowering effects of bitter leaf in boiler chickens fed finishers' mash. Agr. Bio. J. North Am. , 2151-7525.

[59] Patel, S. B. (2004). A novel cholesterol-lowering agent that highlights novel physiologic pathways. Curr. Cardiol. Rep. , 6, 439-42.

[60] Pieper, J. (2003). Overview of niacin formulations: differences in pharmacokinetics, efficacy, and safety. Am. J. Health Sys. Pharm. 60(13 suppl 2): SS14., 9.

[61] Prabhjot, N, Burke, F, Bloesch, A, & Rader, D. (2010). Role of dietary supplements in lowering low-density lipoprotein cholesterol: a review. J. Clin. Lipidol. , 4, 248-58.

[62] Ram, G, & Becker, D. (2011). The role of red yeast rice for the physician. Curr. Atheroscler. Rep., 13, 73-80.

[63] Sabrin, R. M, Ibrahim, G. A, Mohamed, Z. M, & Banjar, K. M. (2013). Natural antihyperlipidemic agents: Current and future perspectives. Phytopharmacol. , 4(3), 492-531.

[64] Safeer, R. S, & Lacivita, C. L. (2000). Choosing drug therapy for patients with hyperlipidemia. Am. Fam. Physician , 61(11), 3371-82.

[65] Saidu, Y, Nwachukwu, F. C, Bilbis, L. S, Faruk, U. Z, & Abbas, A. Y. (2010). Hypoglycaemic and hypolipidemic Effects of root extracts of *Albizzia chevalieri* in alloxan induced diabetic rats. Nig. J. Basic and Appl. Sci. , 18(1), 72-78.

[66] Shamir, R, & Fisher, E. A. (2000). Dietary therapy for children with hypercholesterolemia. Am Fam. Physician. , 61(3), 675-85.

[67] Sodipo, O A, Abdulrahman, F. I, & Sandabe, U. K. (2011). Total lipid profile, faecal cholesterol, very low density lipoprotein cholesterol (VLDL-C), atherogenic index (A.I) and percent atherosclerosis with aqueous fruit extract of *Solanum macrocarpum* in chronic troton-induced hyperlipidemic albino rats. Current Res. J.Bio. Sci. , 4(2), 2026-214.

[68] Stone, N. J. (1994). Secondary causes of hyperlipidemia. Med. Clin. North. Am. , 78, 117-141.

[69] Stone, N. J. (2001). The optimal dietary strategy to manage risk associated with various dyslipidemias. Curr. Cardiol. Rep. , 3, 391-400.

[70] Tenhola, S, Martikainen, A, Rahiala, E, Herrgard, E, Halonen, P, & Voutilainen, R. (2000). Serum lipid concentrations and growth characteristics in 12-year-old children born small for gestational age. Pediatr. Res. ;, 48(5), 623-28.

[71] Toth, P, Dayspring, T, & Pokrywka, G. (2009). Drug therapy for hypertriglyceridemia: fibrates and omega-3 fatty acids. Curr. Atheroscler. Rep., 11, 71-79.

[72] Udem, S. C, Ezeonuegbu, U. C, & Obidike, R. I. (2011). Experimental studies on the hypolipidemic and haematological properties of aqueous leaf extract of *Cleistopholiss patens* Benth & Diets. (Annonacae) in hypercholesterolemic rats. Ann. Med. Health Sci. Res. (1): 115-21

[73] Udenze ECCBraide VB, Okwesilieze CN, Akuodor GC, (2012). Pharmacological effects of *Garcinia kola* seed powder on blood sugar, lipid profile and atherogenic index of alloxan-induced diabetes in rats. Pharmacologia , 3(12), 693-99.

[74] Washington, R. L. (1999). Interventions to reduce cardiovascular risk factors in children and adolescents. Am. Fam. Physician , 59, 2211-18.

[75] World Health Organization and International Diabetes Federation in Europe(1989). Diabetes care and research in Europe; Saint Vincent Declaration. British Med. J. , 299, 1198-1201.

Section 4

Plants with Benefits on Reproductive System

Chapter 11

Garlic and Its Effects on Health with Special Reference to the Reproductive System

Carlo Valente, Guillaume Aboua and
Stefan S. Du Plessis

Additional information is available at the end of the chapter

http://dx.doi.org/10.5772/57191

1. Introduction

Garlic is widely used around the world for its pungent flavour as a seasoning or condiment. From the history, it is known that garlic has been used for more than 7,000 years by humans. Originally the plant was native to central Asia [1], but it has long been used for consumption (raw or cooked) as seasoning in many other parts of the world such as the Mediterranean region, Africa, and Europe. It has specifically been used for its medicinal purposes in ancient Egypt. [2].

The garlic plant's bulb is the most commonly used part of the plant. As mentioned, garlic or more specifically the cloves is believed to have many medicinal properties ranging from positively affecting anything such as high blood pressure (BP) and lowering cholesterol to using it as a treatment for the common cold [3]. Even Hippocrates, Galen, and Dioscorides all mention the use of garlic for many conditions, including parasites, respiratory problems, poor digestion, and low energy [4].

Plants have always been the sources of important medicines since time immemorial. Currently there is a huge movement and emphasis towards scientifically and clinically unlocking the value of traditional phytomedicines in the service of humanity. With this in mind the scope of this chapter is to investigate garlic's effects on human health with special reference to the effect on the reproductive system. The chapter will furthermore aim to explain the mechanisms via which garlic can exert its effect.

2. Garlic: Overview and properties

Allium sativum, or commonly known as garlic, is a vegetable species that can be classified as either a food or a medicinal herb. It is a widely used plant product that is cultivated all over the world. Garlic falls into a family of *Amaryllidaceae* or the genus Allium. Its closest relatives in the onion genus include the onion, shallot, leek, rakkyo and chive [4].

The bulbs are mainly composed of water (approximately 84.09%), organic matter (13.38%) and inorganic matter (1.53%). The leaves consist of more or less the same components with slightly different ratios (water 87.14%, organic matter 11.27% and inorganic matter 1.59%) [5, 6].

The organic matter is mostly carbohydrates while the inorganic matter is compounds such as sulphur and iron. The large number of sulfur compounds contributes to the smell and taste of garlic. Allicin has been found to be the compound most responsible for the "hot" sensation of raw garlic (RG) [7]. Allicin, along with its decomposition products diallyl disulphide and diallyl trisulphide, are major contributors to the characteristic odour of garlic, while other allicin-derived compounds, such as vinyldithiins and ajoene show beneficial *in vitro* biological activity [4].

Despite having a minimal amount of ions and other compounds, those that are present play a very important role in the composition and overall beneficial effects that garlic potentially possesses [8].

When crushed, *Allium sativum* yields allicin, an antibiotic [9] and antifungal compound (phytoncide) discovered by Cavallito and colleagues in 1944. Fresh or crushed garlic also has enzymes, B vitamins, proteins, minerals, saponins, flavonoids, and Maillard reaction products. Furthermore, a phytoalexin (allixin) was found, a nonsulfur compound with a γ-pyrone skeleton structure with antioxidant effects, antimicrobial effect [10]antitumor promoting effects [11], inhibition of aflatoxin B2 DNA binding and neurotrophic effects [11].

There are different variants of the garlic root and each has its own properties that aid with good health. The white (natural) and black (fermented) garlic are just derivatives of how it is prepared, although each has its own unique effects. The white garlic is said to have medicinal properties while the black fermented garlic is more commonly used for cooking. Garlic can further be divided into two main subspecies being Ophioscorodon or hard necked garlic and Sativum or soft necked garlic [12]. Garlic can often be found in 4 forms namely; RG homogenate, garlic powder, aged garlic extract (AGE) and garlic oil.

- The RG homogenate is prepared by collecting garlic cloves and removing several outer layers. The cloves are then blended with distilled water and left for half an hour at 25ºC. The solution is then filtered and a homogenate sample is obtained [13].
- Garlic powder is prepared by pulverising crushed and dehydrated garlic cloves. This is mainly used for cooking purposes.

- AGE is obtained by placing garlic cloves in ethanol for a minimum of 20 months at room temperature. This reduces the concentration of allicin [13]. Which could reduce the medicinal properties of garlic as allicin is said to play a significant role.
- Garlic oil is obtained through a complex steaming and distillation process and is used in cooking or as medicinal oil.

The preparation of the garlic bulb is probably the most important factor in its effectiveness. Fresh garlic is often described as the best preparation to use to get superlative medicinal value out of the herb. Dried or cooked garlic often loses its potency because the amount of allicin present is significantly decreased in the cooking process [3]. Although the active ingredient in garlic is said to be unknown there is a lot of speculation around allicin as being the main constitutive/candidate [3]. More studies on sulphur are currently being done as this could also play a significant role, especially in organically grown garlic. Other studies state that the active ingredients are more directly associated with sulphur-containing amino acids, such as allicin, S-allylcysteine (SAC), S-allylmercaptocysteine (SAMC) S-methylcysteine, diallyl disulphide and sulfoxides [14].

Allicin is a very unstable molecule and breaks down very easily. This is why it is recommended to eat fresh garlic as it contains the highest amount of allicin. It is also the reason for the strong odour that garlic possesses. The more prominent this odour is the higher levels of allicin and beneficial values the bulb is said to have [15]. Due to this instability medical companies have now started to develop garlic supplements that contain Alliin - a stable precursor to allicin. It is only released upon digestion meaning the body will have the added benefit of having a sufficient amount of the favourable metabolite along with the safer more stable option [15].

The preparation of the garlic is of vital importance and studies have shown that each preparation has its own beneficial effects and more importantly its own threshold to when it starts becoming detrimental to the body. 2-5g of RG and 10-15g of boiled garlic provide beneficial effects with regard to prevent cancer development [16]. Likewise a certain amount of garlic supplementation would be beneficial in the male reproductive system. Unfortunately this amount is still unknown.

3. Garlic and human health

Garlic has been considered as a disease preventative food and its effects on the human health have been studied. Garlic infused medicine is on the increase due to the proposed beneficial effects on human health. The effects of garlic on both plant and animal models is best known for its ability to decrease the amount of lipids or free fatty acids, as well as its anti-atherogenic effects in both models [8].

Garlic supplements are now also being widely developed and recent studies have shown just that by mimicking the effect garlic has on the body. Allium products have the potential to reduce the risk of developing cancer or the potential to decrease the risk factors associated with cancers [17]. Research has been done on this and some evidence has been found that it has beneficial effects but there are also studies that show no effect at all [18].

Garlic has shown to have therapeutic effects, but the side effects are poorly investigated. The medicinal effects of garlic on certain diseases and specific systems will subsequently be discussed.

3.1. Effects on cardiovascular system

Cardiovascular disease (CVD) also known as heart disease is becoming an increasingly alarming problem in developing countries as it is the most common form of mortality [14]. Countries such as Spain and the USA have always been associated with heart disease, but developing countries are now showing an increasing trend in developing heart conditions [19]. With risk factors such as hypertension and hypercholesterolemia present, the onset of heart disease becomes more likely [20].

The effects of garlic on the cardiovascular system have been attracting a lot of interest in recent times with the development of modern medicine in particular [3]. An increase in the amount of cholesterol in the body can lead to the formation of atherosclerotic plaques and this is a risk factor for both heart attacks and strokes. Low-density lipoprotein (LDL) cholesterol levels can greatly be reduced without affecting the good High-density lipoprotein (HDL) cholesterol levels. The mode of action is said to be that garlic blocks the liver from making too much LDL because of its bio-active ingredients [15]. The high levels of cholesterol result in an increase in free-radical producing peptides. Reactive oxygen species (ROS) and oxidative stress (OS) levels are also key markers in CVD and by decreasing these levels the onset of heart disease can be delayed. Unfortunately the likeliness of developing heart disease increases with age and decreasing the amount of harmful oxidation in the body would be beneficial.

Garlic can delay the onset of heart disease due to its antioxidant properties. The type of extract used is of vital importance as it will influence the beneficial effects. Garlic reduces the amount of cholesterol in the body and by doing this the heart becomes more protected. Garlic also plays an important role in maintaining the structure and efficacy of endothelial cells and endothelial function [21]. The administration of AGE inhibits the progression of coronary-artery calcification and reduces the risk of a myocardial infarction or a heart attack [20]. Similarly, Allicor (a garlic powder tablet) was given to people suffering from coronary heart disease (CHD). This resulted in decreasing the risk of myocardial infarction, more significantly noted in males as opposed to females [14]. Studies have shown that the most effective way to reduce CVD is to try and reduce all the risk factors. Garlic-based preparations is thought to be promising agents for multifunctional risk reduction, but the mode of action remains slightly obscure [14].

With an increase in age the metabolic parameters of an individual is likely to change and this is evident in the onset of menopause in females. The end of the fertile phase in a woman's life is known as menopause and generally occurs during midlife or typically between the ages of 40 and 50. Together with diabetes, excessive weight, hypertension and endothelial dysfunction, menopause is a well-known risk factor for CVD which could lead to an increase in

http://dx.doi.org/10.5772/57191

metabolic parameters. Evidence shows that the vascular function in postmenopausal women could be affected by the changes in the reproductive hormones. One of the main precautionary measures for postmenopausal women with an increased CVD risk is exercise, however since ancient times garlic has been used as a treatment for CVD. It is said that AGE combined with exercise resulted in greater body weight loss than either AGE or exercise on its own. With the onset of menopause, fat and cholesterol levels are increased as well as the degree of oxidative stress. AGE has shown to reduce all these factors and is more easily absorbed in the body than other garlic preparations [21].

3.2. Effects on blood pressure

Blood pressure or arterial BP is the pressure exerted by circulating blood upon the walls of blood vessels [22]. BP can fluctuate from person to person depending on the individual and their health. A healthy patient should have an ideal BP of 120/80. If the BP exceeds 140/100 the patient is said to be hypertensive and if it is below 90/60 the person is hypotensive [23].

Hypertension and diabetes is said to be lifestyle-related diseases that has become a serious issue for countries previously not associated with it. Asian countries have now started to show a large increase in the amount of people suffering from high BP, with Japan having an estimated total of seven million people living with the disease [24]. Moreover one billion adults worldwide are affected by hypertension with about sixty-five million of them residing in the USA. This has led to approximately 40% of cardiovascular related deaths [25]. Hypertension has been considered to be the most important bio-marker in the onset of CVD.

Anti-hypertensive treatment has not always resulted in the desired effect of reducing the BP and alternative means of medication have now been developed. Garlic supplements and garlic derived products are becoming more and more popular in western medicine. AGE and RG showed to have the highest effect on lowering BP [24]. Interestingly, it is well known that AGE contains less allicin than RG. This has led to more studies being performed in order to establish the compound specifically responsible for lowering of the BP and reducing hypertension. The lowering effect that garlic has on BP is said to be due to the fact that the nitric oxide (NO) system is more active than the renin-angiotensin system. NO and Hydrogen sulphide (H_2S) play major roles in the progression of diseases, both NO and H_2S are considered to be important vasodilators. In a recent study both serum NO and H_2S were measured in diabetic rats and it was shown that chronic administration of garlic normalised both gaseous molecules and reduce BP [26].

It was found that both aged garlic and raw RG produce the same amount of NO implying that nitric oxide synthase (NOS) is the key to lowering BP. Both forms of garlic resulted in an increase in the activation of NOS. An increase in NO will lead to an increase in the relaxation of the blood vessels, and will therefor lead to a decrease in the BP. However, studies have shown that both AGE and RG require at least 3-4 weeks of daily administration before their action is expressed and this suggests that there could be a different mechanism for the lowering of BP [27].

The administration of AGE improved the condition of arteries as well as prevented the stiffening of the blood vessels which is a key marker in aging. By doing this it also improves erythrocytes which are the main component of blood. And therefor improves peripheral circulation and leads to a decrease in erythrocyte deformation. The improvement of blood circulation caused by AGE could be one of the causes of lowering BP, but RG showed to cause an increase in erythrocyte deformation and could lead to anaemia [25]. Garlic's medicinal properties in relation to its ability to lower BP have been studied extensively. It has been shown to significantly reduce BP in hypertensive patients when compared to those receiving a placebo [28]. Chronic feeding of AGE and RG decreased BP. Unfortunately the exact mechanism is not entirely elucidated as of yet. However, RG showed more harmful than beneficial effects. These results suggest that with regard to decrease in hypertension aged garlic would be the better and safer option [24]. It is also a safer treatment to use in conjunction with conventional anti-hypertensive therapy [25].

3.3. Effects on diabetes

Diabetes mellitus, or simply diabetes, is an endocrine disorder that forms part of a group of metabolic diseases characterised by elevated blood sugar levels or an insulin deficiency. Between one and two percent of the global population is affected by diabetes and there are roughly 100 million patients worldwide [29]. The most common form of diabetes is type two diabetes mellitus and comprises 80 percent of all diabetic populations [30]. A predicted increase from 51 to 72 million individuals affected by diabetes is expected in developed countries in the next decade; this translates to an increase of more than 42 percent. Developing countries will however face the brunt of the pandemic as it is expected to show an increase of 170 percent [31].

Diabetes is divided into two categories based on its mechanisms. Type 1 diabetes results from an individual's body failing to produce insulin, and currently requires the person to inject insulin or wear an insulin pump. It is also referred to as insulin-dependent diabetes mellitus (IDDM) or juvenile onset diabetes due to the fact that it is prominent in children [32]. This is a rare case of diabetes in comparison to its counterpart. Type 2 diabetes results from insulin resistance, a condition in which cells fail to use insulin properly, in some cases it is combined with an absolute insulin deficiency. It is also referred to as non-insulin-dependent diabetes mellitus (NIDDM) or adult-onset diabetes [32].

An individual's dietary factors play a key role in both the onset as well as the prevention of diabetes and other metabolic disorders [33]. Garlic is recognised for its therapeutic potential for controlling diabetes and its subsequent metabolic complications. The hypoglycaemic effect that garlic is said to have is attributed to the presence of allicin and sulphur compounds. Studies have shown that the oral administration of RG significantly reduced blood glucose levels and improved insulin sensitivity in garlic treated rats. Administration of aqueous garlic in patients with Type 1 diabetes has been reported to increase insulin sensitivity. Furthermore, metabolic complications such as increased serum-triglyceride, insulin and uric acid levels usually observed in diabetic rats were normalised after garlic administration [30].

http://dx.doi.org/10.5772/57191

Interestingly it has been observed that chronic administration of RG significantly reduced body weight, however the mechanism as to how garlic contributes to a reduction in body wait is still unclear. A study by Elkayam [26] has shown that allicin administered for 2-3 weeks reduced weight gain in fructose fed rats. Together with reducing glucose levels allicin also has the added advantage of decreased weight gain.

Glycation is the spontaneous phenomenon that occurs whenever proteins are exposed to reducing sugars and is depended on the degree and duration of hyperglycaemia in the body. It has been suggested that a direct reaction referred to as the Maillard reaction takes place during hyperglycaemia. This is a reaction that occurs between the sugars and proteins in the body. Advanced glycation end products (AGEPs) are formed when glycated proteins react with dicarbonyl intermediates to form complex heterogeneous, cross-linked and fluorescent molecules. Little is known about the chemistry of AGEPs but AGEPs are said to generate free radicals and lead to oxidative damage and this inevitably leads to diabetic complications [29]. The exact mechanism as to how garlic decreases glycation is uncertain but it is said to be due to decreasing the free radicals in the body, and it also increases anti-oxidant enzymes. Garlic also plays a role in the regulation of the Maillard reaction by inhibiting AGEP production/ formation, but more research is required on the exact mechanism [29].

3.4. Effects on dementia and the brain

Increased homocystein levels damages the endothelial cells that line blood vessels and prompts apoptosis by producing strand breaks in the DNA. This causes thrombotic activity that could result in heart attacks and strokes. Individuals living with dementia have a much higher level of homocystein than healthy people and there is a significant link between high levels of homocystein and loss of cognition. It has also been indicated that the intake of AGE decreases homocystein levels [20, 34].

Studies have also shown that there could be a link between heart diseases and dementia risks [34]. Risk factors such as hypertension, high cholesterol, increasing levels of homocystein, inflammation and oxidative stress are all related to both heart disease and dementia. These risks factors occur in the brain due to an increase in α-β peptide levels or a restriction in the blood supply to tissues. This could then result in cardiovascular or cerebrovascular diseases of which dementia and Alzheimer's disease (AD) is included [20, 34]. In addition to oxidative stress, free radicals such as ROS are closely associated with CVDs, cerebrovascular diseases such as dementia and cancer. It is believed that the damage done to DNA, proteins and lipids are considered of the foremost causes in the commencement and development of the diseases.

Free radicals increase in number when there is an infection, inflammation, hyperhomocysteinemia or exposure to smoking, drugs and radiation [35]. When the LDL cholesterol levels are changed due to oxidative stress and free radicals, the risk of atherosclerosis, cardio and cerebrovascular diseases increase. In addition neuronal apoptosis is triggered which leads to an increase in the risk of brain atrophy and dementia. AGE is known to lower homocystein levels, increase microcirculation and provide protection for endothelial cells from the effects of oxidation. Following a stroke the risk factors of neurodegenerative conditions and CVD include myocardial ischemic or reperfusion injury, AGE can protect the body against this by increasing the production of constitutive NO [20, 34]. AGE has also been shown to possess anti-aging properties, in studies AGE prevented the deterioration of the brain's frontal lobe, and enhanced learning and memory retention.

3.5. Effects on cancer

Cancer or malignant neoplasm is a broad group of diseases involving unregulated cell growth. Cell division and uncontrollable growth of these cells form malignant tumours in individuals living with cancer. These tumours are very likely to invade nearby parts of the body. The lymphatic system or bloodstream may also spread the cancer to more distant parts of the body. However, not all tumours are cancerous. Benign tumours do not invade neighbouring tissues and do not spread throughout the body [36].

There are over 200 different known cancers that affect humans ranging from breast and prostate cancer to colorectal and lung cancer. In the year 2008 approximately 12 million people worldwide were said to be living with cancer and this figure is expected to rise to about 21 million by the year 2030. Lung cancer is responsible for the most deaths closely followed by breast and colorectal cancer [37].

Garlic is said to have chemo-preventive properties and its effects have been closely studied on various cancers. The antitumor effects that garlic potentially possesses are directly attributed to its anti-mutagenic properties [38]. The formations of tumours in vitro and in vivo were shown to be greatly decreased after the administration of fresh garlic, although the mechanism of action is still unknown. The timing and dose of the garlic could be the main factor in inhibition of the pro-carcinogens [38]. A possible mode of action as to how garlic can prevent cancer is by the effects of Diallyl trisulphide (DATS). DATS is a by-product of garlic that exhibits several pharmacological effects (e.g. anti-microbial and CVD), making this compound a promiscuous agent with possible beneficial chemo-prevention properties due to the complex pathways in cancers [39]. Oral ingestion of aged garlic (that is lacking enzymatically produced allicin due to the fact that it was not chopped) reduced 1, 2-dimethylhydrazine induced colon tumours significantly [40]. With specific reference to skin cancer, the treatment results are inconclusive and more research will have to be conducted [41]. Stomach tumours were greatly decreased by administration of AGE. The toxicity of garlic was not directly responsible for the death of cancer cells alone although it does play an important role. Another key role in the prevention of cancers is garlics effect on the immune system. Macrophage activity, NK and killer cells as well as the cytokine TNF were all shown to have increased activity after administration of garlic and this resulted in an increase in antitumor response [42]. Colorectal cancer is the third leading cause of cancer death in the world. In this respect normal garlic cannot be administrated and would need to be introduced as part of a strict diet. The Garlic and low meat diet did however show a decrease in colorectal tumour growth [43].

http://dx.doi.org/10.5772/57191

3.6. Effects on reproductive system

Infertility and especially idiopathic infertility has been on the increase during the last century. Infertility is the inability to conceive after having unprotected sexual intercourse for more than a year of trying [44]. In 19-57% of cases the male is at fault when a couple have infertility concerns [45]. This has led to a lot of research on male fertility and the male reproductive system. Garlic and its effects on the male reproductive system has caused a tremendous amount of interest in the Andrology and reproductive field as some researchers believe it to have a beneficial influence and others believe it to have a detrimental effect on the male reproductive system. The possible reason as to why these discrepancies exist could be due to the preparation and the dosage.

3.6.1. Spermatogenesis and sperm function

In a study performed by Qian and co-workers it was shown that the administration of garlic to rats showed a decrease in sperm quality and functionality. The amount and preparation of garlic will result in a decrease in specific seminal parameters. The crude extract of garlic results in an increase in the percentage of empty seminiferous tubules. It has been reported to reduce membrane disintegration and irreversible immobilization of sperm [46] while at the same time reducing sperm viability [47]. This is the reason as to why some researcher's believe that garlic acts as a natural contraceptive although more research would have to be performed [47]. The majority of data report garlic to have deleterious effects on specifically the male reproductive system. In another study testicular morphological alterations were noted after male adult rats were given 50 mg kg^{-1} of garlic powder for 45-75 days [48]. Hammami and El May (2009) found that garlic improved male sexual dysfunction in direct contrast to the studies previously mentioned which claimed garlic to have a negative impact on male reproductive function. The main difference and possibly the reason between different results could be the lack of standardization between research models and the different amounts of garlic given to test subjects [3].

Spermatogenesis is the process whereby spermatozoa are produced. Needless to say it is a very important process in the male reproductive organs. The production of spermatozoa can be effected by various stimuli. ROS and heat are important in the formation of mature sperm but a large amount of ROS and higher than normal physiological temperatures levels may become hazardous to the spermatozoa.

The daily administration of garlic powder and aqueous garlic to adult rats caused spermicidal effects and spermatogenetic arrest. However, feeding a higher garlic supplementation over a longer period of time to the adult rats caused an increase in Epididymal spermatozoa [3]. Although an animal model was used, comparisons can be linked to a human model to the similarities in the reproductive systems of the respective models. The effect of garlic on spermatogenesis and on testis also yielded contrasting findings. Administration of garlic over a period of time showed to have histological alterations on the cells within the testes. Both the Leydig and Sertoli cells showed lipid droplets along with a decrease in volume. Spermatocytes showed interrupted nuclear development and an increase in apoptosis was also evident [49].

Apoptosis is a physiological term used to explain programmed cell death [50]. Caspase 3 formation is a vital step in the activation of the apoptotic pathway and an increase in crude garlic intake leads to an increase in caspase 3 formation. Apoptosis effects the formation of spermatocytes and spermatids and the testes have shown an increase in apoptotic germ calls after the rat is exposed to crude garlic feeding [51].It was shown that supplementing the diet with crude garlic induced apoptosis in both spermatocytes and spermatids [51]. Dixit & Joshi [48] again noted that treating rats with garlic powder impaired spermatogenesis and led to an early arrest in the development of spermatozoa. This in turn reduced the amount of round spermatids converted into elongated spermatids furthermore impairing spermatogenesis. With regards to the testicular function, garlic and its metabolites have a protective function. The effects of garlic on the testes include prevention of hypogonadism caused by heat and protection against cadmium-induced testicular damage by reversing the alterations in the biochemical parameters [52]. Other beneficial properties are its ability to restore testicular histology and decrease free radicals in the testes which are detrimental when in large amounts.

3.6.2. Hormonal levels and libido

Garlic feeding has both positive and negative effects on testosterone production. It is important to note that between the different studies that were performed, different preparations, amounts and concentrations of garlic were administered. The preparation of the garlic could possibly be the key factor involved in the impact it will have. By administering crude garlic to Rat models it was recorded that there was a decrease in testosterone formation due to the decrease in responsiveness of the leydig cells to the luteinizing hormone. This decrease in responsiveness is due to the histological alteration in the testes (Figure 1). In contrast Oi et al. [53] showed an increase in testosterone levels due to the increase in the luteinizing hormones after administration of 8g of garlic powder. Again, the different preparations of the garlic plant are vital.

Garlic's effects on the reproductive system have led to contradictory results. According to Hammami et al. [51] garlic has been used to improve male sexual dysfunction and this includes impotence. Heated garlic juice is effective in recovering testicular function after experimental hypogonadism, but powder or crude garlic (in large amounts) impairs male reproductive tract functions [51].

Benign prostatic hyperplasia (BHP) is an extremely common condition in older men and can affect the male reproductive system. Milk and other dairy products have been related to an increase in BHP but the results found are very inconsistent. The same trend applies for garlic as studies have shown that cooked garlic can decrease the onset of BPH but RG can increase the onset [54]. Aqueous garlic extract has however shown to improve disease parameters in patients with BPH [55]. Garlic extract also decreases the onset of prostatic cancers and other malignancies [56]. The results are however inconclusive and very contrasting amongst published articles and no real conclusion can be drawn until more research is done on the effects of vegetable- more specific garlic – has on the male reproductive system.

http://dx.doi.org/10.5772/57191

4. Mechanisms

The scientific and pharmacologic explanations for most of the medicinal effects attributed to garlic treatment are still eluding researchers. There is however a few mechanisms via which garlic more than likely exert its effects which are worth mentioning and highly plausible.

4.1. Antioxidant properties

An antioxidant is a molecule that inhibits the oxidation of other molecules in the human body [57]. A chemical reaction known as oxidation occurs when electrons or hydrogen atoms are transferred from a substance to an oxidizing agent. Once this oxidation reaction occurs, free radicals are produced and realised into the body. In turn, these radicals can start chain reactions. Antioxidants terminate these chain reactions by removing free radical intermediates, and inhibit other oxidation reactions [58]. Antioxidants are present in most of the foods we eat and drink like spinach, oranges, whole wheat bread and tea. Garlic is also very rich in antioxidants [59] (Table 1). The powerful odour that fresh garlic possesses is due to the amount of allicin that is present. This odour as well as the unique acquired flavour of garlic has resulted that not every one favours it [20]. This led to the emergence of the AGE. As mentioned previously AGE is obtained via a long and tedious process. The extract obtained through this process does not have the pungent flavour of garlic and is also odourless [60]. This is due to the fact that a large amount of allicin is lost and therefor it loses a lot of its beneficial properties. However, due to the amount of allicin lost, this means that the most prominent component in AGE is the organosulfurs like SAC and SAMC. These compounds are said to have potent antioxidant effects in the body. S-allylcysteine and S-allylmercaptocysteine increase with aging of the garlic. Therefore, the longer the garlic is aged the less allicin it will contain, but the more antioxidant effect it will have. This makes AGE the most potent form of garlic with regards to antioxidant ability.

Oxidative stress is the term used to describe the process that transpires when there are too many free radicals or not enough antioxidant agents in the body [20]. This oxidative damage is often associated with aging and age-degenerative conditions such as dementia and AD. AGE has shown to inhibit this oxidative damaged caused and helps with reducing the risk factor or onset of neurodegenerative disease as well as slowing down the aging process or to be more specific the onset of deteriorating skin. However, the administration of garlic did not decrease the levels of iron mediated oxidative stress [61]. The antioxidant actions of AGE are based on decreasing the amounts of ROS and reactive nitrogen species (RNS) as well as inhibiting LDL oxidation and lipid peroxide formation. An increase in ROS in the body can lead to a host of issues including endothelial dysfunction which is a key marker in the development of cardiac injury. Likewise LDL oxidation could lead to vascular dysfunction and promotes the onset of atherosclerosis and possibly myocardial infarction [20].

A study was done to compare the antioxidant potential of the different garlic preparations. AGE which is predominantly SAC and SAMC was compared to a water extract of fresh garlic containing mostly alliin and RG that contains allicin [62]. AGE had the highest antioxidant effect and surprisingly the other two preparations served more as an oxidant [62]. Although the majority of the antioxidant affects are from the AGE there are incidents where other preparations were used as an antibiotic/antioxidant. A lot of the mechanisms by which garlic acquired its medicinal properties have been specifically ascribed to this potent antioxidant action. It has the ability to stimulate immunological responsiveness and its modulation of prostanoids synthesis. The antioxidant properties of garlic have been studied extensively and it does have a beneficial role in the body. AGE is however more effective in removing free radicals and LDL cholesterol than other preparations of the garlic root, but that does not mean the other preparations aren't important as well.

4.2. Antibiotic properties

Allicin, found in the garlic bulb, serves as a powerful antibiotic which aids the body in inhibiting the growth and reproduction of bacteria [63]. One milligram of allicin is equal to 15 standard units of penicillin [63]. Allicin attacks over 23 types of bacteria, such as staph and salmonella, 60 types of fungi and yeast and is also effective against 17 of the most dangerous fungi [64]. Another example of where allicin serves as a potent antibiotic is in the treatment of Streptolysin O (SLO). SLO is a powerful cytolytic toxin found in almost all group A streptococci. Treatment of SLO with Allicin completely neutralized the haemolytic activity of the bacteria, while the aqueous garlic extract inhibited it altogether [65]. From these results it can be deducted that garlic and its metabolites have antibiotic properties. Extracts of fresh garlic contain antioxidant phytochemicals that prevent oxidative damage.

4.3. NO and H_2S

NO and H_2S play major roles in the progression of diseases, both NO and H_2S are considered to be important vasodilators. In a recent study both serum NO and H_2S were measured in diabetic rats and it was shown that chronic administration of garlic normalised both gaseous molecules [26] and this decreased hypertension by inhibiting certain enzymes such as N omega-nitro-L-arginine-methyl-ester (L-NAME) [66].

5. Conclusion and recommendations

From this review it is evident that garlic certainly has some medicinal properties. Various studies highlighted its cardio protective, antibiotic, anti-hypertensive and cholesterol lowering effects. Some evidence also points to its ability to lower the risk of developing cancer. Not all the research data are as clear and conclusive and certain remain ambiguous. Garlic appears to exert both positive and negative effects on the male reproductive system. Interestingly enough crude garlic (if taken in large amounts) shows the most detrimental and AGE garlic the most beneficial results. The most crucial factor in determining the effects observed is possibly the manner in which the garlic was prepared as well as the amount that is being administered. Interestingly, large amounts are deemed to be more detrimental. Some of the results found showed that the administration of garlic affected testicular function, histological properties and sperm quality [46, 48 & 51]. Hormone levels were subsequently also altered and an increase in testicular tissue apoptosis was recorded [51]. Furthermore crude garlic extracts and garlic juice showed to cause sperm immobilization (administered as 15g/100g and 30g/100g respectively) [51, 67, 68]. More research definitely needs to be performed on the effect of garlic on acrosome and DNA integrity of spermatozoa.

In general it can be said that garlic's therapeutic properties warrants further investigation in order to develop its full treatment potential as a phytotherapeutical agent impacting on human health and used for the treatment of various disease conditions. The specific mechanism of action also need to be identified as it can possible shed more light on and help with the development of more effective pharmacological agents. Additional human studies on AGE and its constituents are needed to elucidate their role in protecting human health, and molecular studies should be intensified to reveal the underlying mechanisms.

Product	Source of commercial sample	Lot#	% Inhibition[2] (SD)
AGE	Kyolic liquid (Mission Viejo)	5LO1	+121.8 (2.73)
A	Garlinase 4000 (Enzymatic Therapy, Green Bay, WI)	213Y46QD	-213.0 (4.67)
B	Garlic powder (McCormick, Baltimore, MD)	0208A	-217.2 (5.20)
C	Quintessence caplet (Pur- Gar, Takoma, WA)	36698	-239.5 (4.85)
D	Quintessence capsule (Pur- Gar, Takoma, WA)	63121	-242.1 (5.15)
E	Garlicin (Nature's Way Product, Springville, UT)	503369	-246.8 (9.24)
F	Kwai (Lichtwerpharma, Berlin, Germany)	94080700	-250.7 (3.01)
G	Garlique (Sunsource HealthProducts, Kihei, HI)	5J0010	-251.0 (10.6)
H	Garlic Time (ArizonaNatural Products,Scottsdale, AZ)	896210	-254.4 (7.14)

[1]Laboratory Report, Wakunaga Pharmaceutical, Hiroshima, Japan, October 1995. Courtesy of Wakunaga of America Company. Garlic products were purchased from stores, as in Freeman and Kodera 1995. Each analysis was performed three times.

[2]Antioxidant properties were measured by the ability of the various products to inhibit the emission of low level chemiluminescence, in a liver microsomal fraction, initiated by t-butyl hydroperoxide (Imai et al. 1994). Inhibition (+) denotes antioxidant activity, resulting from scavenging of reactive oxygen species (ROS) and reflected in the inhibition of light emission. Inhibition (-) denotes prooxidant activity of a product as reflected in an increased light emission, induced by increased ROS activity.

*Table reproduced from "Recent Advances on the Nutritional Benefits Accompanying the Use of Garlic as a Supplement" held November 15–17, 1998 in Newport Beach, CA. The conference was supported by educational grants from Pennsylvania State University, Wakunaga of America, Ltd. and the National Cancer Institute. The proceedings of this conference are published as a supplement to *The Journal of Nutrition 131:1010S–1015S, 2001*.

Table 1. Antioxidant effects of aged garlic extract (AGE) compared with other garlic supplements[1*]

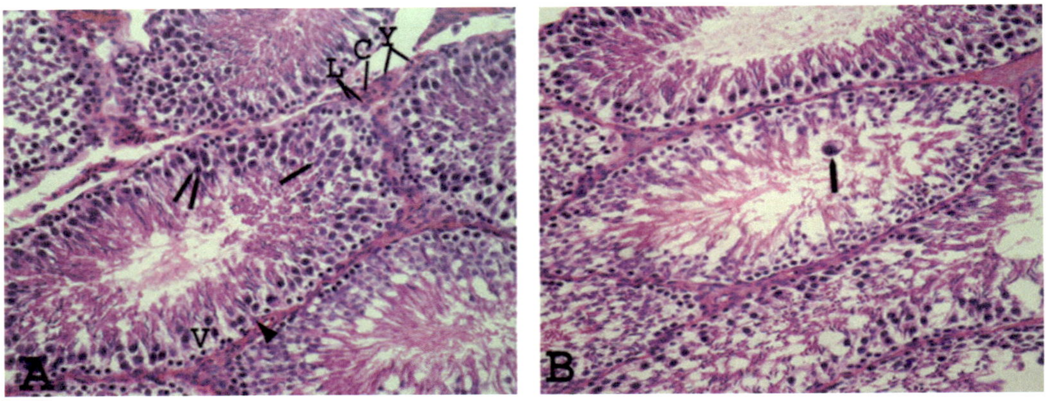

Figure 1. Photomicrographs of sections of testes of albino rats having received 20% of their daily food as crude garlic for two months (subgroup B1) showing: (A) intraepithelial vacuoles of variable sizes (V). Sertoli cell nuclei () on the basal portion of the tubules. Primary spermatocyte nuclei either dividing normally (↑) or with condensed chromatin (↑↑). Some seminiferous tubules possess irregular basal lamina and are separated from each other. Interstitial tissue with Leydig cells (L), plasma cells (c) and lymphocytes (Y) (×200). (B) Giant cell (↑) formation and exfoliation in the lumen of the seminiferous tubules (×200). (Reproduced from Abdelmalik, 2011)

Author details

Carlo Valente[1], Guillaume Aboua[2*] and Stefan S. Du Plessis[1]

*Address all correspondence to: abouay@cput.ac.za

1 Division of Medical Physiology, Faculty of Medicine and Health Sciences, Stellenbosch University, Tygerberg, South Africa

2 Department of Biomedical Sciences, Faculty of Health and Wellness, Cape Peninsula University of Technology, Bellville, South Africa

References

[1] Ensminger AH. Foods & nutrition encyclopedia, Volume 1. CRC Press. 1994; ISBN 0-8493-8980-1. p. 750

[2] Simonetti G, Schuler S., ed. Simon & Schuster's Guide to Herbs and Spices. Simon & Schuster, Inc. ISBN 0-671-73489-X]. 1990

[3] Hammami I, El May M. Impact of garlic feeding(allium sativum) on male fertility, Andrologia 2012; 1-8

[4] Block E. Garlic and Other Alliums: The Lore and the Science. Royal Society of Chemistry. ISBN 0-85404-190-7. 2010

[5] Bilyk A, Sapers GM. Distribution of quercetin and kaempferol in lettuce, kale, chive, garlic chive, leek, horseradish, red radish, and red cabbage tissues. Journal of Agricultural and Food Chemistry 1985;33:226– 33

[6] Abdel-Fattah AF, Edrees M. A study on the composition of garlic skins and the structural features of the isolated pectic acid. Journal of the Science of Food and Agriculture 1972; 23: 871-877

[7] Macpherson LJ, Geierstanger BH, Viswanath V, Bandell M, Eid SR, Hwang S, Patapoutian A. The pungency of garlic: activation of TRPA1 and TRPV1 in response to allicin. Current Biology 2005 24;15: 929-34

[8] Prasad K. Natural products in regression and slowing of progression of atherosclerosis. Current Pharmaceutical Biotechnology 2010; 11:794–800

[9] Focke M, Feld A, Linchtenthaler HK. Allicin, a naturally occurring antibiotic from garlic, specifically inhibits acetyl-CoA synthetase. FEBS Letters 1990; 261: 106- 108

[10] Ankri S, Mirelman D. Antimicrobial properties of allicin from garlic. Microbes and Infection 1999; 2: 125–129

[11] Aaron T. Fleischauer AT, Arab L. Garlic and Cancer: A Critical Review of the Epidemiologic Literature. Journal of Nutrition 2001; 131:1032S–1040S

[12] Hahn, G. Botanical chracterization and cultivation of garlic. In Garlic: The Science and Therapeutic Application of Allium satiVum L. and Related Species, 2nd ed.; Koch, H. P., Lawson, L. D., Eds.; Williams & Wilkins: Baltimore, MD, 1996; 25-36

[13] Kasuga S, Uda N, Kyo E, Ushijima M, Morihara N, Itakura Y. Pharmacologic activities of aged garlic extract in comparison with other garlic preparations. Journal of Nutrition 2001;131:1080–1084

[14] Sobenin I, Pryanishnikov V, Kunnova L, Yevgeny, Rabinovich A, Martirosyan D, Orekhov AN. The effects of time-released garlic powder tablets on multifunctional cardiovascular risk in patients with coronary artery disease. Lipids in Health and Disease 2010; 9:119

[15] Hornick B, Yarnell E. Medical uses for garlic, http://health.howstuffworks.com/wellness/naturalmedicine/alternative/medical-uses-for-garlic-ga.htm (acc on 5th august 2013).

[16] WHO (2002) Traditional Medicine Strategy 2002–2005. WHO, Geneva.

[17] Cerella C, Dicato M, Jacob C, Diederich M. Chemical properties and mechanisms determining the anti-cancer action of garlic-derived organic sulfur compounds. Anticancer Agents Medicinal Chemistry 2011;11:267–271

[18] Kim JY, Kwon O. Garlic intake and cancer risk: an analysis using the Food and Drug Administration's evidence-based review system for the scientific evaluation of health claims. American Journal of Clinical Nutrition 2009; 89:257–264

[19] Fuster B, Kelly BB. Promoting cardiovascular health in the developing world: A critical challenge to achieve global health. Washington, DC: National Academies Press; 2010

[20] Borek C. Garlic Reduces Dementia and Heart-Disease Risk, Journal Nutrition 2006;136: 810S–812S

[21] Seo DY, Lee SR, Kim HK, Baek YH, Kwak YS, Ko TH, Kim N, Rhee BD, Ko KS, Park BJ, Han J. Independent beneficial effects of aged garlic extract intake with regular exercise on cardiovascular risk in postmenopausal women. Nutrition Research Practice 2012;63:226-31

[22] Caro CG. The Mechanics of the Circulation. Oxford [Oxfordshire]: Oxford University Press 1978

[23] Pesola GR, Pesola HR, Nelson MJ, Westfal RE. The normal difference in bilateral indirect blood pressure recordings in normotensive individuals. American Journal of Emergency Medicine 2001; 19: 43–5

[24] Harauma A, Moriguchi T. Aged Garlic Extract Improves Blood Pressure in Spontaneously Hypertensive Rats More Safely than Raw Garlic. Journal of Nutrition 2006;136: 769S–773S

[25] K Ried, Frank OR and Stocks NP. Aged garlic extract reduces blood pressure in hypertensives: a dose–response trial. European Journal of Clinical Nutrition 2013: 67, 64–70

[26] Elkayam A, Mirelman D, Peleg E, Wilchek M, Miron T, Rabinkov A, Oron-Herman M, Rosenthal T. The Effects of Allicin on Weight in Fructose-Induced Hyperinsulinemic, Hyperlipidemic, Hypertensive Rats. American Journal of Hypertension 2003; 16:1053-1056

[27] Ignarro LJ, Buga GM, Wood KS, Byrnes RE, Chaudhuri G. Endothelium derived relaxing factor produced and released from artery and vein is nitric oxide. Proceeding of the National Academy of Sciences USA. 1987; 84: 9265–9

[28] Ried K, Frank OR, Stocks NP, Peter Fakler1 and Sullivan T. Effect of garlic on blood pressure: A systematic review and meta-analysis. BMC Cardiovascular Disorders 2008, 8:13

[29] Saeed M, Nessar A. Antiglycation Properties of Aged Garlic Extract: Possible Role in Prevention of Diabetic Complications, Journal of Nutrition 2006;136: 796S–799S

[30] Padiya R, Khatua TN, Bagul PK, Kuncha M and Banerjee SK. Garlic improves insulin sensitivity and associated metabolic syndromes in fructose fed rats, Nutrition & Metabolism 2011, 8:53

[31] King H, Aubert RE, Herman WH. Global burden of diabetes, 1995-2025: prevalence, numerical estimates, and projections. Diabetes Care 1998, 21:1414-1431

[32] Lambert P, Bingley PJ. What is Type 1 Diabetes? Medicine 2002; 30: 1–5

[33] Carson JF: Chemistry and biological properties of onion and garlic. Food Research International 1987, 3:71-103

[34] Mathew BC, Biju RS. Neuroprotective Effects of Garlic A review. Libyan Journal of Medecine 2008; 23-33

[35] Yao M, Nguyen TV, Pike CJ. {beta}-Amyloid-induced neuronal apoptosis involves c-Jun N-terminal kinase-dependent downregulation of Bcl-w. Journal of Neuroscience. 2005;25:1149–58

[36] Anand P, Kunnumakkara AB, Kunnumakara AB, Sundaram C, Harikumar KB, Tharakan ST, Lai OS, Sung B, Aggarwal BB (September 2008). "Cancer is a preventable disease that requires major lifestyle changes". Pharm. Res. 25 (9): 2097–116

[37] World cancer research fund international http://www.wcrf.org/cancer_statistics/world_cancer_statistics.php (Acc 5th August 2013)

[38] Dorant E, van den Brandt PA, Goldbohm RA, Hermus RJJ, Sturmansd F. Garlic and its significance for the prevention of cancer in humans: a critical view. British Journal of Cancer 1993; 67: 424–429

[39] Antony ML and Singh SV. Molecular Mechanisms and Targets of Cancer Chemoprevention by Garlic-derived Bioactive Compound Diallyl Trisulfide. Indian Journal of Experimental Biology. 2011; 49: 805–816

[40] Katsuki T, Hirata K, Ishikawa H, Matsuura N, Sumi S and Itoh H. Aged Garlic Extract Has Chemopreventative Effects On 1,2-Dimethylhydrazine-Induced Colon Tumors in Rats. Journal of Nutrition 2006, 847S-851S

[41] Wang HC, Pao J, Lin SY, and Sheen L, Molecular mechanisms of garlic-derived allyl sulfides in the inhibition of skin cancer progression, Annals of the New York Academy of Sciences 2012; 1271: 44–52.

[42] Lamm DL, Riggs DR. Enhanced Immunocompetence by Garlic: Role in Bladder Cancer and Other Malignancies, Journal of Nutrition 2001;131: 1067S–1070S

[43] Ngo SNT, Williams DB, Cobiac L, Head RJ. Does Garlic Reduce Risk of Colorectal Cancer? A Systematic Review, Journal of Nutrition 2007,137: 2264–2269

[44] Makar RS, Toth TL. The evaluation of infertility American Journal of Clinical Pathology 2002; 117 (Suppl): S95–103

[45] Wilkes S, Chinn DJ, Murdoch A, Rubin G. Epidemiology and management of infertility: a population-based study in UK primary care. Family Practice 2009; 26:269 – 274.

[46] Qian YX, Shen PJ, Xu RY, Liu GM, Yang HQ, Lu YS, Sun P, Zhang RW, Qi LM, Lu QH. Spermicidal effect in vitro by the active principle of garlic. Contraception 1986 ; 34(3):295-302

[47] Ogbuewu IP, Unamba-Oparah IC, Odoemenam VU, Etuk, IF and Okoli IC, The potentiality of medicinal plants as the source of new contraceptive principles in males. New American Journal of Medical Sciences 2011; 3(6): 255–263

[48] Dixit VP, Joshi S. Effects of chronic administration of garlic (Allium sativum Linn) on testicular function. Indian Journal Experimental Biology 1982; 20:534–536

[49] Hammami I, Nahdi A, Mauduit C, Benahmed M, Amri M, Ben Amar A, Zekri S, El May A, El May MV. The inhibitory effects on adult male reproductive functions of crude garlic (Allium sativum) feeding. Asian Journal of Andrology 2008;10:593–601

[50] Kerr, JF. A histochemical study of hypertrophy and ischaemic injury of rat liver with special reference to changes in lysosomes. Journal of Pathology and Bacteriology 1965; 90 (90): 419–35

[51] Hammami I, Amara S, Benahmed M, El MV, Mauduit M and Mauduit C. Chronic crude garlic-feeding modified adult male rat testicular markers: mechanisms of action. Reproductive Biology and Endocrinology 2009, 7:65

[52] Eteng MU, Onwuka FC, Akpanyung EO, Osuchukwu NC, Bassey SC, Nwankpa P.Reversal of cadmium induced toxicity following dietary supplementation with garlic, ginger and cabbage in male Wistar rats. Journal of Natural Products and Plant Resources 2012; 2 (1):169-174

[53] Oi Y, Imafuku M, Shishido C, Kominato Y, Nishimura S, Iwai Garlic supplementation increases testicular testosterone and decreases plasma corticosterone in rats fed a high protein diet. Journal of Nutrition 2001; 131:2150–2156

[54] Bravi F, Bosetti C, Dal Maso L, Talamini R, Montella M, Negri E, et al. Food groups and risk of benign prostatic hyperplasia urology 67: 73–79, 2006

[55] Galeone C, Pelucchi C, Talamini R, Negri E, Dal Maso L, Montella M, et al.Onion and garlic intake and the odds of benign prostatic hyperplasia. Urology2007;70:672–6

[56] Devrim E and Durak L, Is garlic a promising food for benign prostatic hyperplasia and prostate cancer, Molecular Nutrition and Food Research 2007, 51, 1319 – 1323

[57] Prabhat J, Flather M, Lonn E, Farkouh M, and Yusuf S. "The Antioxidant Vitamins and Cardiovascular Disease: A Critical Review of Epidemiologic and Clinical Trial Data". Annals of Internal Medicine 1995;123(11): 860–872

[58] Helmut S. Oxidative stress: Oxidants and antioxidants. Experimental physiology 1997; 82 (2): 291–5

[59] Rao A, Balachandran B. Role of oxidative stress and antioxidants in neurodegenerative diseases. Nutrition and Neuroscience 2002; 5 (5): 291–309

[60] Moriguchi, T., Saito, H. & Nishiyama, N. Anti-aging effect of aged garlic in inbred brain atrophy model mouse. Clinical Experimental Pharmacology and Physiology 1997; 24: 235–242

[61] Nahdia A,B, Hammamia I, Brasse-Lagnelb C, Pilardb N, Hamdaouic MH, Beaumontb C, El May M, Influence of garlic or its main active component diallyl disulfide on iron bioavailability and toxicity, Nutrition Research 2010; 30 85–95

[62] Imai, J, Ide, N., Nagae, S., Moriguchi, T., Matsuura, H. & Itakura, Y. Antioxidants and free radical scavenging effects of aged garlic extract and its constituents. Planta Medica 1994; 60: 417–420

[63] Pandya K, Solanki B, Maniar K, Gurav N, Bhatt S. Natural herbal supplements- A study on their nutritional value and their phytochemical constituents. International Journal of Pharmaceutical Sciences and Research 2011; 2:1480–94

[64] Ankri S, Mirelman D. Antimicrobial properties of allicin from garlic, Microbes and Infection, 2, 1999, 125–129

[65] Arzanlou M and Bohlooli S. Inhibition of streptolysin O by allicin – an active component of garlic. Journal of Medical Microbiology (2010), 59, 1044–1049

[66] Pedraza-Chaverrí J, Tapia E, Medina-Campos ON, de los Angeles Granados M, Franco M, Garlic prevents hypertension induced by chronic inhibition of nitric oxide synthesis. Life Sciences; 1998; 62 71-77

[67] Chakrabarti K, Pal S, Bhattacharyya AK. Sperm immobilization activity of Allium sativum L. and other plant extracts. Asian Journal of Andrology 2003;5(2):131-5

[68] Abdelmalik SW. Histological and ultrastructural changes in the adult male albino rat testes following chronic crude garlic consumption. Annals of Anatomy 2011; 193: 134–141

Chapter 12

Potentials of Phytotherapeutic Treatment of Erectile Dysfunction

Guillaume Aboua, Claudine Manirafasha,
Boitumelo R. Mosito, Michelle van der Linde and
Stefan S. du Plessis

Additional information is available at the end of the chapter

http://dx.doi.org/10.5772/57174

1. Introduction

Erectile dysfunction (ED) or (male) impotence is a sexual dysfunction characterized by the inability to develop or maintain an erection of the penis [1]. There are various underlying causes, such as a compromised cardiovascular system and diseases such as diabetes and chronic kidney disease (CKD), many of which are medically treatable. The causes of erectile dysfunction may be physiological or psychological [2]. Sexual function includes libido, penile erection, ejaculation, and orgasm. While each of these parameters may be of concern to an individual patient, the vast majority of men complain of ED. Testosterone deficiency frequently is associated with decreased libido and ED. ED is a clinical problem that is underdiagnosed, under-evaluated, and under-treated. The prevalence of ED increases with age, and it is associated with multiple medical conditions including diabetes, hypertension, and heart disease that also increase with age. ED is a highly prevalent and often underreported condition. The prevalence of ED varies in different countries and approximately 100 million men worldwide are estimated to be affected with ED. More than half of US men between the ages of 40 and 70 years are estimated to have ED. The worldwide ED prevalence in men with diabetes ranges from 27% to 75% and it is estimated that the prevalence of ED will double in the next 25 years [3]. There is a strong link between ED and atherosclerotic disease due to the fact that they share similar risk factors. In a study where patients referred for myocardial perfusion single-photon emission computed tomography were screened for ED with a questionnaire, it was found out that 54.8% of the patients had ED. Patients with ED showed more severe coronary heart disease. In diabetic patients, ED has been shown to predict silent coronary artery disease, and in asymptomatic men without cardiovascular risk factors or known vascular disease [4]. Nevertheless, the hypothesis that ED, as a manifestation of autonomic neuropathy, may be linked with the lack of symptoms in a proportion of diabetic patients with silent CAD cannot be excluded [4].

2. Causes of erectile dysfunction

ED arises as a result of a collision of many factors: physical, psychological, physiological and biochemical abnormalities. The exact cause of ED is usually difficult to establish because it normally results from an underlying condition such as diabetes and/or heart disease. ED can also be caused by psychological conditions such as stress, depression and anxiety [5]. The physiological mechanism of erection is a complex neurovascular phenomenon that depends on neural, vascular, hormonal, and psychological factors. Integrated function of these factors is essential for production of a normal erectile response [3]. Recent advances in the understanding of functional anatomy and of neurovascular interactions have improved our understanding of the pathophysiological mechanism of ED [3].

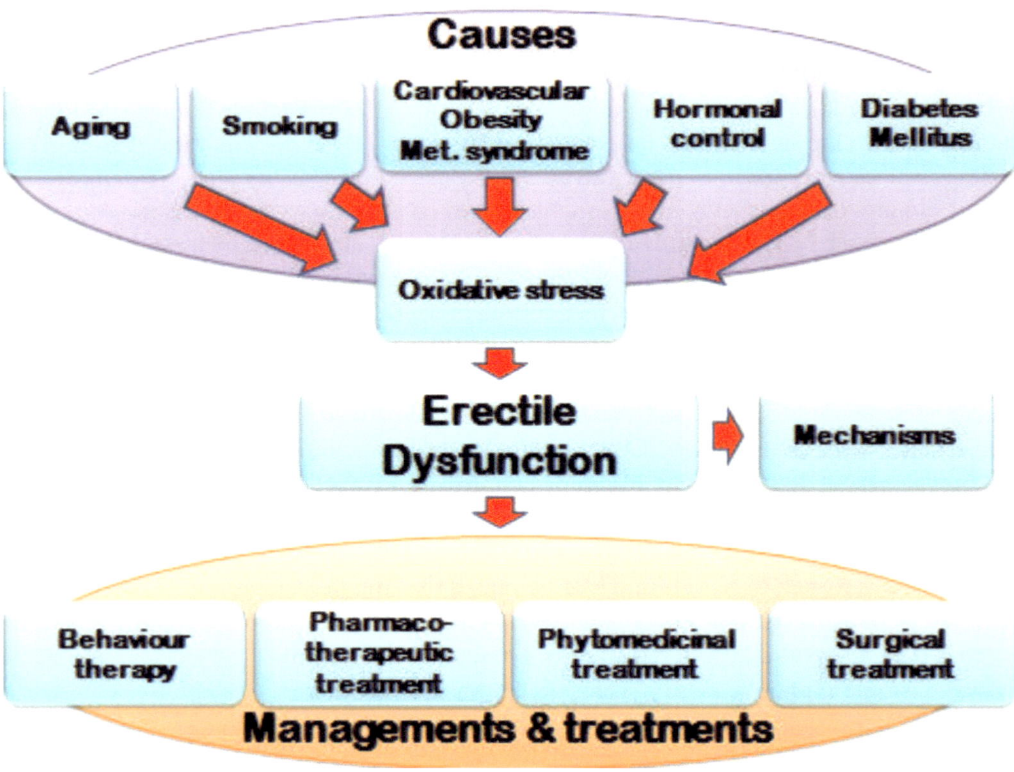

Figure 1. Possible causes, managements and treatment strategies of Erectile Dysfunction

2.1. Aging

Aging has been considered to be one of the major reasons for decreased sexual functions, which are also affected by a change in lifestyle, increased day-to-day stress, depression, diabetes and/or other metabolic and endocrine disorders. Various medications such as antidepressants, tranquilizers, hypnotics, antiandrogens and antihypertensive agents can also lead to the downfall of the sexual functions [6, 7]. There is a close relationship between aging and ED [8]. Research shows that chances of developing ED increase with age and are due to several age-related factors such as a reduction in nonadrenergic noncholinergic nerve endings in the penis and decreased endothelial nitric oxide (eNOS) activity. The decreased activity of eNOS and bioavailability of NO impairs corpus cavernosum relaxation which can be exacerbated by an increased release of vasoconstrictors. These confounding events are responsible for the increase in the contractile tone in the penile vasculature [9]. Testosterone is secreted in a circadian manner in younger men, but diurnal fluctuation is reduced and may disappear in aging men [10]. Whatever the initiating factor of ED, the ultimate common pathological process is damage to smooth-muscle cells and an increase in the accumulation of fibrosis, which decrease the vasodilator response. This increased accumulation of collagen with aging has been observed in both human and rat corporal smooth muscle [11]. The increase in collagen accumulation leads to a decrease in blood flow as measured by peak systolic velocity, and this decrease of blood flow contributes to ED.

As men age, dysfunction of this complex process occurs with an increased incidence and prevalence. The cause of this age-related erectile dysfunction is not well understood and likely involves multifactorial alterations in the cavernosal endothelial cell lining, smooth muscle cells, and synthesis or activity of NO [12].

2.2. Oxidative stress

Oxidative stress (OS) is one of the major contributory factors towards ED. There is a growing interest among researchers regarding the role of oxidative stress in the pathophysiological mechanism of ED. Oxidative stress occurs when there is an imbalance between pro-oxidants and the ability of the antioxidants to scavenge excess reactive oxygen species (ROS) [3]. Penile erectile tissue is formed by 2 dorsal corporal bodies known as the corpora cavernosa. The cavernosal bodies are composed of sinusoidal spaces with a trabecular meshwork. These spaces are lined by endothelium. Neural transmitters, such as acetylcholine, are released from cavernosal nerve endings and stimulate the neuronal NOS (nNOS) enzyme, which leads to the release of NO from the endothelium. Erectile function is mediated by both nNOS and endothelial NOS (eNOS) [13]. NO is the principal mediator of penile erection [13]. Erectile function is dependent on relaxation of the cavernous smooth muscle, and its mechanism of action is dependent on penile smooth muscle relaxation, mediated by NO. Decreased production or absence of NO may play a major role in ED. Production decreases when the availability of substrate for NOS is reduced. NO is a highly reactive free radical that undergoes nonenzymatic reaction with the heme moiety of oxyhemoglobin or that reacts with free radicals, such as superoxide anion, to form peroxynitrite [14]. The relationship between OS in the penis and age related ED has only been recently investigated and it was shown that as one ages, free radicals are produced at a higher rate and their numbers increase in various vascular beds. These mechanisms ultimately produce an ineffective relaxation in cavernosal tissue, which leads to ED. NO interacts with superoxide to form peroxynitrite, which has been reported to play a central role in atherogenesis [14]. Peroxynitrite reacts with the tyrosyl residue of proteins, which inactivates superoxide dismutase (SOD) and Leads to decrease the removal of superoxide [15]. Previous studies have shown that penises from old rats display an increase in nitrotyrosine immunostaining which is a marker for peroxynitrite formation. Due to aging, there is not enough SOD produced to balance superoxide anions produced in aged rat penises, which is why their endothelium and corpus cavernosal smooth muscle display high amounts of superoxide anions as opposed to those of younger animals. Therefore, as extracellular SOD is transferred to aged rats, erectile dysfunction is restored because the superoxide anion formation is reduced [5]. Oxidative and nitrosative stress is associated with infertility, and directly involved in reproductive disorders as diverse as oocyte implantation, endometriosis, and pre-eclampsia in women, and ED, sperm damage and motility in men [16]. NO is reported to decrease the adhesion of platelets and leukocytes to the vascular endothelial cells. A reduced NO concentration aggravates the adhesion of these cells to the endothelium and releases substances (thromboxane A2 and leukotriens) that cause vasoconstriction. These substances further aggravate ED [5].

Hypercholesterolemia is associated with increased ultrastructural predisposition to atherosclerosis and decreased cavernosal smooth-muscle relaxation [17]. Increased cavernosal superoxide levels in hypercholesterolemia may decrease the availability of NO, which may lead to the development of ED. Decreased NO bioavailability in obesity-prone animals has been shown to be due, in part, to increased OS [18]. Oxidative modification of LDL (oxLDL), the major carrier of plasma cholesterol, plays a crucial role in hypercholesterolemia and atherosclerosis development. LDL can undergo oxidative modification by superoxide and peroxynitrite, and it accumulates in atherosclerotic plaques. OxLDL also increases the production of caveolin-1 and its association with eNOS affecting the balance of NO and superoxide generation by eNOS and uncoupling eNOS activity [18]. In human vascular endothelial cells, oxLDL stimulates OS via induction of NAD(P)H oxidase [19].

2.3. The effects of cardiovascular disease, obesity, metabolic syndrome on erectile dysfunction

Obesity is normally associated with generally accepted ED risk factors such as hypertension, hyperlipidaemia, and diabetes but has recently been categorised as an independent cause of ED. An age adjusted BMI has been found to be significantly high in men who have reported severe ED as well as those that are sexually inactive, and this indicates that obesity is a strong predictor of ED. In several analyses from previous studies, obesity remained a major independent predictor of increasingly severe ED [20]. Furthermore, Gazzaruso et al. (2004) suggested that ED could be considered to be the most efficient predictor of silent coronary heart disease (CHD) in a diabetic population, independently of glycometabolic control and ED severity [4]. The interest that is currently being addressed to inflammatory markers is not fortuitous, considered the link between obesity, type II diabetes mellitus and atherosclerotic cardiovascular disease, three pathological conditions increasingly recognized as having an inflammatory genesis, and increasing the risk of ED [21].

Erectile dysfunction represents an early surrogate marker of forthcoming cardiovascular disease (CVD) [22]. It has been hypothesized that ED becomes evident earlier than CVD because the smaller penile arteries reach critical narrowing, with insufficient blood flow, earlier than larger vessels [23].

The recognition of ED, focusing attention on risk profile, could be of help in the prevention of CVD. ED can be used to screen for the presence of hypogonadism, metabolic syndrome, hypertension and silent CVD [24].

Abnormalities of the vasodilator system play an important role in the pathophysiology of ED as it is now recognized as a common cause of ED [25, 26]. Therefore, the earliest events in the development of atherosclerosis (endothelial dysfunction) are similar to the earliest events in the development of ED [27] have suggested that a diagnosis of ED is a sentinel event that should prompt investigation for CHD in asymptomatic men [27] Interestingly enough, Kaiser et al [28] recently reported that subjects with ED but without evidence of clinical cardiovascular disease and free of traditional cardiovascular risk factors present widespread abnormality of endothelial function as has been seen in patients with cardiovascular risk factors. Thus, many patients with ED seem to have a vascular mechanism similar to that seen in atherosclerosis [29].

2.4. Smoking

Several studies were carried out in order to confirm that smoking is an independent risk factor for ED [30]. An example being a study that excluded diabetic patients that was controlled for other factors such as age, trauma history and hypertension concluded that smoking is independently associated with atherosclerosis in the pudendal artery. Tengs and Osgood carried out study in 2001 and reported that 40% of impotent men were current smokers as opposed 28% men in the general population [30]. Cross-sectional studies have reported that smoking is an independent risk factor for ED.

2.5. Diabetes mellitus

Over the years, diabetes mellitus has been known as one of the major direct causes of ED. Research has proved that the probability of ED occurrence is higher in diabetic men than non-diabetic men of the same age and that this difference increases with age. In previous studies, it has been estimated that 50%-75% of men with diabetes have ED [32]. Most of the vascular complications that are linked to both Type l and Type ll diabetes are a result of hyperglycaemia, but the majority of studies apply to Type l diabetes. The impairment of NOS activity and the numerical reduction of nerves containing NOS are the reasons behind diabetes-associated ED. Neurogenic and endothelium controlled relaxation of the smooth muscle as well as the downregulation of mediators downstream from NO such as cGMP and cGMP-dependent protein kinase in the corpus cavernosum are also involved in ED caused by diabetes [33].

ED is an important component of the metabolic or insulin resistance syndrome, as demonstrated by inadequate vasodilation and/or paradoxical vasoconstriction in coronary and peripheral arteries in response to stimuli that release NO [34]. Metabolic actions of insulin to promote glucose disposal are augmented by vascular actions of insulin in endothelium to stimulate production of the vasodilator NO [8]. Metabolic insulin resistance is characterized by pathway specific impairment in PI3K-dependent signalling, which may cause imbalance between production of NO and secretion of ET-1 in the endothelium, leading to decreased blood flow, which exacerbates insulin resistance [17]. Deficiency of endothelial-derived NO is believed to be the primary defect that links insulin resistance and ED. NO deficiency results from decreased synthesis and/or release, in combination with exaggerated consumption in tissues by high levels of reactive oxygen (ROS) and reactive nitrogen (RNS) species, which are produced by cellular disturbances in glucose and lipid metabolism. ED contributes to impaired insulin action, by altering the transcapillary passage of insulin to target tissues. Reduced expansion of the capillary network, with attenuation of microcirculatory blood flow to metabolically active tissues, contributes to the impairment of insulin stimulated glucose and lipid metabolism. This establishes a reverberating negative feedback cycle in which progressive ED and disturbances in glucose and lipid metabolism develop secondarily to the insulin resistance [35]. Studies were done on rats to show that transfer of the adenovirus mediated gene of eNOS to the diabetic rat penis can improve the decreased erectile response by causing an increase in cGMP formation [36]. An additional reason for the decreased eNOS activity in the diabetic rat penis is that there is a reduced L-arginene content. A study was carried out in which diabetic rats were orally administered L-arginine, and results indicated increased endothelium dependent relaxation of cavernosal tissue by improvment of the biosynthesis of NO which ultimately led to an increased erectile response [37].

2.6. Hormonal control on erectile dysfunction

There may be a link between insulin resistance, endothelial dysfunction, metabolism syndrome, ED, and diabetes [35]. Hypogonadism has been shown to be an independent determinant of endothelial dysfunction, thus contributing to vascular pathology, including ED [35]. Testosterone (T) and its metabolites, dihydrotestosterone (DHT) and estradiol (E2), have a critical role in the development and maintenance of normal male genitalia, testes, accessory sex organs, skeletal muscle mass, bone growth mass, male hair patterns, libido and erectile function [38]. Testosterone is also thought to influence central nervous system gender identification [39]. DHT as well as testosterone can maintain libido and erectile function, indicating that estrogen is not required for their maintenance in men [40]. Androgen receptors (ARs) are present in the amygdala, lateral septum, and premamillary bodies in male primates [41]. AR linked brain sites in the hypothalamus, pituitary gland and preoptic areas appear to influence male sexual behaviour. For instance, stimulation of forebrain, hippocampus, and hypothalamic nuclei causes penile erection and/or mating behaviour in laboratory animals [42, 43]. Other studies indicate that the hypothalamic paraventricular nuclei could be the main source of a descending spinal erection pathway to the spinal erection generator [44].

Several studies have shown that acute administration of T induces rapid relaxation in vascular tissues of different species including humans [45, 46] suggesting a non-genomic effect of this hormone on vasomotion [47]. Different mechanisms have been proposed to explain T-induced vasodilatation, [48] but as to which are the effective mechanisms and which are the mediators involved with the T-induced vasorelaxation remain a matter of debate. Testosterone might induce relaxation in human isolated corpora cavernosa strips by activation of smooth muscle adenosine triphosphatesensitive K(+) channels. This finding suggests that T, in addition to its known endothelial action, might regulate erectile function locally by its action on the smooth muscle of the human corpus cavernosum [49 It has been established that different thresholds exist for sexual desire and erectile function in humans, the former being quite higher than the latter [50]. In humans, T deficiency determines a sequence of molecular penile events leading to reduced capacity of smooth muscle and endothelial cells to relax in addition to causing increased sensitivity to contractile factors, that is, alpha-adrenergic agonists and deficiency of NO-induced relaxation during sexual stimulus. Recent evidence in humans suggest that T may directly control the expression and activity of phosphodiesterase type 5 (PDE5) in human corpus cavernosum so that in some selected patients, that is, total-T < 10 nmol/L and/or free-T below 200 nmol/L, androgen supplementation may improve therapeutic efficacy to PDE5-i [8]. Reduced production of testosterone may increase the risk of osteoporosis, sexual dysfunction, fatigue, cardiovascular disease and mood disturbances, and may decrease muscle mass [51]. Hypogonadism may be classified as hypergonadotrophic in cases of testicular failure or hypogonadotrophic in cases of hypothalamic/pituitary failure [51]. Finally, penile NO, the major smooth muscle relaxer responsible for penile erections, is in part regulated by testosterone. To date, it is not known if the peripheral androgenic effects observed in animals also are present in man 52].

3. Mechanisms

Various mechanisms may disturb the regulatory function of eNOS and endothelial NO bioavailability, resulting in vasculogenic ED. As molecular mechanisms of normal erectile function and the pathways leading to vasculogenic ED associated with eNOS are becoming clearer, it seems that eNOS roles in the vascular pathophysiology of the penis are complicated and not always uniform. For example, eNOS phosphorylation in the penis is ineffectively regulated with aging and diabetes, although by different mechanisms. However, increased oxidative stress in the penis seems to be a common component of vasculogenic ED, and activation of the RhoA/ Rho-kinase contractile pathway is seen in several vasculogenic ED states [53].

4. Management and treatments of erectile dysfunction

Erectile dysfunction is a defect of penis reaching and or sustaining erection because of physiological or psychological factors [2]. Different treatments have been proposed including:

- Psychological/behavioural therapy with a trained counsellor aimed at helping people to address feelings of anxiety, fear and guilt that may have an impact on sexual function;
- Pharmacological and drug treatments (e.g testosterone replacement therapy for cases of androgen insufficiency
- Phytomedical treatment
- Surgical treatment

4.1. Behaviour therapy of erectile dysfunction

When there is no obvious medical etiology for ED, psychosocial factors should be explored. The potential clue that psychosocial factors may be a cause is that a man is able to achieve normal erections and orgasm through masturbation or sexual stimulation with a partner other than the "index case" partner with whom he has ED (e.g., a spouse with whom there is substantial conflict). Group or individual cognitive behaviour therapy, psychosexual therapy, including sensate focus technique and therapy aimed at improving relationship difficulties (couple's theraphy) may help to improve sexual dysfunction in men. In some cases, education about medical and psychosocial etiologies of ED in conjunction with a physician reassurance may prove adequate to restore normal male sexual function [54]. Lifestyle interventions focused on modifiable health behaviours may be a safe strategy to improve ED.

4.2. Pharmacotherapeutic treatment of erectile dysfunction

Pharmacology of current and future therapies of erectile dysfunction depend on risk factors and conditions associated with it. Different kinds of administration have been proposed such as intracavernosal administration and non intracavernosal administration [55].

Clinical studies and experimental studies have showed positive and negative effects of the different methods of administration [55]. Pharmacotherapy involves locally acting vasoactive drugs such as papaverin and alprostadil [56] and firstline oral therapy for ED includes phosphodiesterase type 5 (PDE-5) inhibitors such as sildenafil, vardenafil, and tadalafil, which inhibit hydrolysis of the second messenger cyclic guanosine monophosphate (cGMP), the production of which is promoted by NO release within the penile smooth cells [57, 58]. Various centrally acting drugs influence sexual behaviour. In particular, the dopaminergic substance apomorphine is a central enhancer that acts in the paraventricular nucleus of the hypothalamus as a dopamine (D2) receptor agonist, inducing and increasing penile erection responses following sexual stimulation via disinhibition [59].

PDE5 inhibitors have had a tremendous impact on the treatment of ED, but are not always effective (e.g., in patients with diabetes) [55]. Common adverse events with PDE inhibitors include headache (10–16%), flushing (5–12%), dyspepsia (4–12%), nasal congestion (1–10%), and dizziness (2–3%) occurring during treatment [60]. The most successful approach to treat ED has been drugs aimed at mechanisms in the target organ. Despite significant progress, the different mechanisms involved in neurotransmission, impulse propagation, and intracellular transduction of neural signals in penile smooth muscles need further investigation. It should be remembered that most of the pharmacological options for ED treatment do not influence the progress of the underlying pathophysiology and do not cure the disease [55].

Testosterone therapy has been shown to normalize serum testosterone levels in patients with hypogonadism. Testosterone therapy was aimed at maintaining or restoring libido and erectile function; improving or maintaining virilization, muscle mass, strength, and bone density; and to alleviate other symptoms related to hypogonadism. There is some evidence that the addition of type 5 phosphodiesterase inhibitor can potentiate the effects of testosterone replacement in some hypogonadal men [8]. If this is unsuccessful, one should consider other treatments for ED. Because there are a wide range of pharmacotherapy options available, it would be desirable, in many instances, to offer patients an alternative to current pharmacotherapy.

4.3. Effects of phytomedicinal plants on erectile dysfunction

A wide variety of human disorders is currently being treated with the use of plant materials due to their decreased toxicity levels, cost-effectiveness as well as minimized side effects in order to avoid drug resistance caused by pharmacological agents 61- 63].

Plants and herbs are persistently being studied for the identification of novel therapeutic agents. Among the 250,000 higher plant species on earth, more than 80,000 plants have medicinal values [62]. Herbal medicine is still the mainstay of about 75-80% of the global population, mainly in developing countries, for primary health care because of better cultural acceptability, better compatibility with the human body and lesser side effects. The chemical constituents presenting the herbal medicine or plant are a part of the physiological functions of living flora and hence they are believed to have better compatibility with human body [64].

A traditional system of Indian medicine called Ayurveda deals with the sexual dysfunctions in a special category of treatment under the name „*Vajikarna*" or virilification. The system includes the use of aphrodisiacs for erectile dysfunction, spermatogenesis, semenogenesis, and methods of improving defective semen, causes of infertility, reproduction and sexual satisfaction [65].

About 317 phytochemicals are listed for antioxidant potential; 340 plants as aphrodisiac and antioxidants and 40 plants are listed for adaptogenic nature. Ethnobotanical plants contain antioxidant, aphrodisiac and adaptogenic properties [66].

Natural antioxidants are located in different parts of a plant such as wood, bark, stems, pods, leaves, fruit, roots, flowers, pollen, and seeds [67]. Natural products, mainly phytomedicine, or diet ingested by human, are antioxidants capable of terminating the free radical chain reactions [68].

Antioxidant properties in plants are due to the presence of cinnamic acids, coumarins, diterpenes, flavonoids, lignans, monoterpenes, phenylpropanoids, tannins and triterpenes [69]. Phytochemicals like carotenoids, tocopherols, ascorbates and phenols presentin plants are considered strong natural antioxidants and have an important role in health care system. Phenols, a major group with antioxidant properties, comprise subclasses suchphenolic acid, flavonoid, biflavonoid, anthocyanin andisoflavonoid [70]. Adaptogens found in plants modulate response to stress (physical, environmental, or emotional) and help regulate the interconnected endocrine, immune, and nervous systems. This re-regulation of a disordered or highly stressed system is achieved by metabolic regulators such as, catecholamines, glucocorticoids, cortisol, serotonin, nitric oxide (NO), cholecystokinin, corticotrophin-releasing factor (CRF), and sex hormones [71]. *Chlorophytum borivilianum* (Safed Musli) is often referred to as Viagra without the side effects [71]. Safed musli contains saponin and alkaloids which give musli its medicinal properties. Stigmasterol, a form of saponin is very similar in structure to testosterone and consequently can occupy the testosterone receptor sites-doorways to the cells acting like an aphrodisiac. Hecogenin has steroidal-like effects that help to synthesize anabolic hormones. Anabolic hormones allow men to retain nitrogen more readily, which helps form larger more bulging muscle during an erection.

Tribulus terrestris is a herb that has been used in the traditional medicine of China and India for centuries. The active compounds in *Tribulus* are called steroidal saponins. The protective effect of *T. terrestris* for Streptozotocin –induced diabetic rats may be mediated by inhibiting oxidative stress [72]. Oral administration of 100 mg/kg of test drug has proven anabolic effect as evidenced by body weight gain in the body and reproductive organs. Improvement in sexual behaviour of male rats was characterized by increased amount and intromission frequency. Penile erection index (PEI) was also considerably enhanced without any noticeable toxicity. The testosterone level and sperm count also significantly increased. The results are comparable to that of standard drug, sidenafil citrate. Findings of the present study validate the traditional use of *T. terrestris* for its role in enhancing sexual behaviour and potential to be used in the treatment of ED [73].

Ginseng is an essential constituent in traditional Chinese medicine for the treatment of sexual impotence. It is likely that this effect reflects the tonic, restorative and adaptogenic properties. It has been shown that ginsenosides relax rabbit corpus cavernosum and this effect is mediated by nitric oxide, released from endothelial or neural cells. These endothelial and neurogenic effects of ginsenosides in inducing relaxation of the corpus cavernosum may account for the aphrodisiac effect of *Panax ginseng* [74].

Eriosema kraussianum Zulu indigenous plants are effective remedies for the treatment of ED and/or impotence. Five pyranoisoflavones have been isolated from the rootstock of *Eriosema kraussianum* and were screened for smooth muscle relaxation of rabbit penile muscle. The most active of the compounds had an activity of 75% of that found in Viagra. In a test on ED rabbit penile smooth muscle, it showed an activity close to that of Viagra, thus living up to the plant its traditional use [75, 76].

Yohimbine is an alkaloid derived from the African yohimbe tree (*Pausinystalia yohimbe*). It blocks the presynaptic α-2 adrenergic receptors in the brain, leading to reduction of brain and spinal cord norepinephrine levels. Inhibition of sympathetic tone enhances sexual arousal and NO release from penile nerves [77].

4.4. Surgical treatment

Patients who fail to respond to pharmacotherapy or those who want a permanent solution usually have surgical implantations of penile prosthesis. These prosthetics can either be inflatable or malleable, however most patients prefer the inflatable devices because they

http://dx.doi.org/10.5772/57174

provide them with a sense of a natural erection. Inflatable devices are more expensive than malleable devices with satisfaction rates of 70-87% reported from patients after appropriate consultation [78].

Vacuum constriction devices apply negative pressure to the penis in order to draw venous blood into the penis which is then retained by application of a visible constricting band at the base of the penis (a method that seems preferable to older patients) [79]. This method yields a successful erection for intercourse that can be rated as 90%. The satisfaction rates range between 27-94% but about <30% of the patients discontinue use after 2years because of the negative side effects that include penile pain, delayed ejaculation and numbness that occur.

Penile prosthesis can go wrong because there are two major complications involved, namely mechanical failure and infection. Infection rate is therefore reduced by the use of antibiotic prophylaxis or by using implants that are impregnated with antibiotics [80].

5. Conclusion and recommendations

Erectile dysfunction is an increasing global the incidence. ED is also indicative of more serious cardiovascular, psychoactive disorders. Therapeutic interventions that are successful in treating ED may be effective in treating the early stages of conditions that include atherosclerosis, angina, plaque rupture and diabetic angiopathy. One common pathological denominator in both CVD and ED is oxidative stress, that is, the overproduction of ROS, in particular, O^{2-} and H_2O_2.Thus there is direct relationship between oxidative stress, sexual impotency and psychoactive mechanisms that alters nitrogen oxide inhibition mechanisms significantly as stated above. Therefore it is necessary to evaluate potential of natural herbs/ extracts to correct disorders and disabilities evolved in the manifestation of ED. An ideal medicinal plant extract and or natural product will achieve biochemical, physiological, pharmacological responses on erectile dysfunction. However, because of the synergic or antagonistic effects of the contents of the natural plants, herbs or their extract, it would be a worthy to investigate on their bioavailability and properties in order to maximise their use. Moreover, further investigations in the clinical setting and qualify for clinical trials in humans are warranted.

Author details

Guillaume Aboua[1*], Claudine Manirafasha[1], Boitumelo R. Mosito[1], Michelle van der Linde[2] and Stefan S. du Plessis[2]

*Address all correspondence to: abouay@cput.ac.za

1 Department of Biomedical Sciences, Faculty of Health and Wellness, Cape Peninsula University of Technology, Bellville, South Africa

2 Division of Medical Physiology, Faculty of Medicine and Health Sciences, Stellenbosch University, Tygerberg, South Africa

References

[1] Monga M, and Geriatr. The aging penis: Erectile dysfunction. *Geriatric Nephrology and Urology* 1999; 9(1) 27–37

[2] Bosch RJ, Bernard F, Aboseif SR, Steif CG, Lue TF, Tanagho EA. Penile detumescence: characterization of three phases. *Journal of urology* 1991;146(3) 867-71

[3] Agarwal A, Kalyana CN, Rakesh KS, Craig DZ, Rupesh R. Role of Oxidative Stress in the Review Pathophysiological Mechanism of Erectile Dysfunction. *American Society of Andrology* 2006;27(1) 401-402

[4] Gazzaruso C, Giordanetti S, De Amici E. Relationship between erectile dysfunction and silent myocardial ischemia in apparently uncomplicated type 2 diabetic patients. *Circulation* 2004;110:22-26

[5] Bivalacqua TJ, Armstrong JS, Biggerstaff J, Abdel-Mageed AB, Kadowitz PJ, Hellstrom WJ, Champion HC. Gene transfer of extracellular SOD to the penis reduces O2 and improves erectile function in aged rats. *American Journal of Physiology Heart Circulation Physiology* 2003;284:1408–1421

[6] Grimm RHJr, Grandits GA, Prineas RJ, McDonald RH, Lewis CE, Flack JM, Yunis C, Svendsen K, Liebson PR, Elmer PJ, Jeremiah S. Long-term effects on sexual function of five antihypertensive drugs and nutritional hygienic treatment in hypertensive men and women Hypertension. *Hypertension* 1997;29:8-14

[7] Gitlin M. Sexual dysfunction with psychotropic drugs. *Experimental Opinion in Pharmacotherapy* 2004;4:2259-2269

[8] Aversa A, Bruzziches R, Francomano D, Natali M, Gareri P, Spera G. Endothelial dysfunction and erectile dysfunction in the aging man. *International Journal of Urology* 2010;*17:38-47*

[9] Cellek S, Foxwell NA, Moncada S. Two phases of nitrergic neuropathy in streptozotocin-induced diabetic rats. *Diabetes* 2003;52:2353–2362

[10] Morales AM, and Rojas A. Advanced glycation and endothelial functions: A link towards vascular complications in diabetes. *Life Sciences* 2004; 76:715-730

[11] Jevtich MJ, Khawand NY, Vidic B. Clinical significance of ultrastructural findings in the corpora cavernosa of normal and impotent men. *The Journal of Urology* 1990;143(2) 289-293

[12] Seftel AD, Vaziri ND, Ni Z, Razmjouei K, Fogarty J, Hampel N, Polak J, Wang RZ, Ferguson K, Block C. Advanced glycation end products in human penis: elevation in diabetic tissue, site of deposition, and possible effect through iNOS or eNOS. *Urology* 1997;50:1016-1026

[13] urnett AL, Nelson RJ, Calvin DC, Liu JX, Demas GE, Klein SL, Kriegsfeld LJ, Dawson VL, Dawson TM, Snyder SH. Nitric oxide-dependent penile erection in mice lacking neuronal nitric oxide synthase. *Molecular Medicine*, 1996;2(3) 288–296

[14] Beckman JS, and Koppenol WH. Nitric oxide, superoxide, and peroxynitrite: the good, the bad, and ugly. *American Journal of Physiology* 1996;*27: 1424-1437*

[15] Zou H, William J, Xuesong L, Alexis L, Xiaodong W. Apaf-1, a Human Protein Homologous to C. elegans CED-4, Participates in Cytochrome c–Dependent Activation of Caspase-3. *Cell press* 1997;90:405-413

[16] Alderton W, Cooper C, Knowles R. Nitric oxide synthases: structure, function and inhibition. *Biochemistry Journal* 2001;357:593–615

[17] Kim JA, Montagnani, M, Koh KK, Quon MJ. Reciprocal relationships between insulin resistance and endothelial dysfunction: molecular and pathophysiological mechanisms. *Circulation* 2006;113:1888–904

[18] Dobrian D, Davies M, Schriver S. Oxidative Stress in a Rat Model of Obesity-Induced Hypertension. *Hypertension* 2001;37:554-560

[19] Azadzoi KM, Schulman RN, Aviram M, Siroky MB. Oxidative stress in arteriogenic erectile dysfunction. Prophylactic role of antioxidants. *Journal of Urology* 2005;174(1) 386-93

[20] Blanker MH, Bohnen AM, Groeneveld FP. Correlates for erectile and ejaculatory dysfunction in older Dutch men: a community based study. *Journal of American Society* 2001;49:436–442

[21] Esposito K, and Giugliano D. Obesity, the metabolic syndrome, and sexual dysfunction. *International Journal of Impotence Research* 2005;17:391–398

[22] Montorsi P, Ravagnani PM, Galli S. Association between erectile dysfunction and coronary artery disease: matching the right target with the right test in the right patient. *European Urology* 2006;50:721–731

[23] Corona G, Monami M, Boddi V. Male sexuality and cardiovascular risk. A cohort study in patients with erectile dysfunction. *Journal of Sexual Medicine* 2010;8:234-244

[24] Corona G, Forti G, Maggi M. Why can patients with erectile dysfunction be considered lucky? The association with testosterone deficiency and metabolic syndrome. *Aging Male* 2008;11:193–199.

[25] Virag R, Bouilly P, Frydman D. Is impotence an arterial disorder. A study of arterial risk factors in 440 impotent men. *Lancet* 1985;1:181–184

[26] O'Kane PD, Jackson G. Erectile dysfunction: is there silent obstructive coronary artery disease? *International Journal of Clinical Practice* 2001; 55:219–220

[27] Blumentals WA. Should erectile dysfunction be considered as a marker for acute myocardial infarction? *International Journal of Impotence Research* 2004;16:350–353.

[28] Kaiser DR. Impaired brachial artery endotheliumdependent and independent vasodilation in man with erectile dysfunction and no other clinical cardiovascular disease. *Journal of American Cardiology* 2004;43:179–184

[29] Cheitlin MD. Erectile dysfunction. The earliest sign of generalized vascular disease? *Journal of American Cardiology* 2004;43:185–186

[30] Mannino DM, Klevens RM, Flanders WD. Cigarette smoking: an independent risk factor for impotence? *American Journal of Epidemiology* 1994;140

[31] Tengs TO and Osgood ND. The link between smoking and impotence: two decades of evidence. *Prevalence Medicine* 2001;32:447–52

[32] Hakim LS, Goldstein I. Diabetic sexual dysfunction. *Endocrinology Metabolism Clinic North America* 1996;25:379–400

[33] Podlasek CA, Zelner DJ, Bervig TR, Gonzalez CM, McKenna KE, McVary KT. Characterization and localization of nitric oxide synthase isoforms in the BB/WOR diabetic rat. *Journal of Urology* 2001;166:746–755

[34] Cersosimo E, DeFronzo RA. Insulin resistance and endothelial dysfunction: the road map to cardiovascular diseases. *Diabetes Metabolic Research Review* 2006;22:423–36

[35] Akishita M, Hashimoto M, Ohike Y. Low testosterone level is an independent determinant of EDys in men. *Hypertension Res* 2007;30:1029–34

[36] Bivalacqua TJ, Usta MF, Champion HC, Adams D, Namara DB, Abdel-Mageed AB, Kadowitz PJ, Hellstrom WJ. Gene transfer of endothelial nitric oxide synthase partially restores nitric oxide eNOS function/dysfunction in the penis synthesis and erectile function in streptozotocin diabetic rats. *Journal of Urology* 2003;169:1911–1917

[37] Bivalacqua TJ, Usta MF, Champion HC, Leungwattanakij S, Dabisch PA., McNamara DB, Kadowitz PJ, Hellstrom WJ. Effect of combination endothelial nitric oxide synthase gene therapy and sildenafil on erectile function in diabetic rats. *International Journal of Impotence Research,* 2004;16:21– 29

[38] Feldman KW. and Smith DW. Fetal phallic growth and penile standards for newborn male infants. *The Journal of Pediatrics* 1975;86:395–398

[39] Ehrhardt AA. and Meyer-Bhalung WSL. Prenatal Sex Hormones and the Developing Brain: Effects on Psychosexual Differentiation and Cognitive Function. *Annual Review Medicine* 1979;30:417–430

[40] Gooren LGJ. Archives on Sexual Behaviour 1985;14:539–548

[41] Michael RP, Rees HD, Gonsall RW. Sites in the male primate brain at which testosterone acts as an androgen. *Brain Research* 1989;502:11–20

[42] Chen KK, Chan JYH, Chang LS, Chen MT, and Chan SHH. Elicitation of penile erection following activation of the hippocampal formation in the rat. *Neuroscience letters* 1992;141:218–222

[43] Perachio AA, Marr LD, Alexander M. Sexual behavior in male rhesus monkeys elicited by electrical stimulation of preoptic and hypothalamic areas.*Brain Research* 1979;177:127–144

[44] Giuliano F. and Rampin O. *Neuroscience Biobehaviour Review* 2000;24:517–533

[45] Costarella CE, Stallone JN, Rutecki GW, Whittier FC. Testosterone causes direct relaxation of rat thoracic aorta. *Journal of Pharmaceutical Experimental Therapy* 1996;277:349–54

[46] Perusquia M, Hernandez R, Morales MA, Campos MG, Villalon MG. Role of endothelium in the vasodilating effect of progestins and androgens on the rat thoracic aorta. *General Pharmacology* 1996;27:181–5

[47] English KM, Jones RD, Jones TH, Morice AH, Channer KS. Testosterone acts as a coronary vasodilator by calcium antagonist action. *Journal of Endocrinology Investigation* 2002;25:455-8

[48] Tep-areenan P, Kendall DA, Randall MD. Testosterone-induced vasorelaxation in the rat mesenteric arterial bed is mediated predominantly via potassium channels. *British Journal of Pharmacology* 2002;135:735–40

[49] Yildiz O, Seyrek M, Irkilata HC, Yildirim I, Tahmaz L, Dayanc M. Testosterone might cause relaxation of human corpus cavernosum by potassium channel opening action 2009

[50] Isidori AM, Giannetta E, Gianfrilli D. Effects of testosterone on sexual function in men: results of a meta-analysis. *Clinical Endocrinology* 2005;63:381–94

[51] AACE Hypogonadism Task Force. American Association of Clinical Endocrinologists medical guidelines for clinical practice for the evaluation and treatment of hypogonadism in adult male patients – 2002 update. *Endocrinology Practice* 2002;8:439–456

[52] Albrecht-Betancourt A, Hijazi RA, Cunningham GR. Androgen replacement in men with hypogonadism and erectile dysfunction. *Endocrine* 2004;23:143-148

[53] Musicki B. and Burnettl A. eNOS. Function and Dysfunction in the Penis, *Experimental Biological Medicine* 2006;231:154– 165

[54] Heidelbaugh JJ. Management of Erectile Dysfunction. *American Family Physician* 2010;305-312

[55] Andersson KE. Mechanisms of Penile Erection and Basis for pharmacological Treatment of Erectile Dysfunction. *Pharmacological reviews* 2011;63:811–859

[56] Burnett AL. Vasoactive pharmacotherapy to cure erectile dysfunction:fact or fiction? *Urology* 2005;65:224-230

[57] Broderick GA. Oral pharmacotherapy and the contemporary evaluation and management of erectile dysfunction. *Review Urology* 2003;5(7) 9-20.

[58] Omote M. Pharmacological profiles of sildenafil (VIAGRA) in the treatment of erectile dysfunction: *efficacy and drug interaction with nitrate* 1999;114:213-218

[59] Padma-Nathan H, Christ G, Adaikan G, Becher E, Brock G, Carrier S, Carson C, Corbin J, Francis S, DeBusk R, Eardley I, Hedlund H, Hutter A, Jackson G. phosphodiesterase inhibitor therapy for erectile dysunction,Pharmacotherapy for Erectile Dysfunction.*Journal of sexual Medicine*, 2004(2)128-140

[60] Hatzimouratidis K, Amar E, Eardley I, Giuliano F, Hatzichristou D, Montorsi F, Kamtchouing P, Mbongue GYF, Dimo T. Effects of aframomum melegueta and Piper guineense on sexual behaviour of male rats. *Behaviour Pharmacology* 2002;13:243-250

[61] Pari L, Umamaheswari J. Antihyperglycaemic activity of Musa sapientum flowers: effect on lipid peroxidation in alloxan diabetic rats. *Phytotherapy Research* 2000;14:1-3

[62] Ravi A, Mallika A, Venkatesh S, Arunasree MK, Vamshi KI, Madhava RB. Anticancer activity of pupalia lappacea on chronic myeloid leukemia K562 cells. *DARU Journal of Pharmaceutical Sciences* 2012;20:86-90

[63] Malik,J. plants for erectile dysfunction. *International Journal of Natural Product Science* 2011;1:9-14

[64] Sen S, Chakarborty R, Sridhar C, Reddy SR, Biplab De. Free radicals, Antioxidants, diseases and phytomedicines*: current status and future prospect* 2010;3(1) 91-94

[65] Tharakan B. and Manyam BV. Botanical therapies on sexual dysfunctions. *Phytotherapy research* 2005;19:457-463

[66] Mahajan RT, Gajare MS. Manifestation of erectile dysfunction with adaptogenic antioxidant aphrodisiac plants. I*nternational Journal of Pharmacological Biomedical Research* 2012;3(1) 52-68

[67] Chanwitheesuk A, Teerawutgulrag A, Rakariyatham N. Screening of antioxidant activity and antioxidant compounds of some edible plants of Thailand. *Food Chemistry* 2005;92(3) 491-497

[68] Oluwaseun AA, Ganiyu O. Antioxidant properties of methanolic extracts of mistletoes (Viscum album) from cocoa and cashew trees in Nigeria. *African journal of biotechnology* 2008;7(1) 3138-3142

[69] Larkins N, and Wynn A. Veteranary.Clinical :*Small Animals Practice* 2004; 34(1) 291-298

[70] Sule O, Salawu A, Sanni D, Decorti G, Jovana C,Tramer F, Passamonti S, Mulinacci N. Cellular antioxidant activities and cytotoxic properties of ethanolic extracts of four tropical green leafy vegetables. *African Journal of Food Science* 2011;5(4) 267-275

[71] Mahajan GK, Mahajan AY, Mahajan RT. Efficacy of Aphrodisiac Plants towards Improvement in Semen Quality and Motility in Infertile Males. *Journal of Complementary and Integrative Medicine* 2012;9:1-12

[72] Amin AMR, Lotfy M, Shafiullah M, Adeghate E. The protective effect of *tribulus terrestris* in diabetesAnnals of the: *New York Academy of Sciences* 2006;1084:391–401

[73] Singh S, Gupta Y. Aphrodisiac activity of *Tribulus terrestris* in experimental models in rats. *Journal of Men's Health* 2011;8:575-577

[74] Jain A, Bishnoi S, Mandhan V, Sodha R, Jain S. A review on aphrodisiac activities of natural plant extracts. *Recent Advances in Prospects and Potential of Medicinal Plant Proceeding* 2009;12:162-165

[75] Yakubu MT, Akanji MA, Oladiji AT. Male sexual dysunfuction and methods used in assessing medicinal plants with aphrodiasic potentials. *Pharmacogy Review* 2007;1:49-56

[76] Siegfried ED, Marion MH, Orde QM, Jabu TBD, Marion MJJ, Christopher RN natural sexual stimulant. *Phytochemistry* 2002; 59(3) 739-747

[77] Simonsen U, Prieto D, Hernández M, Prejunctional 2-adrenoceptors inhibit nitrergic neurotransmission in horse penile resistance arteries. *Journal urology* 1997;157:23-56

[78] Montague DK, Angermeier KW. Penile prosthesis implantation. *Urology Clinic North America* 2001;28:355–61

[79] Levine LA, Dimitriou RJ. Vacuum constriction and external erection devices in erectile dysfunction. *Urology Clinic North America* 2001;28:335–41

[80] Montorsi F, Rigatti P, Carmignani G. AMS three-piece inflatable implants for erectile dysfunction: a long-term multi-institutional study in 200 consecutive patients. *European Urology* 2000;37:50–5

Chapter 13

Buchu – The Multi-Purpose Ethnomedicinally Important Specie and Its Benefits in the Reproductive System

Bongekile Skosana, Guillaume Aboua and
Stefan S du Plessis

Additional information is available at the end of the chapter

http://dx.doi.org/10.5772/57233

1. Introduction

Indigenous to the Cape region of South Africa [1], Buchu is an aromatic plant known for its essential-oil producing ability and its multiple healing properties. Known taxonomically as Agathosma betulina and Agathosma crenulata [1], its traditional benefits have made their way from Africa to the Western world.

The word "Buchu" originated from the Khoi-San people of southern Africa, and was a word used in reference to any plant that could be dried or powdered [2]. Nowadays, the name Buchu refers to the abovementioned Agathosma species. Previously known as Barosma betulia, the name originates from the word Barosma (Greek) meaning "heavy smell" and the word betulina (Latin) which means "birch-like", a word used in reference to the serrated birch-like appearance of the leaves [3].

There are 150 Agathosma species that are indigenous to South Africa, and of these, A. betulina and A. crenulata are the more renowned herbs [4]. These are used internationally and locally for a variety of medicinal purposes.

Agathosma betulina is a shrub that is well adapted to grow in dry regions [1]. The leaves have round oil glands found scattered across the leaf, which release an aromatic golden oil with a sweet peppermint-like odour [2]. Agathosma crenulata is an aromatic, single-stemmed shrub, which can be found growing in the mountainous regions of the Western Cape [5]. Its dark green leaves release a pale oil with sharp pulegone tones [2].

Fractionation of Buchu by distillation, crystallisation and chromatography releases an oil with many constituents [6]. Agathosma betulina contains the major volatile compounds limonene, menthone, diosphenol and one of its isomers (ψ)-diosphenol, and *l*-pulegone [7]. Aganthosma crenulata contains the same main constistuents, but has trace amounts of diosphenol and larger amounts of *l*-pulegone [7]. These are responsible for the odour, flavour and medicinal properties of Buchu oil [8]. Two monoterpene thiols are accountable for the distinguishing odour of Buchu oil, one being 9-mercapto-*p*-menthan-3-one [6]. This sulphur-containing terpene is essential to the aroma and flavour of the plant [6].

True to its description of being a multi-purpose specie, Buchu has long been used as an antiseptic, an anti-inflammatory agent, for urinary problems including maladies such as haematuria, calculi, kidney disease and infections of the bladder, prostate and urethra [9]. Today it is also used to stimulate perspiration in rheumatic disease and gout, as a digestive tonic [9] which treats cholera and stomach complaints, an antispasmodic, an antipyretic, as a treatment for colds and flu, and most importantly, as a diuretic. In current Pharmacopoeias, it is listed as a diuretic and a urinary tract antiseptic [2]. It is also listed as a treatment for arthritis, cellulite, nausea and diarrhoea, flatulence, prostatitis and UTI's [1, 2, 9].

A number of Buchu preparations are used to deliver it to the body. It may be prepared as a brandy, a tincture (an alcohol or aqueous solution), a tea, or soaked in vinegar [9]. The vinegar can be used for external applications to treat bruises, contusions, sprains and fractures, to clean wounds and to treat rheumatism [10]. The Khoi-San used the plant as an 'antibiotic repellent' to repel insects and mixed it with oil to use as a moisturiser, which was essential in their natural environment and desert climate surroundings [9]. Topical application allowed entry of the active ingredients of Buchu oil through the skin and provided antibacterial and antifungal properties, and also acted as an insect repellent and deodarant [9].

Buchu has a long-standing traditional use, but it has made its way into the fragrance and flavour industries due to its sulphur-containing compounds and sensory properties [2]. It is used to enhance fruit flavours and fragrances, and boost blackcurrant-like flavours. It has a naturally minty, sweet berry, apricot, peach and green herbal taste, and its oils are used in perfumes and colognes [2].

The list of ailments Buchu is capable of counteracting and the multitude of its historical and current uses are what help to define it as an ethnomedicinally important product, making it an outstanding phytomedicine and natural product to stave off illnesses (see Table 1).

2. Pharmacological activity

2.1. Diuretic activity

Diospenol is responsible for the diuretic action of Buchu [3]. There is no explanation of the mechanism of action, but the available literature states that diosphenol acts by irritating the gallbladder, causing the production of urine [18]. Buchu also contains flavonoids that induce urine production [11].

2.2. Antimicrobial activity

Buchu essential oils and extracts were analysed to assess the antimicrobial activity of the plant. The essential oils and extracts were found to be active against the selected pathogens, namely Staphylococcus aureus, Bacillus cereus, Klebsiella pneumonia and Candida albicans [12, 13]. Buchu extracts have a good antibacterial activity, and has been found to be more active against gram positive than gram negative bacteria [12, 13]. Buchu was found to affect the development of biofilms by preventing attachment of bacteria to the polyvinyl chloride surface[2]. This was, however, not the case with the fungus (*C. albicans*), as exposure to the extracts improved the attachment to the surface, allowing the formation of a biofilm [2]. The more well known Buchu species are thus effective against bacteria, but not against fungi. There is, however, a less extensively researched member of the Agathosma family called A. arida that is effective against Candida albicans [1]. Agathosma species have been found to contain coumarins, phenolic substances with benzene and α-pyrone rings [14]. A number of these compounds have been found to be active against microbials by stimulating macrophages, allowing the plant to have an indirect ability to eliminate infection [14].

2.3. Anti-oxidant activity

Free radicals are molecules with one or more unpaired electron(s) [15] that are highly reactive, attacking nearby stable molecules to gain an electron. The two forms of free radicals are reactive oxygen species (ROS) and reactive nitrogen species (RNS) [15]. Free radical scavengers are known as antioxidants, and these assist in keeping free radicals at physiologically homeostatic levels [15]. Polyphenolics in plants are scavengers of free radicals, allowing them to act as anti-oxidants [16]. These compounds act via several mechanisms to reduce free radicals, and make wonderful antioxidants due to the hydrogen donating ability of the phenolic groups [16]. Members of the Agathosma specie have been found to contain flavonoids such as diosmin, hesperidin,rutin, quercitin, mucilage and resins which have extensive anti-oxidant properties[1]. These are some of the compounds that give the Buchu plant its anti-oxidant ability, allowing it to be effective against many ailments that result from an increase in oxidative stress.

2.4. Anti-inflammatory activity

Buchu oil contains limonene, a monoterpene hydrocarbon with anti-inflammatory properties [12, 13]. Essential oils found in Agathosma have been found to inhibit the synthesis of leukotrienes by blocking synthesis of the key enzyme 5-lypoxygenase. By doing so, it reduces inflammation by preventing the initiation and maintenance of the inflammatory process, thereby limiting an infection and preventing its progression [2]. Limonene has also shown to be effective in reducing cyclooxygenase 1 and 2 biosynthesis [2], reducing the proinflammatory agents prostaglandins and leukotrienes from being synthesised, reducing inflammation.

2.5. Toxicity

The Buchu plant should be used at low dosages for most purposes as it contains diosphenol, a compound known to be toxic at higher doses [1]. Pulegone, another compound found in

Buchu, is hepatotoxic [2]. It has been found to reduce the levels of glutathione, a substance used by the liver in several detoxification steps [2], which would allow the accumulation of toxins within the liver. The depletion of glutathione and the excess amounts of pulegone found at high dosages lead to hepatocellular necrosis. Care should thus be taken when Buchu is consumed to ensure that the maximal therapeutic benefits are acquired, without any of the unwanted toxic effects.

3. Buchu and the reproductive system

The benefits of Buchu may be applied to treat ailments of the reproductive system. As previously sited, Buchu is used as a urinary tract antiseptic and as an anti-inflammatory agent [2], thereby reducing the inflammation seen in UTI's and treating infections of the urethra and prostate. Buchu has many direct and indirect effects on the reproductive system via its ability to act as a diuretic, an anti-oxidant, anti-microbial and an anti-inflammatory agent. The ability of Buchu to do this will be looked at in more detail below, focussing on its actions in Benign Prostatic Hypertrophy/Hyperplasia (BPH), prostatitis, in UTI's and on male fertility.

3.1. Benign prostatic hypertrophy/hyperplasia

BPH is the non-malignant enlargement of the prostate, and is the most common benign tumour in men over the age of 60 [17]. BPH has many predisposing factors, which include age, ethnicity, medical and family history and lifestyle factors such as cigarette smoking [17]. Men who have suffered from chronic diseases such as hypertension, coronary artery disease and diabetes mellitus are at risk of developing BPH [17].

The prostate is an exocrine gland [18] composed of fibromuscular tissue in a network of glands embedded in stroma [19]. Androgens are essential to growth of the prostate during early development, purberty and aging [20]. Androgens do not essentially cause BPH, but have been found to play a role in hypertrophy of the prostate along with other factors such as aging, diet, an increase in inflammatory mediators, hormones and oxidative stress [19].

BPH is characterised by nodular overgrowth of the epithelium and fibromuscular tissue [18] of the prostate, with the differentiation of fibroblasts into myofibroblasts being the hallmark of tissue remodelling [18] in the disease. Increased deposition of collagen in the ultrastruscture of the penis and the loss of smooth muscle causes urethral obstruction [21], causing a list of clinical symptoms related to urinary tract obstruction.

The pathophysiology of BPH is multifaceted, with local and endocrine factors being involved [17]. One of the main instigators is age-related changes to sex steroid hormone levels which leads to alterations in the metabolism of androgens locally. This disrupts the growth factor signalling pathways which interact with the stroma/epithelium, promoting tissue remodelling, leading to an increase in the size of the prostate [17]. The remodelled epithelium has an altered production of cytokines and chemoattractants, which encourages inflammation of the prostate and the production of ROS and RNS. With the increased proliferation of stromal and fibromuscular cells comes an increased demand of nutrition and oxygen to be delivered to the prostate [17]. This leads to local tissue hypoxia, promoting neovascularisation to cope with the increased demand for blood flow, and the production of ROS [17]. The increase in ROS leads to further fibroblast to myofibroblast differentiation, perpetuating the cell proliferation cycle and resulting in a further increase in prostate volume.

The roles of other steroidal hormones [20] have been proposed in the pathophysiology of BPH. The reason for this stemmed from the finding that prostatic cells continue to grow, even in the face of declining androgen levels [23]. This led to the rationale that other factors being secreted by the testes may stimulate growth or even sensitize cells of the prostate to the actions of androgens [23]. As men age, the increase in their body weight increases the amount of adipose tissue within the body, leading to an increase in circulating oestrogen levels [24]. This is evident in the levels of free estradiol found circulating in the bloodstream, which remains constant due to the age-related increases in body weight [25, 26]. Adipose tissue causes increased secretion of the enzyme aromatase, which stimulates the conversion of androgen to oestrogen. Increased circulating oestrogen levels stimulate the increased proliferation of cells seen in BPH as oestrogens have been found to increase the number of prostatic epithelial and stromal cells [27, 29]. Oestrogen also has an indirect effect on the increase in prostate volume through its role in mediating the alterations in other circulating serum hormones [20].

The changes seen in androgen levels with age disrupt the interaction of growth factors with prostate cells [22]. The growth of prostate cells is enhanced by the production of growth factors, which are supplied to the prostate via circulation [17] or locally through autocrine production by stromal cells [18]. The locally produced growth factors control cell differentiation and proliferation, and matrix protein production through a network that is interactive, providing for a negative feedback control mechanism that controls normal cell growth [18]. Any disruption in this network leads to abnormal proliferation and stromal hyperplasia [18], which manifects as BPH. Stromal cell proliferation is enhanced by fibroblast growth factors (FGF 1 and 9), insulin-like growth factors (IGF I and II) and transforming growth factor β (TGFβ1) [18]. Expression of these growth factors is upregulated in BPH and are a mechanism which may be altered to reduce accumulation of prostatic cells.

The prostate is located at the neck of the bladder, enveloping the urethra [17]. This location plays a role in the obstructive symptoms seen in patients with BPH, which also correlate with the size of the prostate [17]. There are two components of prostatic enlargement that play a role in obstruction of the bladder outlet which lead to lower urinary tract symptoms, namely static and dynamic [17].

The static component is related to enlargement of the prostate which is attributed to the nodular proliferation classically seen in benign prostatic hypertrophy and hyperplasia [17]. This component accounts for the symptoms related to obstruction of the lower urinary tract seen in cases of BPH. The dynamic component related to the tone of prostatic smooth muscle [17]. Smooth muscle accounts for a rather large percentage of prostatic volume in BPH [17]. These provide binding sites for α_1-adrenoreceptors, making the prostate susceptible to changes in adrenoreceptor signalling. α-adrenergic signalling has a significant influence on survival of stromal cells of the prostate and on the activity of smooth muscle cells in the prostate and the rest of the body [17]. α-adrenergic signalling alters expression of TGFβ1 and extracellular matix turnover [18].

BPH presents clinically with lower urinary tract symptoms such as frequent urination, nocturia (frequent urination at night), the feeling of a full bladder even after voiding, post urination dribbling, weak urine stream and difficulty initiating urination [30]. It is associated with serious morbidity and may lead to complications which include acute urinary retention, and a reduction in the quality of life [17].

3.2. Inflammation in BPH

A substantial number of inflammatory cells and pro-inflammatory cytokines have been found to be involved in prostatic cell proliferation [19]. The prostate is generally populated by a small amount of T and B lymphocytes, mast cells and macrophages [19]. These are chronically activated in BPH and release pro-inflammatory cytokines such as Interleuken 2(IL-2), Interferon gamma (IFN-γ) and TGFβ, which stimulate growth of the fibromuscular stroma [19]. Cytokines released by neighbouring cells stimulate the release of cyclo-oxygenase 2 (COX-2) in prostatic epithelial cells, increasing the cell turnover within the prostate [31, 32].

The local hypoxia stimulated by high cell turnover in BPH brings about the release of ROS which act as inflammatory mediators, causing enlargement of the prostate via stimulating differentiation of fibroblasts to myofibroblasts [33]. Local hypoxia also stimulates the release of growth factors and cytokines by stromal cells, including IL-8, vascular endothelial growth factors, fibroblast growth factors (FGF-2 and 7) and TGFβ [19]. TGFβ regulates stromal cell proliferation and differentiation in BPH, and is a key factor in the control of prostatic growth by androgens [34].

The prostate gland's immune response is mainly a cell mediated one, with regulatory T cells found in the stromal tissue and cytotoxic T cells in the gland's epithelia [35]. The accumulation of activated lymphocytes seen in inflammation of the prostate contributes to the development of BPH by causing tissue destruction and subsequent tissue rebuilding [20]. The cytokines produced may drive growth factor production leading to angiogenesis and cell proliferation as a "wound healing" mechanism [20]. The damage induced by inflammation of the prostate is thus a chronic process of wound healing where the excessive proliferation of prostatic cells leads to a cyclic reactivation of inflammation within the prostate [20]. This hyperproliferation and wound healing leads to the formation of prostatic nodules seen in benign prostatic hypertrophy/hyperplasia [19]. Inflammation leads to prostatic enlargement by stimulating growth of the prostate directly or indirectly by reducing apoptosis [19].

Whilst the mechanism of how inflammation leads to the pathogenesis of BPH is well understood, the origin of the inflammation is not as clearly understood [19]. Numerous aetiologies have been brought forward, including bacterial infections, an autoimmune response, urine reflux combined with chemical inflammation, hormones, diet and any combination of these [19]. The origin thus seems to be multifactorial [19]. It has been proposed that constant injury to epithelial cells leads to the loss of its function as an effective barrier, facilitating the passage and growth of infectious agents, which ultimately leads to further stimulation of the inflammatory response [19].

Inflammation of the prostate increases the risk of urinary retention, which suggests that the inflammatory processes occurring in BPH lead to lower urinary tract symptoms [19].

Prostatic inflammation is a possible target for the prevention and treatment of BPH. Phytotherapy has become a popular treatment modality for BPH, and the anti-inflammatory properties of Buchu may be applied to help alleviate inflammation found in BPH. The presence of essential oils and limonene in buchu oil can inhibit the synthesis of leukotrienes by blocking synthesis of the enzyme 5-LOX[2]. This will reduce inflammation by preventing the initiation and maintenance of inflammatory processes, thereby limiting an infection and preventing its progression[2]. Buchu can also prevent the attachment of bacteria to internal surfaces, inhibiting biofilm formation[2]. The flavonoids found in buchu may also modulate of inflammation and strengthen connective tissue, reducing inflammation and any downstream effects that it may have. The reduction in inflammation can assist in reducing inflammation-induced damage seen in prostatic tissue, putting an end to chronic would healing that is activated to repair the cells damaged by inflammatory processes. It will also diminish inflammation-based tissue remodelling and prevent further enlargement of the prostate.

3.3. Oxidative stress in BPH

Oxidative stress is a condition caused by the imbalance between free radicals and free radical scavengers [15]. Free radicals are molecules with one or more unpaired electron(s) [36] that are highly reactive, attacking nearby stable molecules to gain an electron [15]. The molecule from which the electron was acquired becomes damaged, and it itself may initiate events that lead to damage of surrounding cells [37]. Free radicals are present at physiological concentrations which help maintain homeostasis via their actions as signal transducers [38]. Free radicals come in two common forms, i.e. ROS and RNS [15]. ROS include the superoxide ion, hydrogen peroxide, the peroxyl and the hydroxyl radical [39]. Reactive nitrogen species include nitric oxide, nitrous oxide, peroxynitrite, peroxynitrous acid and the nitroxyl anion, and are considered to be a subsection of ROS [39]. Free radical scavengers are known as antioxidants, and these assist in keeping free radicals at physiologically homeostatic levels [15]. By doing this, they help to prevent any pathological effects that may be activated by the development of oxidative stress, where ROS exceed the number of antioxidants due to increased ROS, decreased levels of antioxidants, or both [15].

The body produces ROS on a daily basis via metabolic processes that occur in a normal cell [40]. ROS are generated endogenously by mitochondria and through metabolic and inflammatory processes, but are also introduced into the body via external sources [40]. Physiological levels of ROS are essential to the regulation of many biological processes [40]. Increased generation of ROS is related to tissue injury and DNA damage, which are processes found in cellular proliferation, aging, infections and mutations in mitochondrial DNA [40]. Increased levels of ROS have also been associated with neoplastic transformation, abnormal cell proliferation and growth [40].

Androgens have been found to increase oxidative stress in the prostate gland [41]. Pathological levels of ROS bring about lipid peroxidation, apoptosis and DNA damage [15]. Lipid peroxidation is one of the main signs of oxidative damage, and has been found to stimulate alterations in membrane structure and has been linked to enzyme inactivation [41]. ROS cause this by abstracting a hydrogen atom from side chains of fatty acids in the cell membrane, initiating lipid peroxidation which has been found to enhance carcinigenesis [41].

Intracellular changes in the levels of ROS occur during proliferative, apoptotic and senescent processes, which can lead to the activation of signalling pathways [40]. As mentioned previously, changes in tissue oxygenation during these processes causes and upregulation of cytokines and growth factors, which trigger prostatic cell proliferation, prostatic growth and inflammation. These processes themselves are a source of oxidative stress, which then leads to further proliferation and the initiation a chronic inflammation. The presence of ROS is thus an essential component in the pathogenesis of BPH when present at high levels within the prostate. This will help reduce ROS levels to physiologically homeostatic levels, allowing them to carry out their functions as signal transducers without activating any pathological mechanisms.

Endogenous antioxidant levels decrease with age [42], and this is compounded by other age-related changes which ultimately lead to the manifestation of BPH. Oxidative stress can lead to cell mutations, which may lead to carcinogenesis and remodelling of the gland's internal structure [43]. BPH is an alternative, benign pathway of unregulated prostatic growth which is encouraged by inflammatory mediators and increased oxidative stress [41]. Management of oxidative stress is thus an imperative step in the management of BPH [41].

Management of oxidative stress is also an important factor in the prevention and treatment of BPH [41]. Buchu is an antioxidant-rich natural remedy that may be used to reduce oxidative stress. The polyphenolics contained within the plant scavenge free radicals, allowing them to act as anti-oxidants[1]. The hydrogen donating ability of the phenolic groups[1] will help reduce the bulid up of ROS. By donating hydrogen groups, these polyphenolics will stabilise free radicals, preventing them from attacking nearby cells to acquire it.

An increase in free radicals stimulates cyclooxygenase(COX) [44], a key enzyme in initiantion of the inflammatory process. Increase COX activity stimulates the production of an array of pro-inflammatory substances called prostaglandins. In patients with BPH and prostatitis there is an increased production of cyclooxygenase 2 (COX-2) and a reduction in the levels of prostaglandin E_1 [44]. Free radical scavengers, particularly hydroxyl radical scavengers, suppress the over expression of COX and prostaglandin synthesis [44]. Ethanolis extracts of Buchu (Agathosma betulina) possess an inhibitory effect on COX-2 synthesis [44]. This inhibition will, as a consequence, suppress the inflammatory response and reduce hypertrophy/hyperplasia and inflammation of the prostate, which is the goal of antioxidant treatment.

Reducing levels of ROS allows Buchu to interrupt the pathogenesis of BPH by reducing tissue injury, DNA damage, neoplastic transformation, and activation of growth factors that lead to abnormal cell proliferation and growth [40]. A diet rich in antioxidants such as vitamins A, C and E may also be prescribed to work in unison with Buchu to reduce oxidative stress.

4. Urinary tract infections

UTI's have a varied incidence that is dependent on age, sex and predisposing factors [45]. UTI's are an uncommon occurrence in healthy young men, but incidence does increase with an increase in age due to predisposing factors and urological abnormalities [45].

The most common cause of UTI'sare bacteria, the most common being Escherichia coli, Klebsiella pneumonia, enterococci and Staphylococcus epidermidis, to name a few [45]. Bacteria causing UTI'sin men have been found to reach the urinary tract via an ascending route [45]. The bacterial flora found around the region of the anus is a reservoir for potential pathogens of the urinary tract [45]. Invasion of the urinary tract is lead by colonisation of the opening of the urethra, followed by adhesion and attachment to the epithelial lining of the urethra, with growth of bacteria on the urethral surface leading to ascension of bacteria into the urinary tract [45]. Invasion of the urethra by bacteria is difficult in men due to the distance between the opening of the urethra and the perianal region where the bacteria causing UTI'sare known to reside, the length of the urethra and the presence of prostatic fluid in the urethra, which is known to have bactericidal activity [45].

Co-infection of the prostate in patients with UTI'sis unknown [45], but a mechanism has been suggested. Reflux of urine into ducts of the prostate lead to the retrograde transfer of bacteria from the urethra into the prostate, bringing about infection of the prostate gland (bacterial prostatitis) [46].

Men with UTI'sare usually predisposed to them by functional or structural abnormalities [47, 49]. Lesions of the urinary tract which predispose men to UTI'sinclude bladder outlet obstruction, bladder stones, stricture of the urethra, cancer of the bladder and kidney stones [50].

Signs and symptoms of UTI'sinclude frequency, pain on urination, flank pain and/or costovertebral angle tenderness, which is tenderness in the area overlying the kidney [45].

Lower UTI'sare related to erectile dysfunction and BPH [51]. This interaction may be affected by extraneous variables such as diabetes, aging and coronary artery diseases such as atherosclerosis, but it was found to be independent of these variables when the co-morbidities were controlled for [51]; the association between lower UTI's(UTI) and erectile dysfunction remains. Men who are found to have more severe lower UTI's have more severe erectile dysfunction [51]. The mechanism that gives rise to this interaction is obstruction of the urethra which is propagated by collagen deposition in the penile ultrastructure and the subsequent loss of smooth muscle [[2]. The loss of smooth muscle leads to the reduction in erectile tissue, resulting in erectile dysfunction.

Buchu has been found to have antimicrobial activity against bacteria that cause urinary tract infections, i.e. Staphylococcus aureus and Klebsiella pneumonia.

Flavonoids found in buchu may modulate inflammation and strengthen connective tissue. They may be used in the acute and long-term use for chronic or recurrent UTI, reducing the symptoms caused by UTI's [52]. The diuretic actions of Buchu will also assist in the reduction of inflammation by helping to flush bacteria out of the urinary tract through its ability to increase urinary output [52], serving to reduce colonisation of the urethra by bacteria, reducing the duration of the UTI.

Buchu may be used in the form of a herbal tincture or a herbal tea. The tincture will deliver adequate quantities of the herb allowing its actions to be distributed throughout the body. The tea will support the herbal action of the tincture and simultaneously increase fluid intake [52].

Buchu may be used alone or in combination with other plants. In combination, the synergistic interactions of the extracts found in buchu and those of other plants will produce a better therapeutic effect in the treatment of a variety of ailments, or, in this instance, in the treatment of UTI's[44]. Antibiotic resistance is rife, and is the cause of a prolonged disease course. A combination of antimicrobial agents helps prevent resistance to antibiotics, increases the spectrum of activity and may even reduce the side effects of therapy [44]. A combination of the plants Agathosma crenulata, Dodonaea viscose and Eucalyptus globules produces a broad spectrum and enhanced antimicrobial activity [44]. Combination of these plants in a 1:1:1 ratio provides additive and synergistic effects [53] where the extracts of each plant act via multiple mechanisms to reduce the number of disease causing microbials. The mixture of bioactive constituents target numerous target sites and work in a synergistic manner [53]. The combination of these plants give an additive anti-inflammatory, anti-fungal, analgesic, antibacterial and antiviral effect [54, 55].

By preventing and reducing colonisation of the urinary tract that leads to urinary tract infections, other co-morbidities associated with UTI's such as erectile dysfunction, prostatitis and erectile dysfunction may be simultaneously prevented.

5. Fertility and ROS

Physiological levels of free radicals are essential in the regulation of sperm maturation, capacitation and hyperactivation, acrosome reaction and sperm-oocyte fusion [15]. ROS can make their way into the seminal plasma where they have a regulatory and a damaging an effect on spermatozoa. Leukocytes and immature spermatozoa are sources of ROS within the seminal plasma [15]. Leukocytes produce ROS as part of their mechanism to clear the body of infections [56], but during an infection, increased production and chemotaxis of leukocytes leads to an increase in ROS and a reduction in the antioxidant called superoxide dismutase [57]. This results in oxidative stress which has negative effects on the function of spermatozoa [15]. The changes in sperm parameters brought about are a reduction in motility and in the fertilisation capacity [58, 59]. The presence of excess cytoplasm in immature spermatozoa leads to activation of the NADPH system, which donates electrons to free radicals [13], allowing them to build up within the seminal plasma. This excess of free radicals leads to an increase in ROS and the disadvantages thereof.

Exogenous sources of ROS allow pathological amounts of ROS to build up within the seminal plasma [15]. Environmental pollutants increase ROS in testes, causing oxidative stress, DNA damage and impaired sperm production [15]. Cigarette smoking allows nicotine to make its way into the seminal plasma, which has been associated with the production of free radicals and a decrease in antioxidant function [15]. Cigarette smoking also increases concentrations of leukocytes in seminal plasma [15]. Excessive intake of alcohol increases ROS while decreasing antioxidants due to increased ethanol metabolism [60]. Spinal cord injury is associated with higher levels of ROS and higher numbers of leukocytes, both of which are known to contribute to oxidative stress, leading to reduces sperm motility and poor sperm morphology [61, 62]. Dilatation of veins in the plexus surrounding the spermatic cord (varicocele) is associated with increased levels of ROS, with a concomitant decrease in sperm function [63]. Higher quantities of nitric oxide have also been found in men with varicocele, and these men have also been found to have higher markers of oxidative stress [64].

As previously stated, ROS have both physiological and pathological roles. Physiological levels of ROS have been found to play a vital role in normal sperm function [15]. ROS are signalling molecules in many processes which allow fertilisation [15]. ROS are essential in sperm maturation as they have been shown to stabilise sperm chromatin, which is required to maintain genetic integrity [15]. Capacitation, a process which occurs in the female genital tract, is a maturation process which gives sperm the ability to gain hyperactive motility and the potential to carry out an acrosome reaction [15]; both of which are vital for fertilisation to take place. Capacitation is a series of molecular changes that brings about membrane hyperpolarisation, protein phosphorylation and an increase in pH and cAMP [65]. Hyperactivation, a subsection of capacitaion, provide spermatozoa with the ability to move through cervical mucous and to penetrate cumulus cells of the oocyte [15]. The acrosome reaction, which is the release of proteolytic enzymes contained within the acrosomal cap, helps to degrade the extracellular matrix of the zona pellucida [65]. This allows spermatozoa to burrow through the zona pellucida, allowing penetration of this layer to permit fusion with the oocyte. Physiological levels of ROS are also essential for sperm-oocyte fusion [15]. Fluidity of the sperm membrane is required to fusion to take place [66]. This is acquired by spermatozoa through capacitation and acrosome reaction [15], processes which are both assisted by the presence of ROS. Membrane fluidity allows sperm to fuse with the oocyte, allowing successful fertilisation.

Pathological levels of ROS are detrimental to sperm function [15]. An imbalance between ROS and antioxidant defence mechanisms results in pathological processes to be initiated. ROS cause damage to proteins, lipid molecules and DNA [67]. Lipid peroxiation causes loss of fatty acids from sperm plasma membranes, which affects the structure and function (i.e. fluidity, transport processed, receptor transduction) of spermatozoa, impairing the functional parameters of sperm and their ability to fertilize [67, 68]. Sperm is usually resistant to DNA damage due to the tight packaging of DNA material and the innate antioxidant defense mechanisms in place [69]. ROS causes DNA damage and leads to infertility. Nitric oxide and hydrogen peroxide have been found to induce DNA damage, which brings about DNA fragmentation and reduced sperm parameters (i.e. motility, and morphology) [70, 73]. The impaired the ability of the Y chromosome to repair DNA strand breaks makes spermatozoa more vulnerable to DNA damage [74]. Damage to cellular components initiates apoptosis. Abnormal spermatozoa are regularly removed via programmed cell death, which is assisted by the presence of ROS [75]. ROS activate mitochondrial release of cytochrome c, which ultimately activates caspases which leads to apoptosis [76, 78]. Hypochlorous acid is also known to oxidise cellular components, directly activating apoptosis [78]. Also, high temperatures within the male reproductive system have been correlated to higher levels of ROS [13].

Antioxidants have been explored as possible therapeutics that may lead to a reduction in levels of ROS [15]. Antioxidant therapy has been shown to reduce oxidative stress, resulting in reduced DNA damage and apoptosis. Antioxidants may be used to keep free radicals at levels that are appropriate for physiological function, while reducing the levels that bring about unwanted pathologies and infertility [15].

Buchu is well known for its antioxidant properties. As discussed above, it has been shown to contain factors which assist in the antioxidant activity of the plant. By using this plant in small therapeutic doses, Buchu may be effective in staving off excess build up of free radicals, decreasing the negative effects on the function of spermatozoa that lead to infertility.

6. Conclusions

Buchu has been utilised in southern Africa for millennia by the Khoi-San people indigenous to the region for a multitude of daily uses and a plethora of ailments. It is a renowned herb whose traditional benefits have made their way from Africa to the Western world. There are 150 Agathosma species that are indigenous to South Africa, and of these, Agathosma betulina and Agathosma crenulata are the most well known. True to its description of being a multi-purpose specie, Buchu has long been used as an antiseptic, and anti-inflammatory, for urinary problems including maladies such as haematuria, calculi, kidney disease and infections of the bladder, prostate and urethra. Buchu's pharmacological profile allows it to be used for its diuretic, antimicrobial, anti-inflammatory and antiseptic purposes. Its uses today have spread beyond its medicinal applications, as this compound has made its way into the fragrance and flavour industries where it is used to enhance fruit flavours and boost fragrances. Buchu's biological profile allows it to be used to alleviate ailments of the reproductive system. Its uses in inflammation, oxidative stress and in the removal of pathogenic species from the body have allowed it to be effective in treating disorders such as BPH and UTI's. Its antioxidant properties may be used to prevent infertility through its potential to help keep ROS/RNS at physiological levels, allowing them to regulate sperm function without allowing pathological levels to be obtained, which can have detrimental effects on the ability to reproduce. Whilst the advantages of using this natural product have been known for a substantial amount of time, the use of Buchu has not made its way into mainsteam markets as definitive research still needs to be done to substantiate its benefits. Because of all its benefits, it would be a worthy task to look into all its properties so that maximal benefit may be obtained from its use.

http://dx.doi.org/10.5772/57233

Author/Study	Findings/Uses of Buchu	Application/Mechanism of action
Moolla *et al*, 2007 Moolla and Viljoen, 2009	Anti-oxidant properties	Members of the Agathosma specie contain flavonoids, i.e. diosmin, hesperidin,rutin, quercitin, mucilage and resins with extensive anti-oxidant properties These compounds act via several mechanisms to reduce free radicals
Cowan MM, 1999 Moolla *et al*, 2007 Lis-Balchin *et al*, 2001 Shwegler, 2003 Viljoen *et al*, 2007	Antibacterial Antimicrobial Antifungal Antibiotic repellent	Buchu essential oils and extracts active against selected pathogens, namely Staphylococcus aureus, Bacillus cereus, Klebsiella pneumonia and Candida albicans. More active against gram positive than gram negative bacteria Affects the development of biofilms by preventing attachment of bacteria Agathosma species found to contain coumarins, phenolic substances with benzene and α-pyrone rings. A number of these compounds have been found to be active against microbials by stimulating macrophages
Lis-Balchin *et al*, 2001 Moolla and Viljoen, 2009	Urinary problems haematuria calculi kidney disease infections of the bladder, prostate, urethra	Oil distilled from Buchu leaves has therapeutic properties and major uses, including the treatment of kidney and urinary tract infections, as well as haematuria and prostatitis
Watt and Breyer-Brandwijk, 1962 Gentry HS, 1961 Eaton CL Simpson, 1988	Diuretic properties	Diospenol is responsible for the diuretic action of Buchu. Diosphenol acts by irritating the gallbladder, causing the production of urine. Buchu contains flavonoids that induce urine production
Moolla *et al*, 2007 Moolla and Viljoen, 2009 Lis-Balchin M *et al*, 2001 Bajpayee P *et al*, 2012 Grieve M, 1937	Arthritis, Rheumatism Nausea and diarrhoea Flatulence	The Agathosma species has been many applications, among these are its uses in the treatment of arthritis and rheuamtism through its ability to reduce uric acid. Buchu has been listed as a treatment for stomach ailments and for relief from nausea, diarrhoea and flatulence
Grieve M, 1937 Van Wyk *et al*, 1997	Bruises, contusions, sprains, fractures Cleans wounds	A number of Buchu preparations are used to deliver it to the body. It may be soaked in vinegar and used as an external application to treat bruises, contusions, sprains and fractures Used as an antiseptic to clean wounds

Moolla *et al*, 2007 Moolla and Viljoen, 2009	Fragrant Aromatic Deodorant Enhances fruit flavours, enhances blackcurrant flavours	Two monoterpene thiols are accountable for the distinguishing odour of Buchu oil, one being 9-mercapto-*p*-menthan-3-one. This sulphur-containing terpene is essential to the aroma and flavour of the plant Buchu has a naturally minty, sweet berry, apricot, peach and green herbal taste, and its oils are used in perfumes and colognes
Viljoen *et al*, 2006 Moolla *et al*, 2007	Anti-inflammatory	Buchu oil contains limonene, a monoterpene hydrocarbon with anti-inflammatory properties. Essential oils found in Agathosma found to inhibit the synthesis of leukotrienes by blocking synthesis of the key enzyme 5-lypoxygenase Limonene also shown to be effective in reducing cyclooxygenase 1 and 2 biosynthesis

Table 1. Table showing the diverse uses and properties of Buchu, which are the properties which help to define Buchu it as an ethnomedicinally important product

Author details

Bongekile Skosana[1], Guillaume Aboua[2] and Stefan S du Plessis[1]

1 Division of Medical Physiology, Faculty of Medicine and Health Sciences, Stellenbosch University Tygerberg, South Africa

2 Faculty of Health and Wellness, Department of Biomedical Sciences, Cape Peninsula University of Technology, South Africa

References

[1] Moolla A, Van Vuuren SF, Van Zyl RL, Viljoen AM. Biological activity and toxicity profile of 17 Agathosma (Rutaceae) species. South African Journal of Botany 2007;73:588-592

[2] Moolla A, Viljoen AM. 'Buchu' – Agathosma betulina and Agathosma crenulata (Rutaceae): A review. Journal of Ethnophatmacology 2009;119:413-419

[3] Gentry HS. Buchu, a new cultivated crop in South Africa. Economic Botany 1961;15(4):326-331

[4] Goldblatt P, Manning J. 2000. Cape Plants: A Conspectus of the Cape Flora of South Africa. National Botanical Institute of South Africa, Pretoria

[5] Van Wyk B-E, Gericke N. 2000. People's Plants. Briza Publications, Pretoria, South Africa

[6] Kaiser R, Lamparsky D, Schudel P. Analysis of buchu leaf oil. Journal of Agriculture and Food Chemistry 1975;23(5):943-950

[7] Fluck AAJ, Mitchel WM, Perry HM. Composition of Buchu Leaf Oil. Journal of the Science of Food and Agriculture 1961:290-292

[8] Van Wyk, B.-E. The potential of South African plants in the development of new medicinal products. South African Journal of Botany 2001;77:912-929

[9] Lis-Balchin M, Hart S, Simpson E. Buchu (Aganthosma betulina and A. Crenulata, Rutaceae) essential oils: their pharmacological action on guinea-pig ileum and antimicrobial activity on microorganisms. Journal of Pharmacy and Pharmacology 2001;53:579-592

[10] Grieve, M. 1937. A Modern Herbal. Jonathan Cape, London pp 133-134

[11] Diuretic diet pills http://dietpillshelp.com/diuretic-diet-pills/ Accessed 2 August 2013

[12] Moolla, A., Van Vuuren, S.F., Van Zyl, R.L., Viljoen, A.M. Biological activity and toxicity profile of 17 Agathosma (Ruataceae) species. South African Journal of Botany 2007;73:588–592

[13] Viljoen,A.M.,Moolla,A.,VanVuuren, S.F.,VanZyl, R.L., Başer, K.H.C., Demirci, B., Özek, T. The biological activity and essential oil composition of 17 Agathosma (Rutaceae) species. Journal of Essential Oil Research 2006;18: 2–16

[14] Cowan, M.M. Plant products as antimicrobial agents. Clinical Microbiology Reviews 1999;12:564–582

[15] Kothari S, Thompson A, Agarwal A, du Plessis SS. Free radicals: Their beneficial and detrimental effects on sperm maturation. Indian Journal of Experimental Biology 2010;48:425-435

[16] Yen, G.C., Hsieh, C.L. Anti-oxidant activity of extracts from Du-zhong (Eucommia ulmoides) toward various lipid peroxidation models in vitro. Journal of Agricultural and Food Chemistry 1998;46:3952–3957

[17] Ziada A, Rosenblum M, Crawford ED. Benign prostatic hyperplasia: an overview. Urology 1999; 53:1-6

[18] Eaton CL. Aetiology and pathogenesis of benign prostatic hyperplasia. Current opinion in urology 2003;13:7-10

[19] Bostanci Y, Kazzazi A, Momtahen S, Laze J, Djavan B. Correlation between benign prostatic hyperplasia and inflammation. Current Opinion in Urology 2013;23:5-10

[20] Briganti A, Capitanio U, Suardi N et al. Benign prostatic hyperplasia and its aetiologies. European Urology Supplements 2009;8:865-871

[21] Ozayar A, Zumrutbas AE, Yaman O. The relationship between lower urinary tract symptoms (LUTS), diagnostic indicators of benign prostatic hyperplasia (BPH), and erectile dysfunction in patients with moderate to severely symptomatic BPH. International Urology and Nephrology 2009;40:933-939

[22] Sampson N, Madersbacher S, Berger P. Pathophysiology and therapy of benign prostatic hyperplasia. Wiener Klinische Wonchenschrift 2008;120(13-14):390-401

[23] Grayhack JT: Changes with aging in human seminal vesicle fluid fructose concentration and seminal vesicle weight. Journal of Urology 1961;86:142

[24] Vermeulen A, Kaufman JM, Goemaere S, van Pottelberg I. Estradiol in elderly men. Aging Male 2002;5:98–102

[25] Stettner M, Kaulfuss S, Burfeind P, et al. The relevance of estrogen receptor-beta expression to the antiproliferative effects observed with histone deacetylase inhibitors and phytoestrogens in prostate cancer treatment. Mol Cancer Ther 2007;6:2626–33

[26] Thomas JA, Keenan EJ. Effects of estrogens on the prostate. J Androl 1994;15:97–9

[27] Rittmaster RS, Fleshner NE, Thompson IM. Pharmacological approaches to reducing the risk of prostate cancer. Eur Urol 2009;55:1064–74

[28] Bonkhoff H, Berges R. The evolving role of oestrogens and their receptors in the development and progression of prostate cancer. Eur Urol 2009;55:533–42

[29] Gilleran JP, Putz O, DeJong M, et al. The role of prolactin in the prostatic inflammatory response to neonatal estrogen. Endocrinology 2003;144:2046–54

[30] Blaivas JG: Obstructive uropathy in the male. Urologic Clinics of North America 1996;23:373–384

[31] Kramer G, Marberger M. Could inflammation be a key component in the progression of benign prostatic hyperplasia? Current Opinion in Urology 2006;16:25–29

[32] Wang L, Yang JR, Yang LY, Liu ZT. Chronic inflammation in benign prostatic hyperplasia: implications for therapy. Medical Hypotheses 2008; 70:1021–1023

[33] Yoo TK, Cho HJ. Benign prostatic hyperplasia: from bench to clinic. Korean Journal of Urology 2012; 53:139–148

[34] Descazeaud A, Weinbreck N, Robert G, et al. Transforming growth factor beta-receptor II protein expression in benign prostatic hyperplasia is associated with prostate volume and inflammation. British Journal of urology International 2011; 108:E23–E28

[35] Bostwick DG, de la Roza G, Dundore P, Corica FA, Iczkowski KA. Intraepithelial and stromal lymphocytes in the normal human prostate. Prostate 2003;55:187–93

[36] Agarwal A, Prabakaran C, Allamaneni S. What an andrologist/urologist should know about free radicals and why. Urology 2006;2:67

[37] Agarwal ACM, Abdelrarazik H, Sharma RK. Oxidative stress management iin patients with male or female factor infertility. Handbook of Chemiluminescent Methods in Oxidative Stress Assessment. 2008:195

[38] De Lamirande E, Jiang H, Zini A, Kodama H, Gagnon C. Reactive oxygen species and sperm physiology. Reviews of reproduction 1997;2:48

[39] Sikka SC. Relative impact of oxidative stress on male reproductive function. Current Medical Chemistry 2001;8:835

[40] Savas M. Oxidative Stress in Benign Prostate Hyperplasia. Oxidative stress in applied basic research and clinical practice 2012:591-615

[41] Manzoor A, Suhail N, Mansoor T, Banu N, Ahmad S. Evaluatuion of oxidative stress and DNA damage in Benign Prostatic Hyperplasia patients and comparison with controls. Indian Journal of Clinical Biochemistry 2012;4:385-388

[42] Mchedlidze MG, Shioshvili TI. Influence of antioxidants on the development of benign prostatic hyperplasia. Georgian medical news 2006;140:23-27

[43] Calò LA, Pagnin E, Davis PA, Lodde M, Mian C Semplicini A, Pycha A. Effect of doxazosin on oxidative stress-related proteins in benign prostatic hyperplasia. Urologica Internationalis 2006;76(1):36-41

[44] Steenkamp V, Gouws MC, Gulumian M, Elgorashi EE, van Staden J. Studies on antibacterial, anti-inflammatory and antioxidant activity of herbal remedies used in the treatment of benign prostatic hyperplasia and prostatitis. Journal of Ethnopharmacology 2006;103:71-75

[45] Ulleryd P. Febrile urinary tract infection in men. International Journal of Antimicrobial Agents 2003;22:S89-S93

[46] Blacklock NJ. The anatomy of the prostate: relationship with prostatic infection. Infection 1991;19(Suppl 3):S111-4

[47] Ronald AR. Current concepts in the management of urinary tract infections in adults. Medical Clinics of North America 984;68:335-49

[48] Schaeffer AJ. Urinary tract infection in men-state of the art. Infection 1994;22(Suppl 1):19-21

[49] Nicolle LE. A practical guide to antimicrobial management of complicated urinary tract infection. Drugs and Aging 2001;18:243-54

[50] Ulleryd P, Zackrisson B, Aus G, Bergdahl S, Hugosson J, Sandberg T. Selective urological evaluation in men with febrile urinary tract infection. British Journal of Urology International 2001;88:15-20

[51] Ozayar A, Zumrutbas AE, Yaman O. The relationship between lower urinary tract symptoms (LUTS), diagnostic indicators of benign prostatic hyperplasia (BPH), and erectile dysfunction in patients with moderate to severely symptomatic BPH. International Urology and Nephrology 2009;40:933-939

[52] DiPasquale R. Effective use of herbal medicine in urinary tract infections. Journal of Dietary Supplements, 2009;5(3):219-229

[53] Al-Bayati, FA. Synergistic antibacterial activity between Thymus valgaris and Pimpinella anisum essential oils and methanol extreacts. Journal of Ethnopharmacology 2008;116:403-406

[54] Gatie M, Gebre-Mariama T, Rietz R, Hohne C, Huschkad C, MSchmidtkee M, Abetaf a, Neuberb RHH. Evaluation of the anti-microbial and anti-inflammatory activities of the medicinal plants Dodonaea viscose, Rumex nervosus and Rumex abyssinicus. Fitoterapia 2003;74:139-143

[55] Patel M, Coogan MM. Antifungal activity of the plant Dodonaea viscose var. Angustifolia on candida albicans from HIV-infected patients. Journal of Ethnopharmacology 2008;139:81-89

[56] Tremellen K. Oxidative stress and male fertility – a clinical perspective. Human Reproduction Update 2008;14:243

[57] Blake DR, Allen RE, Lunec J. Free radicals in biological systems – a review orientated to inflammatory processes. British medical Bulletin 1987;43:371

[58] Wolff H, Politch JA, Martinez A, et al. Leukocytospermia is associated with poor semen quality. Fertility and Sterility 1990;53:528

[59] Maruyama DK Jr, Hale RW, Rogers BJ. Effects of white blood cells on the in vitro penetration of the zona-free hamster eggs by human spermatozoa. Journal of Andrology 1985;6:127

[60] Koch OR, Pani G, Borello S et al. Oxidative stress and antioxidant defences in ethanol-induced cell injury. Molecular Aspects of Medicine 2004;25:191

[61] Padron OF, Bracket NL, Sharma RK et al. Seminal reactive oxygen species and sperm motility and morphology in men with spinal cord injury. Fertility and Sterility 1997;67:1115

[62] de Lamirande E, Leduc BE, Iwasaki A, Hassouna M, Gagnon C. Increased reactive oxygen species formation in semen of patients with spinal cord injury. Fertility and Sterility 1995;63:637

[63] Mitropoulos D, Deloconstantinos G, Zervas A et al. Nitric oxide synthase and xanthine oxidase activates in the spermatic vein of patients with varicocoele: a potential role for nitric oxide in sperm dysfunction. Journal of Urology 1996;156:1952

[64] Mehraban D, Ansari M, Keyhan H et al. Comparison of nitric oxide concentration in seminal fluid between infertile patients with and without varicocoel and normal fertile men. Urology Journal 2005;2:106

[65] O'Flaherty C, de Lamirande E, Gagnon C. Positive role of reactive oxygen species in mammalian sperm capacitation: triggering and modulation of phosphorylation events. Free Radical Biology and Medicine 2006;41:528

[66] Aitken RJ. The cell biology of fertilization. Advances in Experimental Medicine and Biology 1997;424:291

[67] Agarwal A. Oxidative stress and human reproduction. Oxidative Stress, Disease and Cancer. Roswell Park Cancer Institute (New York) 2006:687

[68] Sikka SC, Rajasekaran M, Hellstrom WJ. Role of oxidative stress and antioxidants in male fertility. Journal of Andrology 1995;16:464

[69] Twigg J, Irvine DS, Houston P et al. Iatrogenic DNA damage induced in human spermatozoa during sperm preparation: protective significance of seminal plasma. Molecular Human Reproduction 1998;4:439

[70] Sawyer DE, Mercer BG, Wiklendt AM, Aitken RJ. Quantitative analysis of gene-specific DNA damage in human spermatozoa. Mutation Research 2003;529:21

[71] Agarwal A, Said TM. Oxidative stress, DNA damage and apoptosis in male fertility: a clinical approach. British Journal of Urology International 2005;95:503

[72] Amiri I, Sheikh N, Najafi R. Nitric oxide level in seminal plasma and its relation with sperm DNA damages. Iranian Biomedical Journal 2007;11:259

[73] Irvine DS, Twigg JP, Gorman EL et al. DNA integrity in human spermatozoa: relationships with semen quality. Journal of Andrology 200;21:33

[74] Cocuzza M, Sikka SC, Athayde KS, Agarwal A. Clinical relevance of oxidative stress and sperm chromatin damage in male fertility: an evidence based analysis. International Brazilian Journal of Urology 2007;33:603

[75] Sakkas D, Marierhoz E, Manicardi G et al. Origin of DNA damage in ejaculated human spermatozoa. Reviews of Reproduction 1999;4:31

[76] Agarwal A, Makker K, Sharma R. Clinical relevance of oxidative stress in male factor fertility: an update. American Journal of Reproductive Immunology 2008;59:2

[77] Wang X, Sharma RK, Sikka SC et al. Oxidative stress is associated with increased apoptosis leading to spermatozoa DNA damage in patients with male factor fertility. Fertility and Sterility 2003;80:531

[78] Said TM, Paasch U, Glander HJ, Agarwal A. Role of caspases in male infertility. Human Reproduction Update 2004;10:39

[79] Ishii T, Matsuki S, Iuchi Y et al. Accelerated impairment of spermatogenic cells in SOD1-knockout mice under heat stress. Free Radical Research 2005;39:697

[80] Bajpayee P, Kumar K, Sharma et al. Prostatitis: Prevalence, health impacts and quality improvement strategies. Acta Poloniae Pharmaceutica 2012;69(4):571-579

Chapter 14

Antioxidant -Rich Natural Products and Diabetes Mellitus

Ayodeji B. Oyenihi, Nicole L. Brooks,
Oluwafemi O. Oguntibeju and Guillaume Aboua

Additional information is available at the end of the chapter

http://dx.doi.org/10.5772/57192

1. Introduction

Diabetes mellitus (DM) is one of the most common metabolic disorders worldwide with an estimated 143 million people suffering from the disease [1]. This number may double by 2030 [2]. Although understanding of the pathophysiological processes involved in DM has increased, with great feats achieved in the management of DM, yet serious diabetic complications still confront patients and physicians [3]. Diabetes mellitus is characterized by chronic hyperglycemia (very high blood glucose levels) and disturbances of carbohydrate, fat and protein metabolism associated with absolute or relative deficiency in insulin secretion or insulin action [4-5]. On the basis of aetiology and clinical presentation, DM is classified into two; type 1 diabetes mellitus also called insulin-dependent diabetes mellitus (IDDM) and type 2 which is the non-insulin dependent diabetes mellitus (NIDDM). The effects of DM include long term damage, dysfunction and failure of various organs, especially the eyes, kidneys, livers, hearts, and blood vessels [6].

In the treatment of diabetes, many oral hypoglycemic agents like sulfonylureas, meglitinides, thiazolidines, D-phenylalanine and α-glucosidase inhibitors are used in addition to insulin treatment action along with appropriate diet and exercise [5]. However, none can be termed as an ideal one, due to their toxic side effects and sometimes diminution in response after prolonged use [7]. The limitations and side effects associated with existing synthetic oral hypoglycemic agents had necessitated the search for newer drugs. As a result, natural agents from plants and plant products have been the alternative target to source for new antioxidant and antidiabetic agents based on their traditional use.

2. Hyperglycemia and oxidative stress

A relationship has been established between hyperglycemia, oxidative stress and numerous pathways which can lead to the development of diabetic complications. Four of these pathways are very important: activation of protein kinase C isoforms, increased hexosamine pathway flux, increased advanced glycation end-product (AGE) formation [8-9], and increased aldose-reductase pathway flux [10]. Oxidative stress has been implicated to play a central role in these pathways. Oxidative stress occurs as a result of excessive formation of reactive oxygen species (ROS) and reactive nitrogen species (RNS) collectively described as free radicals. Free radicals are highly unstable and have the ability to attract electrons from macromolecules such as carbohydrates, protein, lipid and DNA [11]. Excessive ROS can cause structural deterioration and instability of the macromolecules, consequently affecting proper cellular signaling pathways, gene regulation and function [12]. Although, the human system has check-in mechanisms to deal with oxidative damage and free radical formation through endogenous and exogenous antioxidants, however, when the rate of formation of ROS overwhelms the detoxifying ability of the antioxidants, oxidative stress can occur [11, 13-14].

The increase in oxidative stress in diabetes mellitus could be attributed to elevated blood glucose levels, which upon auto-oxidation generates free radicals and damages the cell membrane through peroxidation of membrane lipids [15] and protein glycation [16]. Chronic hyperglycemia results in oxidative stress via auto-oxidation of glucose in the presence of transition metals [17]; decreased activities of antioxidant enzymes such as superoxide dismutase (SOD) and glutathione peroxidase [18]; increased oxidative phosphorylation [19], glycosylation of proteins [17]; and activation of the hexosamine pathway [20]. Hyperglycemia-induced oxidative stress has been demonstrated to result in beta cell dysfunction and death [21-22], as well as in fibrosis of pancreatic islets [23-24]. It has also been established that hyperglycemia increases mitochondrial ROS production, which could represent a key event in the development of diabetic complications [19, 25].

Hyperglycemia has been reported to induce oxidative insult and apoptosis in diabetic liver and renal tubular cells [26-27]. Hyperglycemia leads to increased levels of ROS and D-glucose which has been shown to be capable of inducing apoptosis through the activation of Bax-caspase pathway [28]. Caspases are a family of cysteine proteases known to be the effectors of apoptosis. Upon activation of Bax by free radicals, caspases are activated, which alter mitochondrial function by reducing the electrochemical gradient across the mitochondrial membrane leading to the release of mitochondrial cytochrome C into cytoplasm [28-29]. Studies had shown that movement of Bax into the mitochondrial membrane is accompanied by a significant increase in the activities of caspase-3 and caspase-9 [30-32].

3. Levels of antioxidant action

The antioxidants acting in the defense systems act at different levels such as preventive, radical scavenging, repair and de novo, and the fourth line of defense, i.e., the adaptation.

According to Lobo *et al.* [33], the first line of defense is the preventive antioxidants, which suppress the formation of free radicals. Although the precise mechanism and site of radical formation in vivo are not well elucidated yet, the metal-induced decompositions of hydroperoxides and hydrogen peroxide must be one of the important sources. To suppress such reactions, some antioxidants reduce hydroperoxides and hydrogen peroxide beforehand to alcohols and water, respectively, without generation of free radicals and some proteins sequester metal ions. Glutathione peroxidase, glutathione-s-transferase, phospholipid hydroperoxide glutathione peroxidase (PHGPX), and peroxidase are known to decompose lipid hydroperoxides to corresponding alcohols. PHGPX is unique in that it can reduce hydroperoxides of phospholipids integrated into biomembranes. Glutathione peroxidase and catalase reduce hydrogen peroxide to water.

The second line of defense is the antioxidants that scavenge the active radicals to suppress chain initiation and/or break the chain propagation reactions. Various endogenous radical-scavenging antioxidants are known: some are hydrophilic and others are lipophilic. Vitamin C, uric acid, bilirubin, albumin, and thiols are hydrophilic, radical-scavenging antioxidants, while vitamin E and ubiquinol are lipophilic radical-scavenging antioxidants. Vitamin E is accepted as the most potent radical-scavenging lipophilic antioxidant.

The third line of defense is the repair and de novo antioxidants. The proteolytic enzymes, proteinases, proteases, and peptidases, present in the cytosol and in the mitochondria of mammalian cells, recognize, degrade, and remove oxidatively modified proteins and prevent the accumulation of oxidized proteins.

The DNA repair systems also play an important role in the total defense system against oxidative damage. Various kinds of enzymes such as glycosylases and nucleases, which repair the damaged DNA, are known [33].

There is another important function called adaptation where the signal for the production and reactions of free radicals induces formation and transport of the appropriate antioxidant to the right site [34].

4. Antioxidants and diabetes mellitus treatment

The human system employs the use of endogenous enzymatic and non-enzymatic antioxidant defense systems against the onslaught of free radicals and oxidative stress [35-36]. Enzymatic antioxidants include superoxide dismutase, catalase, glutathione peroxidase, glutathione reductase. Non-enzymatic antioxidants include vitamins A, C, and E, glutathione, alpha-lipoic acid, carotenoids, and coenzyme Q. Other antioxidants include biflavonoids, minerals (copper, zinc, manganese, and selenium), and cofactors (folic acid, vitamins B1, B2, B6 and B12). These antioxidants work synergistically with each other using different mechanisms against different free radicals and stages of oxidative stress [37]. Hyperglycemia has been reported to impair the endogenous antioxidant defense systems in many ways during diabetes in addition to generating free radicals [18, 38]. The involvement of hyperglycemia-mediated oxidative damage in diabetes mellitus has led to the hypothesis that drugs that improve glycemic index and/or oxidative stress will be beneficial in the treatment of diabetes mellitus and its complications.

Majority of the drugs currently used in the treatment of diabetes mellitus have antioxidant activities in addition to their primary pharmacological activity. For example, aminoguanidine has been shown to exhibit free radical scavenging properties and inhibit lipid peroxidation [39-43] although clinical trials were discontinued in Europe and in the United States due to its long term toxicity. Troglitazone lowered hydroperoxides and decreased SOD activity in type 2 diabetic rats [44]. Glibenclamide, a sulphonylureas in addition to its glucose lowering effect possesses antioxidant properties due to its ability to restore liver catalase and superoxide dismutase in diabetic rats [45]. Also, repaglinide used in the treatment of type 2 diabetes mellitus exhibited antioxidant properties and inhibited protein peroxidation by upregulating glutathione reductase and glutathione levels in diabetic rabbits in addition to its insulin releasing effects [46].

Several *in vivo* studies have been carried out to ascertain the effects of antioxidants on experimental diabetic models [47-53]. Most of these studies reported the beneficial role of antioxidants against specific biomarkers of oxidative stress and provided the foundation for clinical trials embarked on later [54-60]. Majority of the studies were not designed specifically to assess the effects of antioxidant use in diabetic patients and none has been carried out yet on antioxidant-rich plant products despite the large evidence supporting its use. Medicinal plants and antioxidant-rich plant products definitely hold promise in this area in the near future.

5. Role of flavonoids in diabetes mellitus

The presence of polyphenolic compounds such as flavonoids, phenols, flavonols, and proanthocyanidins in plants is associated with the antioxidant and antidiabetic potentials [61]. A number of studies have reported on the beneficial effect of flavonoids in diabetes mellitus [62-63]. Examples of flavonoids include quercetin, rutin, diosmin, luteolin, lycopene, catechins and cinnamic acids.

5.1. Quercetin

Quercetin (3,3',4',5-7-penta- hydroxyflavone), belongs to the class flavonol, a member of the flavonoid family and is widely distributed in plants. Quercetin and rutin are the flavonoids most abundantly consumed in foods [64]. Sources of quercetin include brassica green vegetables, carrots, berries, onions, apple, legumes, green tea, citrus fruits, red wines etc [65]. Quercetin has been shown to prevent oxidative stress [66] by different mechanisms, including scavenging free radicals [67], inhibiting xanthine oxidase [68], lipid peroxidation, and chelating metal ions [69]. Quercetin is a powerful antioxidant, proven by *in vitro* [70] and *in vivo* studies [71]. Quercetin ameliorated the damage caused by oxidative stress in pancreatic tissues in rats, by directly quenching lipid peroxides and indirectly enhancing the production of endogenous antioxidants [72].

http://dx.doi.org/10.5772/57192

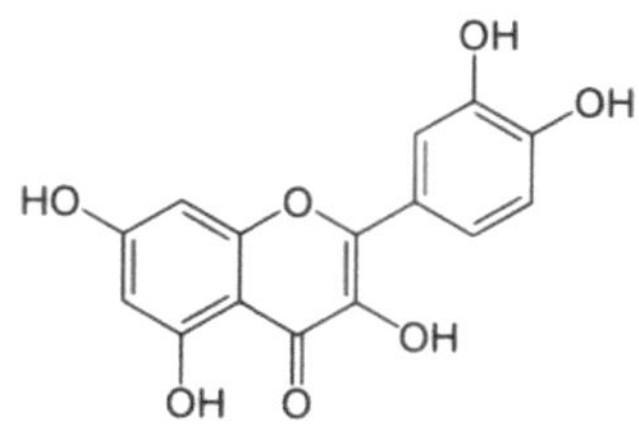

Figure 1. The chemical structure of quercetin.

Quercetin reduces intestinal glucose absorption by inhibiting GLUT 2 in CaCo-2 intestinal cells [73-74]. Quercetin has been extensively investigated in diabetic rat models in recent times. It decreases the fasting blood glucose and improves glucose tolerance [75]; protects against oxidative damage and preserves pancreatic beta cell integrity [76]. Kobori *et al.* [77] reported that quercetin alleviated diabetic symptoms and liver injury in diabetic patients. Quercetin blocks tyrosine kinase thereby interfering with insulin signaling and the propagation of the biological actions of the hormone [78-79]. Quercetin elevated insulin secretion in insulin-secreting cell line induced by glucose and glibenclamide [80] by mediating ERK1/2 pathway [81]. Insulin resistance was improved in genetically obese Zucker rats upon administration of quercetin [82]. Quercetin also reduced maltose-induced postprandial hyperglycemia in type 2 diabetic patients by inhibiting intestinal alpha glucosidase activity [83]. Several mechanisms of action of quercetin in diabetes have been postulated and those included: decreases lipid peroxidation, increases antioxidant enzymes activity like superoxide dismutase (SOD), glutathione peroxidase (GPX), and catalase [76]. Other mechanisms are inhibition of insulin-dependent activation of phosphoinositol-3 kinase (PI-3K) [84], increase adiponectin levels [85], and decrease the intestinal maltose activity [27].

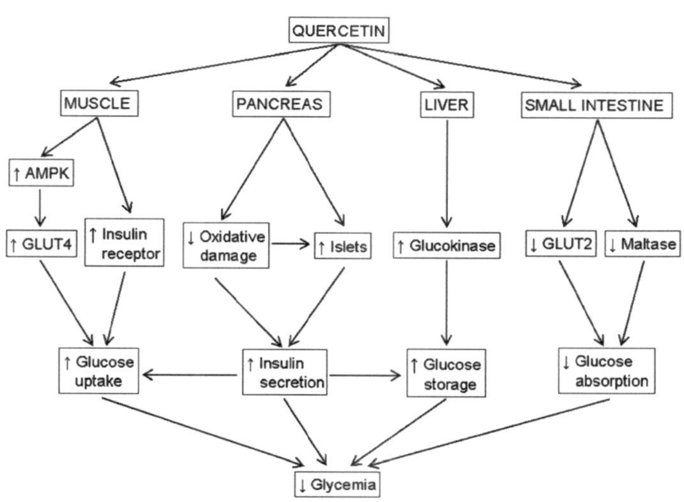

Figure 2. Proposed mechanisms for anti-diabetic effects of Quercetin. Reproduced from Portillo *et al.,* (2011).

5.2. Rutin

Rutin {2-(3,4-dihydroxyphenyl)-5,7-dihydroxy-3-[α-Lrhamnopyranosyl-(1→6)-β-D-gluco pyranosyloxy]-4*H*chromen-4-one} is abundantly present in onions, apples, tea and red wine [86]. The name rutin originated from the plant *Ruta graveolens*. Rutin exhibits multiple pharmacological activities including antibacterial, antitumour, antidiabetic, antiinflammatory, antidiarrhoeal, antiulcer, antimutagenic, myocardial protecting, vasodilator, immunomodulator and hepatoprotective activities [87]. It is a potent antioxidant and anti-inflammatory agent that has the potential to provide a lot of health benefits [88].

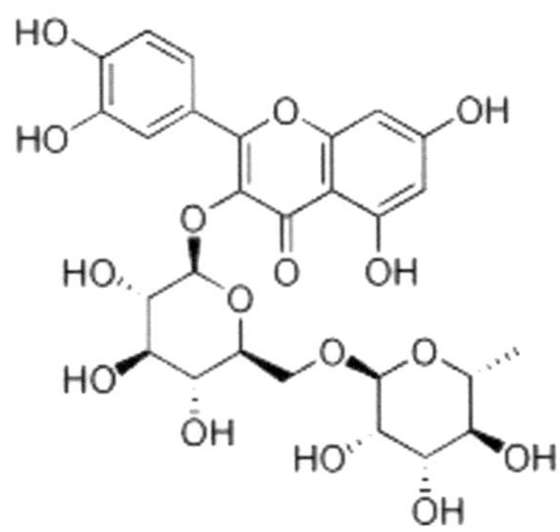

Figure 3. The chemical structure of rutin.

Rutin by its ability to scavenge free radicals and to inhibit lipid peroxidation, prevents streptozotocin-induced oxidative stress and protects pancreatic beta cells resulting in increased insulin secretion and decreased blood glucose levels. Rutin effectively reduced the increased levels of thiobarbituric acid reactive substances and hydroperoxides in the diabetic state *in vivo* [89] and *in vitro* [90]. Rutin reduces hyperglycemia and dyslipidemia while inhibiting the progression of liver and heart dysfunction in diabetic rats [91]. It also significantly decreases elevated reactive oxygen species while increasing endogenous antioxidant enzymes in kidney of diabetic rats and may consequently control or prevent the development of diabetic nephropathy [92]. When Rutin supplementation tablets (500mg) was administered simultaneously with their regular medication for 60 days to patients with type 2 diabetes mellitus, the hypertension, total cholesterol and low-density lipoproteins (LDL) were markedly attenuated. Rutin also decreased the levels of fasting blood glucose, systolic and diastolic blood pressure and improved lipid profiles in the diabetic subjects [93]. Rutin found in *Morus alba* leaves, possesses significant, dose-dependent antidiabetic activity in a type 2 diabetic rat model [94].

5.3. Diosmin

Diosmin (3′,5,7-trihydroxy-4′-methoxyflavone 7-rutinoside) is a naturally occurring flavonoid glycoside that can be isolated from various plant sources or derived by dehydrogenation of the corresponding flavanone glycoside Hesperidin, that is abundant in the pericarp of various citrus fruits [95]. Diosmin was first isolated in 1925 from *Scrophularia nodosa*. Diosmin is

http://dx.doi.org/10.5772/57192

considered to be a vascular-protecting agent used to treat chronic venous insufficiency, hemorrhoids, lymphedema, and varicose veins. Diosmin exhibits anti-inflammatory, antioxidant, and anti-mutagenic properties [95-97]. Clinical studies have demonstrated that diosmin can be used to treat venous leg ulcers and hemorrhoids [98]. Also, its anti-inflammatory and anti-apoptotic activity has been demonstrated in neuronal cells [99].

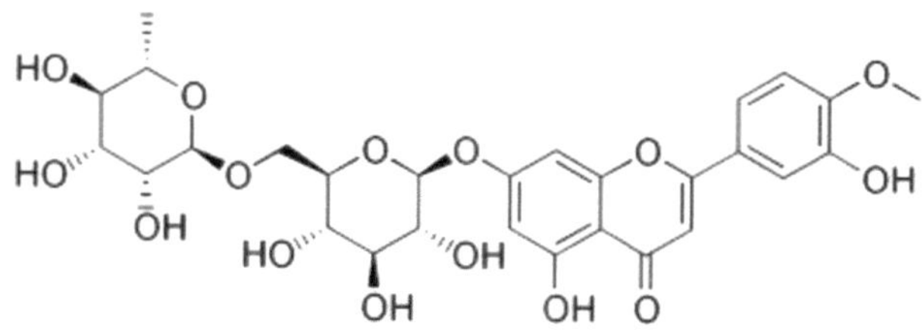

Figure 4. The chemical structure of diosmin.

Diosmin was found to be capable of normalizing capillary filtration rate and prevent ischemia in diabetics [100-101]. Diosmin has been shown to improve factors associated with diabetic complications. A decrease in hemoglobin A1c as well as an increase in glutathione peroxidase was observed in type 1 diabetic patients after an intervention with a diosmin-containing flavonoid mixture [102]. Diosmin and hesperidin are known to lower hepatotoxicity induced by carbon tetrachloride (CCl4) and lipopolysaccharides (LPS), minimize oxidation stress caused by nicotine, reduce blood sugar and cholesterol, and inhibit carcinogenesis of the bladder and colon [31, 103-106]. Administration of diosmin for 45 days significantly lowered plasma glucose level, increased the activities of hepatic key enzymes such as hexokinase and glucose-6-phosphate dehydrogenase in addition to decreasing glucose-6-phosphatase and fructose-1,6-bisphosphatase concentrations in streptozotocin-nicotinamide treated rats exhibiting its antihypeglycemic properties [107]. Diosmin lowered plasma glucose and increased plasma insulin levels in diabetic rats by ameliorating the oxidative stress induced by streptozotocin and nicotinamide. Activities of antioxidant enzymes (superoxide dismutase, catalase, glutathione peroxidase, and glutathione s-transferase), vitamin C, vitamin E and reduced glutathione were increased while lipid peroxidation was reduced in liver and kidney of diabetic rats upon treatment with diosmin. Diosmin was also recently reported to possess antihypertensive property by increasing the activities of antioxidant enzymes,, reducing reactive oxygen species and normalizing marker enzymes in serum and tissues (liver, kidney, heart, aorta) when rats were made hypertensive by deoxycorticosterone acetate (DOCA) salt [108].

5.4. Luteolin

Luteolin (3′,4′,5,7-tetrahydroxyflavone) is a flavonoid widely distributed in the plant kingdom including several such as *Reseda luteola L., Achillea millefolium L, Chamomillae requtita, Cynara scolymus, Thymus vulgaris, Limonium sinuatum* [109]. Luteolin has a variety of pharmacological activities, including anti-mutagenic, anti-tumorigenic [110], anti-inflammatory [111], anti-hypertensive [112], and anti-oxidative [113] properties. It is thought to play an important role in the human body as an antioxidant, a free radical scavenger, an agent in the prevention of inflammation, a promoter of carbohydrate metabolism, and an immune system modulator [114]. The antioxidant activity of luteolin and its glycosides has been associated with their capacity to scavenge reactive oxygen and nitrogen species [115-116], to chelate transition metals that may induce oxidative damage through the Fenton reaction [117] to inhibit prooxidant enzymes [118] and to induce antioxidant enzymes [119-120]. The antioxidant activity of luteolin has been investigated *in vitro* and *in vivo* [121-122].

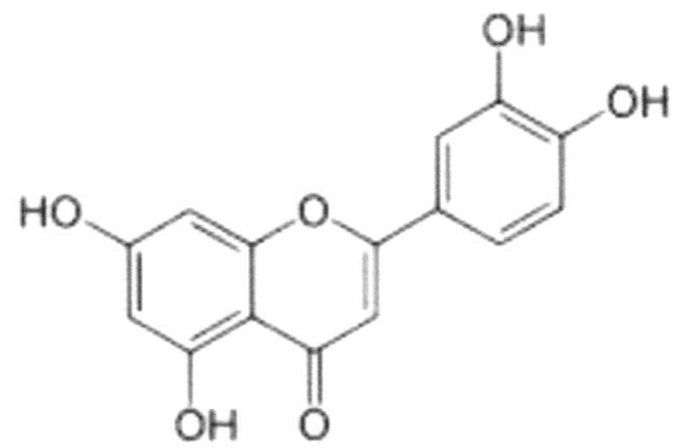

Figure 5. The chemical structure of luteolin.

The antidiabetic property of luteolin was reported by Zarzuelo *et al* [123] where a significant decrease in glycemia levels (> 50%), a 2.5-fold increase in insulin blood levels, elevated pancreatic insulin and DNA content were observed. Luteolin is reported to inhibit alpha-glucosidase and alpha-amylase suggesting that it can suppress postprandial hyperglycemia in patients with non-insulin dependent diabetes mellitus [124]. Recently, luteolin was found to influence insulin action and production of adipokines/cytokines in adipocytes by activating the PPARγ pathway suggesting its role in preventing insulin resistance and type 2 diabetes mellitus [125].

5.5. Lycopene

Lycopene is a carotenoid present in tomatoes (*Lycoperisicon esculentum*). It can be found in many fruits and vegetables like water melon, pawpaw and pink grape fruit. Lycopene is a potent antioxidant according to *in vitro* and human studies, inactivating hydrogen peroxide and nitrogen dioxide [126] and reducing the susceptibility of lymphocyte DNA to oxidative damage [127]. The presence of many conjugated double bonds in lycopene may account for its antioxidant properties [128]. Lycopene quenches singlet oxygen and traps peroxyl radicals [129]. The singlet quenching ability has been reported to be twice as high as that of beta carotene and 10 times higher than that of alpha tocopherol and butylated hydroxyl toluene (BHT) [130-132]. Lycopene is also a potent neuroprotective [133], anti-proliferative, anti-cancer [134], anti-inflammatory [135] and hypocholesterolemic agent [136]. The mechanisms of action against reactive species for lycopene has been proposed to be by adduct formation, electron transfer to radicals and allylic hydrogen attraction [137-141].

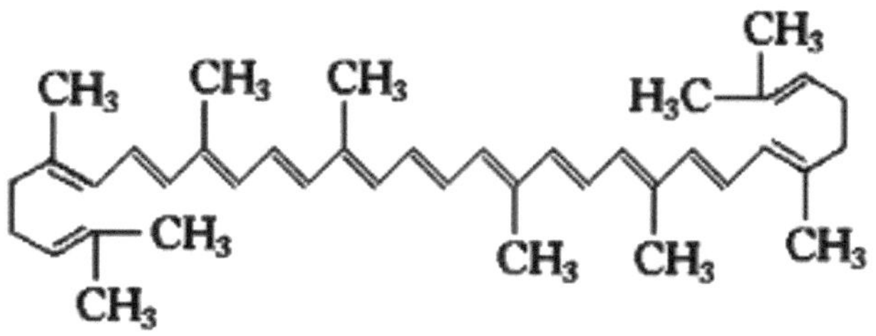

Figure 6. The chemical structure of lycopene.

Lycopene values in serum were found to be significantly lower in patients suffering from type-2 diabetes and impaired glucose metabolism [142-143]. Also, according to data from phase I of the Third National Health and Nutrition Examination Survey (1988-1991), lycopene was found to be inversely related to fasting serum insulin suggesting a possible role for lycopene in the pathogenesis of insulin resistance and diabetes [144]. Lycopene was also found to be useful in the management of neuropathy, a complication of diabetes mellitus, by attenuating cold allodynia and thermal hyperalgesia in streptozotocin induced diabetic rats [145].

5.6. Catechins

Tea (*Camellia sinensis* L) is the most widely consumed beverage in the world, next to water [146-147]. Tea contains catechins, polyphenolic compounds belonging to the flavonoid family. The most important catechins in green tea are: epigallocatechin gallate (EGCG), epigallocatechin (EGC), epicatechin gallate (ECG) and epicatechin (EC) [148]. The antioxidant properties of catechins have been well documented [149-155]. The mechanisms of action of catechins may include free radical scavenging [149-150, 152-153], chelating metal ions to form inactive complexes [150, 152, 156-157], transferring electrons rapidly to ROS induced radical sites on DNA [158] and forming stable semi-quinone free radicals [150]. Catechins also increase the body's endogenous antioxidants to reduce oxidative damage and decrease lipid peroxidation biomarkers in several tissues in rats [158]. Apart from their antioxidant properties, catechins are also anti-carcinogenic, anti-tumorigenic, anti-mutagenic, anti-proliferative, anti-inflammatory, anti-allergic, anti-hypertensive and chemopreventative [159].

In diabetes mellitus, the effects of catechins *in vitro* and *in vivo* studies were investigated [160-163]. In rat models of diabetes, catechins have been demonstrated to have ameliorative effects on biomarkers of oxidative stress on diabetic erythrocytes [164] and on erythrocyte Na/H antiport [165].

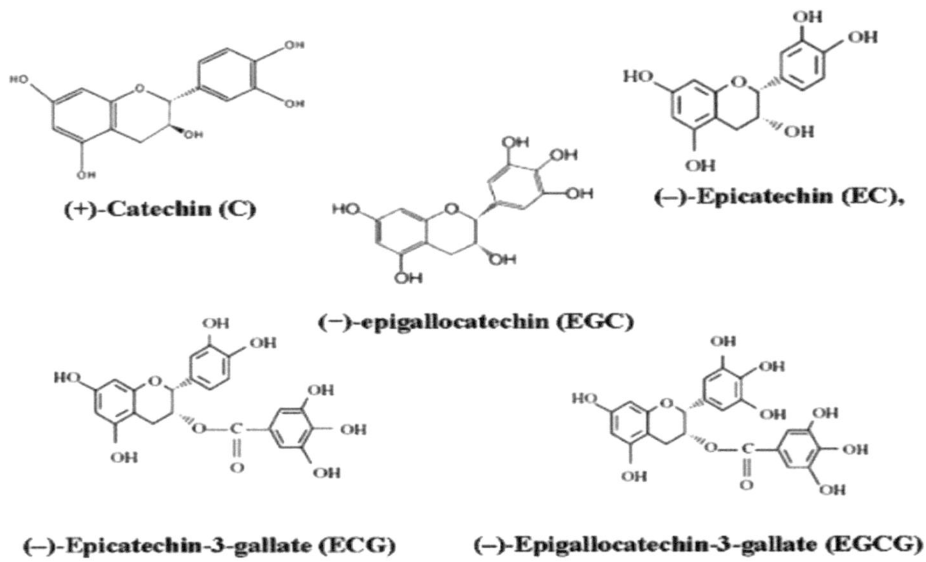

Figure 7. The chemical structure of catechins

5.7. Cinnamic acids

Cinnamon, used extensively since ancient times in food as a herb or spice, has been shown to ameliorate the symptoms of metabolic syndromes, such as insulin resistance and elevated levels of glucose and lipids [166]. Cinnamon bark contains cinnamic acid, cinnamaldehyde and cinnamic alcohol [167]. Cinnamic acid has been reported to exhibit several pharmacological properties including hepatoprotective [168], antioxidant [169] and anti-diabetic properties [170].

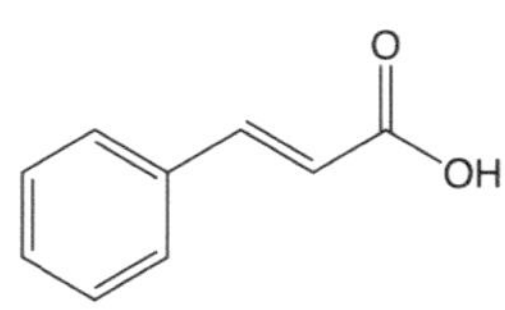

Figure 8. The chemical structure of cinnamic acid.

Cinnamic acid was recently reported to be capable of preventing advanced glucated end-products (AGEs)-mediated diabetic complications. It inhibited the formation of AGEs in a bovine serum albumin (BSA)/fructose system, as well as reduced the levels of fructosamine, the formation of N-(carboxymethyl) lysine (CML) and the level of amyloid cross beta-structure [167]. Sinapic acid is a 4-hydroxy-3, 5-dimethoxy cinnamic acid derivative. It is widely distributed in edible plants such as cereals, nuts, oil seeds and berries [171]. Sinapic acid is a potent antioxidant [172]. Sinapic acid possesses potential anti-hyperglycemic effects, through an increase in insulin production associated with a subsequent increase in the activity of

http://dx.doi.org/10.5772/57192

glcolytic enzyme, hexokinase and decrease in the activity of gluconegoenic enzymes, glucose-6-phosphatase and fructose-1, 6-bisphosphatase [173].

6. Selected antioxidant-rich natural plants with antidiabetic potentials

6.1. *Sclerocarya birrea*

Sclerocarya birrea (Family : Anacardiaceae) is a medium-size-to-large deciduous tree widely used for the treatment of proctitis, dysentery, and diarrhea in South Africa and Africa at large and its antimicrobial and antiparasitic properties has been documented [174-175]. *Sclerocarya birrea* is widely used as traditional remedy against diabetes in Africa [176] and has a significant hypoglycemic effect [177]. The methanolic extracts of different parts of the tree such as the leaves, fruit juice, roots and stem-bark has antioxidant properties [61] due to high contents of flavonoids and polyphenolic compounds.

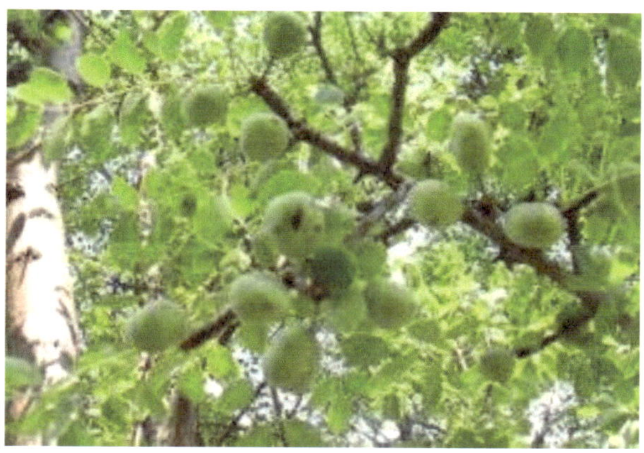

Figure 9. *Sclerocarya birrea* plant

6.2. *Prosopis glandulosa*

Prosopis glandulosa (Family: Fabaceae) commonly known as Honey mesquite is a small to medium height tree or shrub that is thorny and branching near the ground found mostly in southern parts of India. The bark and leaves are used by the tribes and native medical practitioners to treat various ailments such as leprosy, dysentery, bronchitis, asthma, leucoderma, piles, and tremors of the muscles, tumors, eye diseases and rheumatism [178]. It is commonly found in the dry, arid regions of the northern and north-western Cape of South Africa. Literature studies have indicated that the plant contains flavan-3-ol dimer, mesquitol [179-180] and catechin [181]. Phytochemical screening of leaves from *Prosopis glandulosa* indicates the presence of alkaloids, glycosides, flavonoids, phenolic compounds, steroids and terpenoids [182].

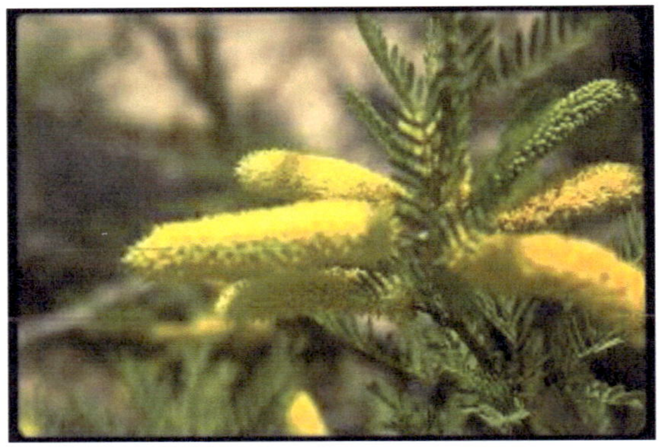

Figure 10. *Prosopis glandulosa* plant

6.3. *Tamarindus indica*

Tamarindus indica Linn (Family: caesalpiniaceae) is a plant that grows naturally in tropical and subtropical regions and has become an important plant for food, herbs in many parts of the world [183]. Literature studies reported *Tamarindus indica* as a traditional medicine for the management of diabetes mellitus in human and experimental animals [184-185]. Siddhuraju [183] reported the potential antioxidant activity of *Tamarindus indica* seeds isolating the antioxidant components 2-hydroxy-30,40-dihydroxyacetophenone, methyl 3,4- ihydroxybenzoate, 3,4-dihydroxyphenylacetate and oligomeric proanthocyanidins. Phenolic compounds such as procyanidin B2, epicatechin, procyanidin trimer, procyanidin tetramer, procyanidin pentamer, procyanidin hexamer, polymeric tannins, polymeric tannins are also present in the seeds of *Tamarindus indica* [186]. It has been postulated that the antidiabetic property of *Tamarindus indica* observed in experimental animals may be due to the presence of the antioxidant-rich compounds [187].

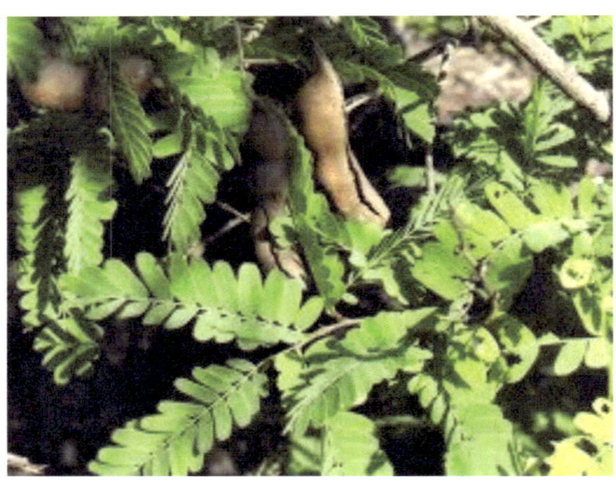

Figure 11. Tamarindus indica plant

http://dx.doi.org/10.5772/57192

7. Conclusion

The pathophysiology of most of the diseases affecting mankind today (*diabetes mellitus* inclusive) seems to have a common denominator, namely oxidative stress. Although, it is a wide topic with several theories, mechanisms, sites and targets of action, reactive oxygen species (ROS) have been implicated in the management of many diseases. As a result, antioxidants have received overwhelming attention in recent years with many outstanding achievements. Most therapeutic agents and drugs are either antioxidants or act primarily to prevent the formation of excess ROS. Therefore it is not surprising to note that natural products with antioxidant properties from plant origin are again gaining prominence in research circles all over the world.

Currently, a lot of therapeutic agents with different modes of action have been designed to combat hyperglycemia; the efficacy and effectiveness of these agents are limited due to several reasons. Individual agent with particular mechanism of action can only act on part of the pathogenic process and only to a partial extent [188-189]. Also, several defects in the pathophysiology of diabetes remain unresolved, and therefore, result in the inability to single out a drug target to focus on as human systems are too interwoven and complex to be fully understood through conventional experimental protocols [190]. However, combination of natural products and phytomedicines from different plants present in most traditional medicines appears to take a different, more holistic approach. These medicinal preparations contain a variety of natural products that act synergistically on a variety of targets through different mechanisms fighting the disease in a more efficient manner. Consequently, the conventional, unidirectional therapeutic method in the management of diabetes seems to be gradually replaced by a more holistic, multidimensional approach

Author details

Ayodeji B. Oyenihi[1], Nicole L. Brooks[2], Oluwafemi O. Oguntibeju[3] and Guillaume Aboua[4]

1 Department of Biochemistry, School of Life Sciences, University of KwaZulu-Natal, Durban, South Africa

2 Department of Wellness Sciences, Faculty of Health & Wellness Sciences, Cape Peninsula University of Technology, Bellville, South Africa

3 Oxidative Stress Research Centre, Departments of Biomedical Sciences, Faculty of Health and Wellness Sciences, Cape Peninsula University of Technology, Bellville, South Africa

4 Department of Biomedical Sciences, Faculty of Health and Wellness Sciences, Cape Peninsula University of Technology, Bellville, South Africa

References

[1] King H, Aubert R.E, and Herman W.H. Global burden of diabetes, 1995-2025: prevalence, numerical estimates, and projections. Diabetes Care. 1998;21(9):1414-1431.

[2] Harris M.I, Flegal K.M, Cowie C.C, Eberhardt M.S, Goldstein D.E, Little R.R, Wiedmeyer H.M, and Byrd-Holt D.D. Prevalence of diabetes, impaired fasting glucose, and impaired glucose tolerance in U.S. adults. The Third National Health and Nutrition Examination Survey, 1988-1994. Diabetes Care. 1998;21:518-524.

[3] Tiwari A.K., and Rao J.M. Diabetes mellitus and multiple therapeutic approaches of phytochemicals: Present status and future prospects. Current Science. 2002;83(1): 30-37.

[4] Jayakar B. and Suresh B. Antihyperglycemic and hypoglycemic effect of Aporosa lindleyana in normal and alloxan induced diabetic rats. Journal of Ethnopharmacology. 2003;84: 247-249.

[5] Bastaki S. Diabetes mellitus and its treatment. International Journal of Diabetes and Metabolism 2005;13:111-134.

[6] Bennett P.H and Knowler W.C. Definition, diagnosis and classification of Diabetes Mellitus and glucose homeostasis: Joslin's Diabetes Mellitus. In: Kahn CR, WEIR GC, KING GL, JACOBSON AM, MOSES AC, SMITH RJ editors. Lippincott, Williams and Wilkins 2005: 331-339.

[7] Chattopadhyay R.R. A comparative evaluation of some blood sugar lowering agents of plant origin. Journal of Ethnopharmacology. 1999;67:367–372.

[8] Vlassara H and Palace M.R. Diabetes and advanced glycation endproducts. Journal of Internal Medicine. 2002;251:87-101.

[9] Peppa M, Uribarri J, and Vlassara H. The role of advanced glycation end products in the development of atherosclerosis. Current Diabetes Reports. 2004;4: 31-36

[10] Rolo A.P and Palmeira C.M. Diabetes and mitochondrial function: role of hyperglycemia and oxidative stress. Toxicology and Applied Pharmacology. 2006;212:167-178.

[11] Valko M., Leibfritz D., Moncola J., Cronin M.T.D., Mazura M., and Telser J. Free radicals and antioxidants in normal physiological functions and human disease. The International Journal of Biochemistry and Cell Biology. 2007;39:44–84.

[12] Pop-Busui R, Sima A, Stevens M. Diabetic neuropathy and oxidative stress. Diabetes/ Metabolism Research and Reviews. 2006;22:257-273.

[13] Ridnour L.A., Thomas D.D., Mancardi D., Espey M.G., Miranda K.M., Paolocci N., Feelisch M., Fukuto J., and Wink D. A. The chemistry of nitrosative stress induced by nitric oxide and reactive nitrogen oxide species. Biological Chemistry. 2004;385:1-10

[14] Halliwell B. Free radicals and antioxidants - quo vadis? Trends in Pharmacological Sciences. 2011;32:125-130.

[15] Baynes J.W and Thorne S. Role of oxidative stress diabetic complications: a new perspective on an old paradigm. Diabetes, 1999;48: 1-9.

[16] Baynes W. Chemical modification of protein by lipids in diabetes. Clinical Chemistry and Laboratory Medicine 2003;41: 1159-1165.

[17] Wolff S.P., Bascal Z.A. and Hunt J.V. "Autoxidative glycosylation": free radicals and glycation theory. Progress in Clinical and Biological Research. 1989;304:259-75.

[18] Blakytny, R. and Harding, J. J. Glycation (non-enzymic glycosylation) inactivates glutathione reductase. Biochemical Journal, 1992;288:303-7.

[19] Nishikawa T., Edelstein D., Du X. L, Yamagishi S., Matsumura T., Kaneda Y., Yorek M.A, Beebe D., Oates P.J., Hammes H.P., Giardino I. and Brownlee M. Normalizing mitochondrial superoxide production blocks three pathways of hyperglycaemic damage. Nature. 2000;404:787-90.

[20] Kaneto H., Xu G., Song K., Suzuma K., Bonner-Weier S., Sharma A. and Weier G. C. Activation of the hexosamine pathway leads to deterioration of pancreas b-cells function through the induction of oxidative stress. Journal of Biological Chemistry. 2001;276:31099-31104.

[21] Donath M. Y.; Gross D. J.; Cerasi E. and Kaiser N. Hyperglycemia-induced b-cell apoptosis in pancreatic islets of Psammomys obesus during development of diabetes Diabetes. 1999;48:738-44.

[22] Robertson R.P, Harmon J, Tran P.O, Tanaka Y, and Takahashi H. Glucose toxicity in beta cells: type 2 diabetes, good radicals gone bad, and the glutathione connection. Diabetes. 2003;52:581–587.

[23] Hayden M.R. Islet amyloid and fibrosis in the cardiometabolic syndrome and type 2 diabetes mellitus. Journal of the Cardio-metabolic Syndrome. 2007;2:70-5.

[24] Hong O., Lee S., Rhee M., Ko S., Cho J., Choi Y., Song K., Son H. and Yoon K. Hyperglycemia and hyperinsulinemia have additive effects on activation and proliferation of pancreatic stellate cells: possible explanation of islet-specific fibrosis in type 2 diabetes mellitus. Journal of Cell Biochemistry. 2007;101:665-75.

[25] Kiritoshi S, Nishikawa T, Sonoda K, Kukidome D, Senokuchi T, Matsuo T, Matsumura T, Tokunaga H, Brownlee M and Araki E. Reactive oxygen species from mitochondria induce cyclooxygenase-2 gene expression in human mesangial cells: potential role in diabetic nephropathy. Diabetes. 2003;52 :2570–2577.

[26] Stitt-Cavanagh E., MacLeod L, and Kennedy C.R.J. The Podocyte in Diabetic Kidney Disease. The ScientificWorld JOURNAL. 2009;9:1127–1139.

[27] Kim Y.J, Kim Y.A, Yokozawa T.. Pycnogenol modulates apoptosis by suppressing oxidative stress and inflammation in high glucose-treated renal tubular cells. Food and Chemical Toxicology. 2011;49:2196–2201.

[28] Green D.R and Reed J.C. Mitochondria and apoptosis. Science 1998;281:1309–1312.

[29] Liu X, Kim CN, Yang J, Jemmerson R and Wang X. Induction of apoptotic program in cell-free extracts: requirement for dATP and cytochrome C. Cell. 1996;86:147–157.

[30] Fraser A. and Evans G. A. license to kill. Cell. 1996;85:781–784.

[31] Yang J, Liu X, Bhalla K, Kim C.N, Ibrado A.M, Cai J, Peng T.I, Jones D.P and Wang X. Prevention of apoptosis by Bcl-2: release of cytochrome c from mitochondria blocked. Science. 1997;275:1129–1132.

[32] Nakagami H, Morishita R, Yamamoto K, Taniyama Y, Aoki M, Yamasaki K, Matsumoto K, Nakamura T, Kaneda Y and Ogihara T. Hepatocyte growth factor prevents endothelial cell death through inhibition of bax translocation from cytosol to mitochondrial membrane. Diabetes. 2002;51:2604–2611.

[33] Lobo V. Patil A. Phatak A. and Chandra N. Free radicals, antioxidants and functional foods: Impact on human health. Pharmacognosy Reviews. 2010;4:118–126.

[34] Niki E. Antioxidant defenses in eukaryotic cells. In: Poli G, Albano E, Dianzani MU, editors. Free radicals: From basic science to medicine. Basel, Switzerland: Birkhauser Verlag;. 1993;365–73

[35] Harris, E.D. Regulation of antioxidant enzymes. Journal of Nutrition. 1992;122:625-626.

[36] Jacob R.A. The integrated antioxidant system. Nutrition Research. 1995;15:755-766.

[37] Maritim A, Sanders R, Watkins J.I. Effects of alpha-lipoic acid on biomarkers of oxidative stress in streptozotic-induced diabetic rats. Journal of Nutrition and Biochemistry. 2003;14(5):288-294.

[38] Saxena A.K, Saxena P, Kale R.K and Baquer N.Z. Impaired antioxidant status in diabetic rat liver: Effect of vanadate. Biochemical Pharmacology. 1993;45:539–542.

[39] Biegelsen E.S and Vita J.A. Human studies of antioxidants and vascular function. In: Keaney Jr. JF, editor. Oxidative stress and vascular disease. Dordrecht: Kluwer Academic Publishers: 1999;213-243.

[40] Gaziano J.M. Antioxidants and cardiovascular disease. In: Keaney Jr. JF, editor. Oxidative stress and vascular disease. Dordrecht: Kluwer Academic Publishers: 1999;245-258.

[41] Kern T.S, Tang J, Mizutani M, Kowluru R.A, Nagaraj R.H, Romeo G., Podesta F., and Lorenzi M. Response of capillary cell death to aminoguanidine predicts the develop-

ment of retinopathy: comparison of diabetes and galactosemia. Investigative Ophthalmology and Visual Science. 2000;41: 3972-3978.

[42] Dobsak P., Courderot-Masuyer C., Siegelova J, Svacinova H., Jancik J.,Vergely-Vanriessen C., Rochette. Antioxidant properties of aminoguanidine: a paramagnetic resonance test Scripta Medica (BRNO). 2001;74 (1): 45–50.

[43] El-Shazly A.M, Mahmoud A.M, and Darwish N.S. Potential prophylactic role of aminoguanidine in diabetic retinopathy and nephropathy in experimental animals. Acta Pharmaceutica. 2009;59: 67–73.

[44] Fukui T, Noma T, Mizushige K, Aki Y, Kimura S, and Abe Y. Dietary troglitazone decreases oxidative stress in early stage type II diabetic rats. Life Sciences. 2000;66:2043–2049.

[45] Elmali E, Altan N, and Bukan N. Effect of the Sulphonylurea glibenclamide on liver and kidney antioxidant enzymes in streptozocin-induced diabetic rats. Drugs. 2004;5:203–8

[46] Gumieniczek A, Hopka H, Rolinski J, Bojarska-Junak A. Antioxidative and anti-inflammatory effects of repaglinide in plasma of diabetic animals. Pharmacology Research 2005;

[47] Mekinova D, Chorvathova V, Volkovova K, Staruchova M, Grancicova E, Klvanoca J, and Ondreicka R. Effect of intake of exogenous vitamins C, E and beta-carotene on the antioxidative status in kidneys of rats with streptozotocin-induced diabetes. Nahrung. 1995;39(4):257-261.

[48] Kocak G, Aktan F, Canbolat O, Ozogul C, Elberg S, Yildizoglu-Ari N, and Karasu C. Alpha-lipoic acid treatment ameliorates metabolic parameters, blood pressure, vascular reavtivity and morphology of vessels already damaged by streptozotocin-diabetes. Nutrition and Metabolism. 2000;13:308-318.

[49] Obrosova I, Fathallah L, and Greene D. Early changes in lipid peroxidation and antioxidative defense in rat retina. European Journal of Pharmacology. 2000;398:139-146.

[50] Cinar M, Ulker S, Alper G, and Evinc A. Effect of dietary vitamin E supplementation on vascular reactivity of thoracic aorta in streptozotocin-diabetic rats. Pharmacology. 2001;62(1):56-64.

[51] Maritim A, Sanders R, Watkins J.I. Effects of alpha-lipoic acid on biomarkers of oxidative stress in streptozotic-induced diabetic rats. Journal of Nutrition and Biochemistry. 2003;14(5):288-294.

[52] Rauscher F, Sanders R, and Watkins J.I. Effects of coenzyme Q10 treatment on antioxidant pathways in normal and streptozotocin- induced diabetic rats. Journal of Biochemistry and Molecular Toxicology. 2001;15:41-46.

[53] Kedziora-kornatowska K, Szram S, Kornatowski T, Szadujkis-Szadurski L, Kedziora J, and Bartosz G. Effect of vitamin E and vitamin C supplementation of antioxidative

state and renal glomerular basement membrane thickness in diabetic kidney. Experimental Nephrology. 2003;95:134-143.

[54] Ziegler D, Hanefeld M, Ruhnau K..J, Meissner H.P, Lobisch M, Schutte K, and Gries F.A Treatment of symptomatic diabetic peripheral neuropathy with the anti-oxidant alpha-lipoic acid. A 3-week multicentre randomized controlled trial (ALADIN Study). Diabetologia. 1995;38(12):1425-1433.

[55] Reljanovic M, Reichel G, Rett K, Lobisch M, Schuette K, Moller W, Tritschler H.J, and Mehnert H. Treatment of diabetic polyneuropathy with the antioxidant thioctic acid (alpha-lipoic acid): a two year multicenter randomized double-blind placebo-controlled trial (ALADIN II). Alpha Lipoic Acid in Diabetic Neuropathy. Free Radical Research. 1999;31(3):171-179.

[56] Ziegler D, Hanefeld M, Ruhnau K, Hasche H, Lobisch M, Schutte K, Kerum G, and Malessa R. Treatment of symptomatic diabetic polyneuropathy with the antioxidant alpha-lipoic acid: a 7- month multicenter randomized controlled trial (ALADIN III Study). ALADIN III Study Group. Alpha-Lipoic Acid in Diabetic Neuropathy. Diabetes Care. 1999;22(8):1296-1301.

[57] Skyrme-Jones R.A, O'Brien R.C, Berry K.L, and Meredith I.T. Vitamin E supplementation improves endothelial function in type I diabetes mellitus: a randomized, placebo-controlled study. Journal of the American College of Cardiology. 2000;36(1): 94-102.

[58] Gaede P, Poulsen H.E, Parving H.H, and Pedersen O. Double-blind, randomized study of the effect of combined treatment with vitamin C and E on albuminuria in Type 2 diabetic patients. Diabetes and Medicine. 2001;18(9):756-760.

[59] Lonn E.M, Yusuf S, Dzavik V, Doris C.I, Yi Q, Smith S, Moore-Cox A, Bosch J, Riley W.A, Teo K.K. Effects of ramipril and vitamin E on atherosclerosis : The study to evaluate carotid ultrasound changes in patients treated with ramipril and vitamin E (SECURE). Circulation. 2001;103(7):919-925.

[60] Beckman J.A, Goldfine A.B, Gordon M.B, Garrett L.A, Keaney J.F Jr, and Creager M.A. Oral antioxidant therapy improves endothelial function in Type 1 but not Type 2 diabetes mellitus. American Journal of Physiology. 2003;285(6):2392-2398.

[61] Mariod A.A., Matthaus B., and Hussein I. H. “Antioxidant properties of methanolic extracts from different parts of Sclerocarya birrea,” International Journal of Food Science and Technology. 2008;43:921–926,

[62] Adaramoye O.A. and Adeyemi E.O. Hypoglycaemic and hypolipidaemic effects of fractions from Kolaviron, a biflavonoid complex from Garcinia kola in streptozotocin- induced diabetes mellitus rats. Journal of Pharmacy and Pharmacology. 2006;58:121-128.

[63] Rauter A.P., Martins A., Borges C., Mota-Filipe H., Pinto R., Sepodes B. and Justino J. Antihyperglycaemic and protective effects of flavonoids on streptozotocin-induced diabetic rats. Phytotherapy Research. 2010;24(2): S133-S138.

[64] Nakamura T, Kaneda Y and Ogihara T. Hepatocyte growth factor prevents endothelial cell death through inhibition of bax translocation from cytosol to mitochondrial membrane. Diabetes. 2002;51: 2604–2611.

[65] Hakkinen S.H., Karenlampi S.O., Heinonen I.M., and Mykkanen H. Content of the flavonols quercetin, myricetin, and kaempferol in 25 edible berries. Journal of Agriculture and Food Chemistry. 1999;47:2274-2279.

[66] Larocca L.M., Teofili, L., Sica, S., Pierelli L., and Menichella G. Quercetin inhibits the growth of leukemic progenitors and induces the expression of transforming growth factor-B1 in these cells. Blood. 1995;85:3654-3661

[67] Cox D., Whichelow M.J, and Prevost T.A. Antioxidant effects of flavonoids. Public Health Nutrition. 2000;3:19-29.

[68] Chang W.S, Lee, Y.J, Lu, F.J. and Chiang, H.C. Inhibitory effects of flavonoids on xanthine oxidase. Anticancer Research. 1993;13:2165-2170.

[69] Chen Y.T, Zheng R.L., Jia Z.J. and Ju Y. Flavonoids as superoxide scavengers and antioxidants. Free Radical Biology and Medicine. 1990;9:19-20.

[70] Fiorani M., Guidarelli A., Blasa M., Azzolini C., Candiracci M., Piatti E., and Cantoni O. Mitochondria accumulate large amounts of quercetin: prevention of mitochondrial damage and release upon oxidation of the extra-mitochondrial fraction of the flavonoid. Journal of Nutrition and Biochemistry. 2010;21:397-404.

[71] Meyers K.J., Rudolf J.L. and Mitchell A.E. Influence of dietary quercetin on glutathione redox status in mice. Journal of Agriculture and Food Chemistry. 2008;56:830-836.

[72] Abd El-Baky A.E. Quercetin protective action on oxidative stress, sorbitol, insulin resistance and beta cells function in experimental diabetic rats. International Journal of Pharmaceutical Studies and Research 2011;2(2)11-18.

[73] Kwon O, Eck P, Chen S, Corpe C.P, Lee J.H, Kruhlak M, and Levine M. Inhibition of the intestinal glucose transporter GLUT2 by flavonoids. Federation of American Societies for Experimental Biology Journal. 21: 2007;366-77.

[74] Manzano S and Williamson G. Polyphenols and phenolic acids from strawberry and apple decrease glucose uptake and transport by human intestinal Caco-2 cells. Molecular Nutrition and Food Research. 2010;54:1773-80.

[75] Vessal M, Hemmati M, and Vasei M. Antidiabetic effects of quercetin in streptozocin-induced diabetic rats. Comparative Biochemistry and Physiology Part C: Toxicology. 2003;135:357-64.

[76] Coskun O, Kanter M, Korkmaz A, and Oter S. Quercetin, a flavonoid antioxidant, prevents and protects streptozotocin-induced oxidative stress and β-cell damage in rat páncreas. Pharmacology Research. 2005;51: 117-23.

[77] Kobori M, Masumoto S, Akimoto Y, and Takahashi Y. Dietary quercetin alleviates diabetic symptoms and reduces streptozotocininduced disturbance of hepatic gene expression in mice. Molecular Nutrition and Food Research. 2009;53: 859-68.

[78] Elberg G, Jinping L, Leibovitch A, and Shechter Y. Non-receptor cytosolic protein tyrosine kinases from various rat tissues. Biochimica et Biophysica Acta. 1995;1269:299-306.

[79] Portillo M.P., Aguirre L, Arias N, Macarulla M. T, and Gracia A. Beneficial Effects of Quercetin on Obesity and Diabetes. The Open Nutraceuticals Journal. 2011;4: 189-198.

[80] Youl E, Bardy G, Magous R, Cros G, Sejalon F, Virsolvy A, Richard S, Quignard J.F, Gross R, Petit P, Bataille D, and Oiry C. Quercetin potentiates insulin secretion and protects INS-1 pancreatic b-cells against oxidative damage via the ERK1/2 pathway. British Journal of Pharmacology. 2010;161(4):799-814.

[81] Longuet C, Broca C, Costes S, Hani E.H, Bataille D, and Dalle S. Extracellularly regulated kinases (p44/42 mitogen-activated protein kinases) phosphorylate synapsin I and regulate insulin secretion in the MIN6 beta-cell line and islets of Langerhans. Endocrinology. 2005;146: 643-54.

[82] Rivera L, Morón R, Sánchez M, Zarzuelo A, and Galisteo M. Quercetin ameliorates metabolic syndrome and improves the inflammatory status in obese zucker rats. Obesity. 2008;16:2081-7.

[83] Hussain S.A, Ahmed Z.A., Mahwi T.O., and Aziz T.A. Quercetin Dampens Postprandial Hyperglycemia in Type 2 Diabetic Patients Challenged with Carbohydrates Load International Journal of Diabetes Research. 2012;1(3): 32-35.

[84] Steward L.K, Wang Z, Ribnicky D, Soileau J.L, Cefalu W.T, and Gettys T.W. Failure of dietary quercetin to alter the temporal progression of insulin resistance among tissues of C57BL/6J mice during the development of diet-induced obesity. Diabetologia. 2009;52: 514-23.

[85] Wein S, Behm N, Petersen R.K, Kristiansen K, Wolffram S. Quercetin enhances adiponectin secretion by a PPARℵ independent mechanism. European Journal of Pharmaceutical Sciences. 2010;41:16-22.

[86] Hertog M.G., Hollman P.C., Katan M. B. and Kromhout D. Intake of potentially anticarcinogenic flavonoids and their determinants in adults in The Netherlands. Nutrition and Cancer. 1993;20:21–29.

[87] Janbaz K.H., Saeed S.A. and Gilani A.H Protective effect of rutin on paracetamol- and CCl4-induced hepatotoxicity in rodents. Fitoterapia. 2002;73: 557–563.

[88] Navarro-Núñez L., Lozano M.L, Palomo M, Martínez C, Vicente V, and Castillo J, "Inhibits Platelet Adhesion and Thrombus Formation and Synergizes with Aspirin in the Suppression of the Arachidonic Acid Pathway", Journal of Agriculture and Food Chemistry. 2008;56(9): 2970–6.

[89] Kamalakkannan N and Prince P.S.M. Antihyperglycaemic and Antioxidant Effect of Rutin, a Polyphenolic Flavonoid, in Streptozotocin-Induced Diabetic Wistar Rats. Basic, Clinical Pharmacology and Toxicology. 2006;98: 97–103.

[90] Kozlov A.V., Ostrachovitch E.A. and Afanas'ev I.B. Mechanism of inhibitory effects of chelating drugs on lipid peroxidation in rat brain homogenates. Biochemical Pharmacology. 1994;47:795–799.

[91] Fernandes H., Angélica A., Lourenzi E., Novelli B., Okoshi K., Okoshi M.P, Di Muzio B.P., Guimarães J.F.C, Fernandes A Jnr. Influence of rutin treatment on biochemical alterations in experimental diabetes. Biomedicine and pharmacotherapy. 2010;64(3): 214-219.

[92] Alsaif M.A. Beneficial Effects of Rutin and Vitamin C Coadministration in a Streptozotocin-Induced Diabetes Rat Model of Kidney Nephrotoxicity. Pakistan Journal of Nutrition. 2009;8 (6):745-754.

[93] Sattanathan K., Dhanapal C.K.,and Manavalan R. LDL lowering properties of rutin in diabetic patients. International Journal of Pharma and Bio sciences. 2010;1(4): 0975-6299.

[94] Hunyadi A, Martins A, Hsieh T.J, Seres A, Zupko′ I. Chlorogenic Acid and Rutin Play a Major Role in the In Vivo Anti-Diabetic Activity of Morus alba Leaf Extract on Type II Diabetic Rats. PLoS ONE 2012;7(11): e50619. doi:10.1371/journal.pone.0050619.

[95] Carmada L., Distefano V., DelBosco S.F., and Schillaci D. Antoproliferative activity of citrus juices and HPLC evaluation of their flavonoid composition. Fitoterapia. 2007;78:426-429.

[96] Galati E.M, Monforte M.T, Kirjavainen S, Forestieri A.M, and Trovato A. Il Farmaco, 1994;49:709.

[97] Crespo M.E, Galvez J, Cruz T, Ocete M.A, and Zarzuelo A. Antiinflammatory activity of diosmin and hesperidin in rat colitis induced by TNBS. Planta Medica. 1999;65:651-653.

[98] Hitzenberger G. Therapeutic effectiveness of flavonoids shown on the example of DaflonC4 500 mg. Wein. Med. Wochenschr. 1997;174:409.

[99] Rezai-Zadeh K, Douglas Shytle R, Bai Y, Tian J, Hou H, Mori T, Zeng J., Obregon D., Town T., and Tan, J. Flavonoid-mediated presenilin-1 phosphorylation reduces Alzheimer's disease beta-amyloid production. Journal of Cellular and Molecular Medicine. 2009;13:574-88.

[100] Lacombe C, Lelievre J.C, Bucherer C, and Grimaldi A. Activity of Daflon 500 mg on the hemorheological disorders in diabetes. International Angiology. 1989;8:45-48.

[101] Valensi P.E, Behar A, De-Champvallins M.M, Attalah M, Boulakia F.C, and Attali J.R. Effects of a purified micronized flavonoid fraction on capillary filtration in diabetic patients. Diabet Med. 1996;13:882-888.

[102] Manuel Y, Keenoy B, Vertommen J, and De Leeuw I. The effect of flavonoid treatment on the glycation and antioxidant status in type 1 diabetic patients. Diabetes Nutrition and Metabolism. 1999;12:256-263.

[103] Tanaka T. Makita H., Kawabata K., Mori H., Kakumoto M and Satoh K. Carcinogenesis. 1997;18: 957.

[104] Tirkey N, Pilkhwal S, Kuhad A, and Chopra K. Hesperidin, a citrus bioflavonoid, decreases the oxidative stress produced by carbon tetrarchloride in rat liver and kidney. BMC Pharmacology. 2005;5:2.

[105] Jung U.J, Lee M.K, Park Y.B, Kang M.A and Choi M.S. Effect of citrus flavonoids on lipid metabolism and glucose-regulating enzyme mRNA levels in type-2 diabetic mice. International Journal of Biochemistry and Cell Biology. 2006;38:1134-1145.

[106] Kaur G, Tirkey N, Chopra K. Beneficial effect of hesperidin on lipopolysaccharide-induced hepatotoxicity. Toxicology. 2006;226: 152-160.

[107] Pari L. and Srinivasan S. Antihyperglycemic effect of diosmin on hepatic key enzymes of carbohydrate metabolism in streptozotocin-nicotinamide-induced diabetic rats, Biomedicine and Pharmacotherapy. 2010;64(7):477-481.

[108] Silambarasan T and Raja B. Diosmin, a bioflavonoid reverses alterations in blood pressure, nitric oxide, lipid peroxides and antioxidant status in DOCA-salt induced hypertensive rats. European Journal of Pharmacology. 2012;679(1): 81-89.

[109] Kraft K. Artichoke leaf extract—recent findings reflecting effects on lipid metabolism, liver and gastrointestinal tracts. Phytomedicine. 1997;4(4), 369-378.

[110] Ross J.A and Kasum C.M. Dietary flavonoids: bioavailability, metabolic effects, and safety. Annual Review of Nutrition. 2002;22:19-34.

[111] Choi J.S, Choi Y.J, Park S.H, Kang J.S, and Kang Y.H. Flavones mitigate tumor necrosis factor-alpha-induced adhesion molecule upregulation in cultured human endothelial cells: role of nuclear factor-kappa B. Journal of Nutrition. 2004;134:1013–9.

[112] Loizzo M.R, Said A, Tundis R, Rashed K, Statti G.A, Hufner.A., and Menichini.F. Inhibition of angiotensin converting enzyme (ACE) by flavonoids isolated from Ailanthus excelsa (Roxb) (Simaroubaceae). Phytotherapy Research. 2007;21:32–6.

[113] Ma X, Li Y.F, Gao Q, Ye Z.G, Lu X.J, Wang H.P, Jiang, H.D., Bruce, I.C. and Xia, Q. Inhibition of superoxide anionmediated impairment of endothelium by treatment with luteolin and apigenin in rat mesenteric artery. Life Sciences. 2008;83:110–7.

[114] Xu K., Liu B., Ma Y., Du J., Li G., Gao H., Zhang Y. and Ning Z. Physicochemical Properties and Antioxidant Activities of Luteolin-Phospholipid Complex. Molecules. 2009;14:3486-93.

[115] Horvathova K., Chalupa I., Sebova L., Tothova D., Vachalkova A. Protective effect of quercetin and luteolin in human melanoma HMB-2 cells. Mutation Research. 2005;565:105-12.

[116] Odontuya G., Hoult J.R., and Houghton P.J. Structure-activity relationship for antiinflammatory effect of luteolin and its derived glycosides. Phytotherapy Research. 2005;19: 782-6.

[117] Cheng I.F. and Breen K. On the ability of four flavonoids, baicilein, luteolin, naringenin, and quercetin, to suppress the Fenton reaction of the iron-ATP complex. Biometals. 2000;13:77-83.

[118] Hu C, and Kitts D.D. Luteolin and luteolin-7-O-glucoside from dandelion flower suppress iNOS and COX-2 in RAW264.7 cells. Molecular and Cellular Biochemistry. 2004;265:107-113.

[119] Wruck C.J., Claussen M., Fuhrmann G., Romer L., Schulz A., Pufe T., Waetzig V., Peipp M., Herdegen T., Gotz M.E. Luteolin protects rat PCl2 and C6 cells against MPP+ induced toxicity via an ERK dependent Keap1-Nrf2-ARE pathway. Journal of Neural Transmission. 2007;72:57-67.

[120] Choi B.M, Lim D.W, Lee J.A, Gao S.S, Kwon D.Y, and Kim B.R. Luteolin suppresses Cisplatin-induced apoptosis in auditory cells: possible mediation through induction of heme oxygenase-1 expression. Journal of Medicinal Food. 2008;11:230-6.

[121] Qiusheng Z., Yuntao Z., Rongliang Z., Dean G., Changling L. Effects of verbascoside and luteolin on oxidative damage in brain of heroin treated mice. Pharmazie. 2005;60:539-43.

[122] Manju V., Balasubramaniyan V., Nalini N. Rat colonic lipid peroxidation and antioxidant status: the effects of dietary luteolin on 1,2-dimethylhydrazine challenge. Cellular and Molecular Biology Letters. 2005;10: 535-51.

[123] Zarzuelo A., Jiménez I., Gámez M.J., Utrilla P., Fernadez I., Torres M.I., and Osuna I. Effects of luteolin 5-O-b-rutinoside in streptozotocin-induced diabetic rats. Life Sciences. 1996;58, 2311–2316.

[124] Kim J. S., Kwon C. S., and Son K. H. Inhibition of alpha-glucosidase and amylase by luteolin, a flavonoid. Bioscience, Biotechnology and Biochemistry. 2000;64(11): 2458-61.

[125] Ding L, Jin D, and Chen X. Luteolin enhances insulin sensitivity via activation of PPARγ transcriptional activity in adipocytes. Journal of Nutrition and Biochemistry; 2010;21(10): 941-7.

[126] Bohm F, Tinkler J.H, and Truscott T.G. Carotenoids protect against cell membrane damage by the nitrogen dioxide radical. Natural Medicine. 1995;1:98-99.

[127] Porrini M and Riso P. Lymphocyte lycopene concentration and DNA protection from oxidative damage is increased in women after a short period of tomato consumption. Journal of Nutrition. 2000;130:189-192.

[128] Arab L. and Steck S. Lycopene and cardiovascular disease. American Journal of Clinical Nutrition. 2000;71: 1691S-5S.

[129] Kuhad A., Sethi R. and Chopra K. Lycopene attenuates diabetes-associated cognitive decline in rats. Life Sciences. 2008;83:128–134.

[130] Agarwal S, and Rao A.V. Tomato Lycopene and Its Role in Human Health and Chronic Diseases. Canadian Medical Association Journal. 2000;163(6) : 739.

[131] Basuny A.M, Mostafat D.M. and Azouz A. Supplementation of polyunsaturated oils with lycopene as natural antioxidant and antipolymerization during heating process. Minia Journal of Agricultural Research and Development. 2006;26: 449-469.

[132] Basuny A.M, Gaafar A.M. and Arafat S.M. Tomato lycopene is a natural antioxidant and can alleviate hypercholesterolemia. African Journal of Biotechnology. 2009;23: 6627-6633.

[133] Hisao G, Fong T.H, Tzu N.H, Lin K.H, Chou D.S, and Sheu J.R. A potent antioxidant, lycopene, affords neuroprotection against microglia activation and focal cerebral ischemia in rats. In Vivo. 2004;18: 351- 356.

[134] Gunasekera R.S, Sewgobind K., Desai S., Dunn L, Black H.S., McKeehan W.L, and Patil B. Lycopene and lutein inhibit proliferation in rat prostate carcinoma cells. Nutrition and Cancer. 2007;58:171–177.

[135] Akbaraly N.T, Faure H., Gourlet V., Favier A. and Berr, C. Plasma carotenoid levels and cognitive performance in an elderly population: Results of the EVA Study. Journals of Gerontology, Series A, 2007;62: 308–316.

[136] Riso P., Visioli F., Grande S., Guarnieri S., Gardana C., Simonetti P., Porrini M. Effect of a tomato-based drink on markers of inflammation, immunomodulation, and oxidative stress. Journal of Agriculture and Food Chemistry. 2006;54, 2563–2566.

[137] Krinsky N.I. Carotenoids as antioxidants. Nutrition. 2001;17: 815-817.

[138] Mortensen A., Skibsted L.H., Truscott T.G. The interaction of dietary carotenoids with radical species. Archives of Biochemistry and Biophysics. 2001;385, 13–19.

[139] oung A.J. and Lowe G.M. Antioxidant and prooxidant properties of carotenoids. Archives of Biochemistry and Biophysics. 2001;385, 20–27.

[140] El-Agamey A., Lowe, G.M., McGarvey D.J., Mortensen A., Phillip D.M, Truscott T.G., Young A.J. Carotenoid radical chemistry and antioxidant or pro-oxidant properties. Archives of Biochemistry and Biophysics. 2004;430:37–48.

[141] Krinsky N.I and Johnson E.J. Carotenoid actions and their relation to health and disease. Molecular Aspects of Medicine. 2005;26: 459–516.

[142] Polidori M.C., Mecocci P., Stahl W., Parente B., Cecchetti R., Cherubini A., Cao P., Sies H., Senin U. Plasma levels of lipophilic antioxidants in very old patients with Type 2 diabetes. Diabetes/Metabolism Research and Reviews. 2000;16:15–19.

[143] Coyne T, Ibiebele T.I, Baade P.D, Dobson A, McClintock C, Dunn S, Leonard D, Shaw J. Diabetes mellitus and serum carotenoids: Findings of a population-based study in Queensland, Australia. American Journal of Clinical Nutrition. 2005;82: 685–693.

[144] Ford E.S, Will J.C, Bowman B.A, and Narayan K.M. Diabetes mellitus and serum carotenoids findings from the Third National Health and Nutrition Examination Survey. American Journal of Epidemiology. 1999;149:168-176.

[145] Kuhad A., and Chopra K. Lycopene ameliorates thermal hyperagesia and cold allodynia in STZ-induced diabetic rat. Indian Journal of Experimental Biology. 2008;46:108-111.

[146] Krul C, Luiten-Schuite A, Tenfelde A, van Ommen B, Verhagen H, and Havenaar R. dAntimutagenic activity of green tea and black tea extracts studied in a dynamic in vitro gastrointestinal model. Mutation Research. 2001;474:71–85.

[147] Schmidt M, Schmitz H.J, Baumgart A, Guedon D, Netsch M.I, Kreuter M.H, Schmidlin C.B, and Schrenk, D. Toxicity of green tea extracts and their constituents in rat hepatocytes in primary culture. Food Chemistry and Toxicology. 2005;43:307– 14.

[148] Sutherland B.A., Rosanna M.A., Rahman, Appleton I. Mechanisms of action of green tea catechins, with a focus on ischemia-induced neurodegeneration Journal of Nutritional Biochemistry. 2006;17:291– 306.

[149] Ruch R.J, Cheng S.J, and Klaunig J.E. Prevention of cytotoxicity and inhibition of intercellular communication by antioxidant catechins isolated from Chinese green tea. Carcinogenesis. 1989;10:1003–8.

[150] Guo Q, Zhao B, Li M, Shen S, and Xin W. Studies on protective mechanisms of four components of green tea polyphenols against lipid peroxidation in synaptosomes. Biochim Biophys Acta; 1996;1304:210– 22.

[151] Sawai Y and Sakata K. NMR analytical approach to clarify the antioxidative molecular mechanism of catechins using 1,1- diphenyl-2-picrylhydrazyl. Journal of Agriculture and Food Chemistry. 1998;46:111 –4.

[152] Kashima M. Effects of catechins on superoxide and hydroxyl radical. Chemical and Pharmaceutical Bulletin (Tokyo). 1999;47:279– 83.

[153] Nanjo F, Mori M, Goto K, and Hara Y. Radical scavenging activity of tea catechins and their related compounds. Bioscience Biotechnology Biochemistry.1999;63:1621–3.

[154] Zhao B, Guo Q, and Xin W. Free radical scavenging by green tea polyphenols. Methods in Enzymology. 2001;335:217–31.

[155] Sang S, Tian S, Wang H, Stark R.E, Rosen R.T, Yang C.S, and Ho C.T. Chemical studies of the antioxidant mechanism of tea catechins: radical reaction products of epicatechin with peroxyl radicals. Bioorganic and Medicinal Chemistry. 2003;11:3371– 8.

[156] Grinberg L.N, Newmark H, Kitrossky N, Rahamim E, Chevion M, and Rachmilewitz E.A. Protective effects of tea polyphenols against oxidative damage to red blood cells. Biochemistry and Pharmacology. 1997;54:973– 8.

[157] Seeram N.P and Nair M.G. Inhibition of lipid peroxidation and structure–activity-related studies of the dietary constituents anthocyanins, anthocyanidins, and catechins. Journal of Agriculture and Food Chemistry. 2002;50:5308– 12.

[158] Anderson R.F, Fisher L.J, Hara Y, Harris T, Mak W.B, Melton L.D, and Packer J.E. Green tea catechins partially protect DNA from hydroxyl radical induced strand breaks and base damage through fast chemical repair of DNA radicals. Carcinogenesis; 2001;22:1189– 93.

[159] Skrzydlewska E, Ostrowska J, Farbiszewski R, and Michalak K. Protective effect of green tea against lipid peroxidation in the rat liver, blood serum and the brain. Phytomedicine. 2002;9:232– 8.

[160] Anderson R.A and Polansky M.M. Tea enhance insulin activity. Journal of Agriculture and Food Chemistry. 2002;50: 7182-7186.

[161] Sabu M.C, Smitha K, and Kuttan R. Anti-diabetic activity of green tea polyphenols and their role in reducing oxidative stress in experimental diabetes. Journal of Ethnopharmacology. 2002;83:109-116.

[162] Tsuneki H, Ishizuka M, Terasawa M, Wu J.B, Sasaoka T, and Kimura I. Effect of green tea on blood glucose levels and serum proteomic patterns in diabetic (db/db) mice and on glucose metabolism in healthy humans. BMC Pharmacology. 2004;4:18-27.

[163] Fukino Y, Shimbo M, Aoki N, Okubo T, and Iso H. Randomized controlled trial for an effect of green tea consumption on insulin resistance and inflammation markers. Journal of Nutritional Science and Vitaminology (Tokyo); 2005;51:335-342.

[164] Rizvi S.I, Abu Zaid M, Anis R, and Mishra N. Protective role of tea catechins against oxidation-induced damage of type 2 diabetic erythrocytes. Clinical and Experimental Pharmacology and Physiology. 2005;32:70–75.

[165] Rizvi S.I, and Abu Zaid M. Impairment of sodium pump and Na/H exchanger in erythrocytes from NIDDM patients. Effect of tea catechins. Clinica Chimica Acta. 2005;354: 59–67

[166] Qin B., Panickar K.S., and Anderson R.A. Cinnamon: Potential role in the prevention of insulin resistance, metabolic syndrome, and type 2 diabetes. Journal of Diabetes Science and Technology. 2010;4: 685–693.

[167] Sirichai A., Weerachat S., Aramsri M., Sathaporn N., and Sirintorn Y. Cinnamic Acid and Its Derivatives Inhibit Fructose-Mediated Protein Glycation. International Journal of Molecular Sciences. 2012;13:1778-1789.

[168] Lee E.J., Kim S.R., Kim J., and Kim Y.C. Hepatoprotective phenylpropanoids from Scrophularia buergeriana roots against CCl4-induced toxicity: Action mechanism and structure-activity relationship. Planta Medica. 2002;68: 407–411.

[169] Natella F., Nardini M., Di, Felice M., and Scaccini C. Benzoic and cinnamic acid derivatives as antioxidants: Structure-activity relation. Journal of Agriculture and Food Chemistry.1999;47:1453–1459.

[170] Liu I.M., Hsu F.L, Chen C.F, and Cheng J.T. Antihyperglycemic action of isoferulic acid in streptozotocin-induced diabetic rats. British Journal of Pharmacology. 2000;129: 631–636.

[171] Shahidi F. and Naczk M. Cereals, legumes and nuts. In " Phenolics in Food and Nutra ceuticals, CRC press, Boca Raton, 2004;17-166.

[172] Nenadis N., Lazaridou O. and Tsimidou M. Use of reference compounds in antioxidant activity. Pancreas. 2007;15(3): 246-50.

[173] Kanchana G., Shyni W.J, Rajadurai M. and Periasamy R. Evaluation of Antihyperglycemic Effect of Sinapic Acid in Normal and Streptozotocin-Induced Diabetes in Albino Rats. Global Journal of Pharmacology. 2011;5(1): 33-39.

[174] Masoko P., Mmushi T. J., Mogashoa M. M., Mokgotho M. P., Mampuru L. J., and Howard R.L. "In vitro evaluation of the antifungal activity of Sclerocarya birrea extracts against pathogenic yeasts," African Journal of Biotechnology. 2008;7: 3521–3526.

[175] Njume C., Afolayan A. J., Green E., and Ndip R. N. "Volatile compounds in the stem bark of Sclerocarya birrea (Anacardiaceae) possess antimicrobial activity against drug-resistant strains of Helicobacter pylori. International Journal of Antimicrobial Agents. 2011;38(4): 319-324

[176] Dieye A.M, Sarr A, Diop S.N, Ndiaye M, Sy G.Y, Diarra M, Rajraji G.I, Ndiaye S.A and Faye B. Medicinal plants and the treatment of diabetes in Senegal: survey with patients. Fundamental and Clinical Pharmacology. 2008;22: 211–216.

[177] Dimo T., Rakotonirina S.V., Tan P.V., Azay J, Dongo E, Kamtchouing P, and Cros G. Effect of Sclerocarya birrea (Anacardiaceae) stem bark methylene chloride/methanol extract on streptozotocin-diabetic rats. Journal of Ethnopharmacology. 2007;110: 434–438.

[178] Kirtikar, K. R. and Basu, B. D. Indian Medicinal Plants, Bishen Singh Mahendra Pal Singh, Dehradun,, 1998;2(7):22462247.

[179] DeFeudis F.V, Papadopoulos V and Drieu K. Gingko biloba extracts and cancer: a research area in its infancy. Fundamentals of Clinical Pharmacology. 2003;17: 405- 17.

[180] Takeoka G.R and Dao L.T. Antioxidant constituent of almond [Prunus dulcis (Mill.) D.A. Webb.] hulls. Journal of Agriculture and Food Chemistry. 2003;51: 496-501.

[181] Van Rensburg W.J, Ferreira D, Malan E and Steenkamp J.A. Tyrosinase catalysed biphenyl construction from flavan-3-ol substrates. Phytochemistry. 2000;53: 285-92.

[182] Kumar R.S, Rajkapoor B, Perumal P, Dhanasekaran T, Josea M.A. and Jothimanivannan C. Antitumor Activity of Prosopis glandulosa Torr. on Ehrlich Ascites Carcinoma (EAC) Tumor Bearing Mice. Iranian Journal of Pharmaceutical Research. 2011;10: 505-510.

[183] Siddhuraju P. Antioxidant activity of polyphenolic compounds extracted from defatted raw and dry heated Tamarindus indica seed coat. LWT Food Science and Technology. 2007;40:982-990.

[184] Maiti R, Das U.K and Ghosh D (). Attenuation of Hyperglycemia and Hyperlipidemia in Streptozotocin- Induced Diabetic Rats by Aqueous Extract of Seed of Tamarindus indica. Biological and Pharmaceutical Bulletin. 2005;28:1172-1176.

[185] Martinello F, Soaresm S.M and Franco J.J. Hypolipidemic and antioxidant activities from Tamarindus indica L. pulp fruit in hypercholestromic hamsters. Food and Chemical Toxicology. 2006;44:810-818.

[186] Sudjaroen Y, Haubner R, Wu°rtele G, Hull W.E, Erben G, Spiegelhalder B, Changbumrung S, Bartsch H and Owen R.W (). Isolation and structure elucidation of phenolic antioxidants fromTamarind (Tamarindus indica L.) seeds and pericarp. Food and Chemical Toxicology. 2005;43:1673-1682.

[187] Mahmoudzades-Sagheb H, Heidari Z, Shahraki M and Moudi B. A stereological study of effects of aqueous extract of Tamarindus indica seeds on pancreatic islets in Streptozotocin-induced diabetic rats. Pakistan Journal of Pharmaceutical Sciences. 2010;23:427-434.

[188] Lebovitz, H.E. Postprandial hyperglycemic state: importance and consequences. Diabetes Research and Clinical Practice. 1998;40: S27–S28.

[189] DeFronzo R.A. Pharmacologic Therapy for Type 2 Diabetes Mellitus. Annals of Internal Medicine. 1999;131:281-303.

[190] Bailey C.J. Potential new treatments for type 2 diabetes. Trends in Pharmacological Sciences. 2000;1(7):259-65

Section 5

Antihypertensive Plant

Chapter 15

Potential Role of *Parkia biglobosa* in the Management and Treatment of Cardiovascular Diseases

O.B.L. Alinde, A.J. Esterhuyse and O.O. Oguntibeju

Additional information is available at the end of the chapter

http://dx.doi.org/10.5772/57229

1. Introduction

Non-communicable diseases (NCD), also known as chronic diseases represent one of the most serious health challenges of the 21st century. According to the World Health Organisation (WHO), global mortality due to NCD is projected to reach 55 million of deaths in the next 20 years, with 25 million of death caused by cardiovascular diseases (CVD) [1-3]. This is drawing a particular attention to the importance of intensifying research in the area aiming at fighting CVD through prevention and treatment. In a recent report of the WHO, CVD already accounted for 48% of NCD deaths [1]. Additionally, hypertension has been estimated to be the major risk factor for CVD morbidity and mortality, causing 51% of stroke deaths and 45% of coronary heart diseases deaths [1, 3]. Furthermore, CVD is increasing in the low- and middle-income with Sub-Saharan African countries recording the highest rate of hypertension [1-3]. It has been observed that these countries record an increase in the overall rate of hypertension mainly because of severe financial constraints for its management and control [1, 4].

With the prevalence of hypertension in the world's death rate, new approaches to investigate the treatment and management of this disease are highly in demand in order to reduce the overall rate of adult mortality from CVD. Quest for solutions has open doors to research in the field of alternative and complementary medicine as an effective, safe, simple and inexpensive strategy. Medicinal plants and fruits and vegetables are reputed for their excellent health-enhancing bioactive micronutrients, their cost-effectiveness and their widespread bioavailability [5-9]. While some medicinal plants have been investigated in hypertension research, many remain a mystery [5-9]. Therefore, the interest of this review is to summarize the findings of recent studies on the potential cardioprotective effect of *Parkia biglobosa*, a locally available medicinal West African plant that has been reported to display anti-inflammatory, antimicrobial, antioxidant, anti-cancer and hypotensive activities in its diverse parts [10-14]. In this chapter, a brief explanatory overview of hypertension and its implication in CVD will be given followed by a summary of potential ability of *Parkia biglobosa* to modulate health, especially CVD.

2. Hypertension

Hypertension, also known as raised blood pressure (BP), is a chronic medical condition and a slow progressive disease defined by a mean systolic BP (SBP) of at least 140 mm Hg and/or a diastolic BP (DBP) of at least 90 mm Hg [4, 15- 16]. In the USA, the seventh report of the Joint National Committee (JNC 7) on Prevention, Detection, Evaluation, and Treatment of High Blood Pressure has classified measured BP into different schemes and introduced a new classification referred to as "Prehypertension" [15]. Prehypertension was not defined as a disease-state but represented BP measurements of individuals at high risk of developing hypertension (Table 1). Hypertension has been classified into primary hypertension or essential hypertension (EH) and secondary hypertension (SH). They have respectively unknown and known aetiology.

JNC 7 category	Blood pressure (mm Hg)	
	SBP	DBP
Normal	lower than 120	lower than 80
Prehypertension	120 to 139	80 to 89
Hypertension	140 or higher	90 or higher
Stage 1	140 to 159	90 to 99
Stage 2	160 or higher	100 or higher

Table 1. JNC 7 Classification of blood pressure [4, 15]

Hypertension is a major public health problem responsible for 51% of stroke deaths and 45% of coronary heart diseases deaths [1, 3]. It represents the leading global risk factor of mortality, about 12.8% of global death [3] and is also reported to affects both man and woman [17]. Additionally, the prevalence of hypertension is reported to increase with body weight and advancing age [2, 15-16, 18]. Conversely, hypertension in children has been reported, especially, in overweight and obese children [19]. It has been observed that Black men and women have the highest prevalence of total hypertension [15-16]. Furthermore, while the large proportion of the population suffers from EH (90-95%), only 5-10% among the cases suffers from SH [20-24]. It has been reported that most individuals have an uncontrolled hypertension because the disease is predominantly a "silent" disease which is asymptomatic [17]. Epidemiological studies estimated that in the United States, one in five adult remains unaware of his diseased-state [16]. Nonetheless, with the rise of campaign aimed at increasing hypertension awareness and treatment, the prevalence of uncontrolled hypertension is declining in developed countries, when compared to developing countries [16, 18]. Actually, the low- and middle-income countries, especially Sub-Saharan African countries record an increase in the overall rate of hypertension mostly because of the severe financial constraints, limited set of health services, low access to facilities and low level of awareness, control, treatment campaigns [4].

2.1. Aetiology of essential hypertension

The aetiology of EH remains a mystery. Even though, EH is the commonest form of hypertension (90% - 95% of all cases), the underlying defects triggering its onset are not known. This explains the difficulty in finding a definite cure. It has been theoretically proposed (Mosaic Theory of Dr Irvine Page) that the aetiology of EH is multifactorial with genetic, environmental, anatomical, adaptive, neural, endocrine, humoral, haemodynamic risk factors and that those different risk factors interlink together to cause hypertension [25-27]. Some of these risk factors are described below:

2.1.1. Environmental risk factors

Various dietary habits and unhealthy lifestyle have also been identified to play a major role in the pathogenesis of hypertension such as:

- Pollutants
- Use of tobacco,
- Chronic consumption of alcohol,
- Lack of weight maintenance (sport inactivity),
- Adoption of diets characterised by high intake of glucose, high intake of saturated fat and cholesterol, high intake of salt (exceeding 5.8 grams daily) [6, 28].

The consequences of this adopted lifestyle give the rise to metabolic and physiological alterations which mediate the pathogenesis of hypertension and promotes other deleterious conditions such as hyperglycaemia (principal characteristic of diabetes) and hyperlipidaemia (principal characteristic of obesity) [29].

2.1.2. Hereditary risk factors

Genetic factors are thought to play a prominent role in the development of essential hypertension, especially genetic abnormalities of the baroreceptor system. However, the genes for hypertension have not yet been identified.

The baroreceptor system consists of nerves ending receptors sensitive to stretch, pulse rate and pressure changes of the blood vessels [30]. They are present on the wall of large arteries such as the aortic arch and the carotid sinus (Figure 1). They stand as the first line of neural control system over blood pressure fluctuation and constitute a short term regulation of BP [31-33]. With a significant change in BP, baroreceptors transmit impulses to central nervous system (CNS) to activate a "feedback" mechanism from autonomous nervous system called baroreceptor reflex or baroreflex. The baroreceptor autonomous reflex restores the BP to normal values [30-33]. It has been reported that that lack of baroreflex sensitivity is associated with the presence of a family history of hypertension [32, 34]. This shows that hypertension could be initiated from specific hereditary genetic abnormalities involving baroreceptors sensitivity [32, 34].

In addition, hereditary genetic abnormalities of the neuroendocrine regulation of baroreceptors have similarly been recognised as predictors of EH. For instance, studies have related overexpression of Chromogranin A (Cg A) in plasma, adrenal medulla and sympathetic neurons to essential hypertension in both clinical and experimental models [25, 35]. Similarly, Cg A loci genetic polymorphism was related to hypertension [36]. Chromogranin A is a prohormone stored and released with catecholamine (epinephrine, norepinephrine and dopamine) by exocytosis [37-38]. It is believed that Cg A influence sympathetic tone since it is a prohormone for active peptides with regulatory properties, namely vasostatin, pancreastastin and catestatin [37, 39]. Catestatin exhibits catecholamine release-inhibitory function and may function as a vasodilator [40-41]. Decreased circulating level of catestatin has been related to EH because it increases adrenergic pressor response by no longer exerting antagonism to neuronal nicotinic acetylcholine receptor [40-41].

Several genetic factors can affect the renin-angiotensin-aldosterone system and indirectly result in hereditary hypertension. For instance, deficient formation of kinin components (proteins that act locally to induce vasodilatation) in the body may also lead to hypertension and development of CVD. Renal kinin-kallikrein system helps to excrete excess sodium from the biological system [42]. Therefore, a reduction in renal expression of kinin-kalllikrein system can also be identified as a genetic factor for hypertension as a result of accumulation of sodium in the body. Consequently, diminished urinary kallikrein (sub-group of serine protease) excretion could represent a genetic marker of hereditary hypertension [42-43].

2.1.3. Haemodynamic, endocrine, neural, anatomical risk factors

The cardiovascular system ensures the supply of blood to all organs and tissues via distensible blood vessels such as arteries, veins and capillaries of the circulatory system (peripheral and pulmonary). Blood pressure represents the force with which the blood pushes against the wall of the arteries. At physiological level, factors such as blood volume, cardiac output, diameter of artery lumen, and elasticity of artery determine BP [44-45]. In addition, different systems contribute to the short-term and long-term regulation of BP such as:

- The nervous system baroreceptor reflex [46].
- The humoral secretion of vasoconstrictors and vasodilators substances such as acetylcholine, atropine [47].
- The kidneys regulation of BP via renal body fluid feedback, namely the renin-angiotensin-aldosterone system and the pressure natriuresis [31, 43].

Therefore, any molecular and physiological dysfunction affecting the regulation of BP can be associated with the pathogenesis of hypertension such as dysfunctions of the renin angiotensin system (RAS), dysfunctions in electrolytes homeostasis, dysfunctions of the endocrine system and increased arterial resistance [25, 48]. For example, the renin angiotensin system (RAS) is a central system involved in the regulation of BP and electrolytes homeostasis. Briefly, with a decrease in BP, kidneys prorenin are converted into active renin. Active renin cleaves the hepatic precursor protein angiotensinogen into the inactive angiotensin I (Ang I) [43, 49]. Then, the angiotensin converting enzyme (ACE) hydrolyses two principal molecules. Firstly, ACE cleaves the inactive Ang I to give active vasoconstrictor hormone Angiotensin II (Ang II). Angiotensin II, not only increases BP by constricting blood vessels but also causes the adrenal gland to release aldosterone, a hormone which increase BP through renal retention of sodium and water (increase of blood volume) and decrease excretion of potassium [42-43, 49]. Secondly, ACE which is a kininase II interact with the kinin-kalllikrein system and inactivate the vasodilator bradikinin by releasing pentapeptide Arg-Pro-Pro-gly-Pheo and tripeptide Ser-Pro-Phe fragments [42]. Therefore, failure to regulate the activated RAS at different level could lead to hypertension. Another example of system dysfunction involved the failure to regulate the increased activity of norepinephrine [48].

2.2. Aetiology of secondary hypertension

The aetiology of SH has been often identified with an underlying illness which indirectly increases BP. It has also been demonstrated that SH can emerge from drugs intake and health conditions such as pregnancy [15, 20, 50-52] (Table 2). Therefore, the treatment of SH is associated along with the treatment of the identified underlying factors.

Causes	Examples	
Renal diseases	RENAL PARENCHYMAL DISEASES: •Glomerulonephritis •Polycystic kidney diseases •Diabetic nephropathy •Hydronephrosis •Chronic kidney disease (CKD)	RENOVASCULAR DISEASES/RENAL ARTERY STENOSIS •Atherosclerotic renal artery diseases •Fibromuscular dysplasia •Renal artery embolism •Arteriovenous malformation of the renal artery
Vascular diseases	•Coarctation of aorta •Aortoarteritis	
Endocrinal and metabolic diseases	•Primary aldosteronism (Conn Syndrome), •Primary sodium retention (Liddle's Syndrome) •Cushing syndrome •Pheochromocytoma	
Neurological diseases	•Brain tumours •Encephalitis	
Drugs	•Oral contraceptive pills •Non-steroidal anti-inflammatory medications •Drug Abuse (Cocaine, Alcohol)	

Table 2. Causes of secondary hypertension [52]

2.3. Molecular mechanisms involved in the pathogenesis of hypertension

Previous studies have shown the involvement of excessive reactive oxygen species (ROS) in the pathophysiology of CVD [53-56]. At a molecular level, oxidative stress (Oxs) has been identified to have major implication in the development of clinical and experimental hypertension [57-59]. It was demonstrated that chronic glutathione depletion induced severe elevation of arterial BP [60]. The lack of endogenous antioxidant enzymes worsens oxidative stress and can indirectly promote the risk of hypertension. For example, a recent research supports the influence of genetic polymorphism of antioxidant enzymes in increasing the risk of hypertension [61]. Likewise, [62] in Taiwan demonstrated that manganese superoxide dismutase (MnSOD) polymorphism significantly increased the risk of hypertension.

Inflammation and lipid peroxidation are central to the development of multiple CVD and are mediated by a variety of cell types including macrophages, lymphocytes, endothelial cells and vascular smooth muscles cells [63-65]. The multiple cell types which participate in vascular inflammation produce various pro- and anti-inflammatory cytokines and specific membrane receptors allowing them to transmit their effects to the cells. Studies place a strong emphasis on the role of oxidative stress in the pathophysiology of hypertension through promotion of chronic inflammation [66]. In fact, the rise of Oxs in the vasculature decreased bioavailability of nitric oxide (NO). This leads to endothelial dysfunction due to the loss of vasodilation of blood vessels [58, 67-69]. In addition, oxidative stress coupled with hyperlipidaemia and hypercholesterolemia in the vasculature gives rise to atherosclerosis by oxidation of lipids in the vessels. Atherosclerosis is an inflammatory disease leading to increased arteriolar resistance and increased large artery stiffness and obstruction of blood vessels and subsequent ischemia [70].

2.4. Consequences of hypertension

The continuous high pressure exerted on the arteries wall causes long term damages to both blood vessels and organs. In fact, when hypertension is not timely acknowledged and controlled, damages to organs can become severe and fatal [15, 51-52]. Numerous complications resulting from hypertension are illustrated in Table 3.

2.5. Orthodox therapeutic approaches to managing/treating hypertension

Although, no definite cure has been found to treat essential hypertension, many approaches have been used to manage and control its incidence; in particular lifestyle changes and the use of medications. Lowering salt and alcohol intake, lowering consumption of saturated fats and cholesterol rich food and practising regular exercise are important steps taken towards control of BP [17]. However, these steps are often associated with prescription of anti-hypertensive medication. Many types of anti-hypertensive drugs have been developed over the years such as diuretics, ACE inhibitors, angiotensin II receptor-blocker, calcium channel blockers, alpha and beta blockers [71-73]. Even though a wide variety of anti-hypertensive drugs are effective to control and manage hypertension, they are not without considerable side effects [74-75]. Additionally, the cost of medication is not

http://dx.doi.org/10.5772/57229

End Organ	CVD Damages	Complications/ Consequences
Heart	•Acute coronary syndrome, •Ischaemic heart diseases •Myocardial infarction, •Atrial fibrillation, •Arrhythmias, •Coronary artery disease, •Left ventricular hypertrophy leading to chronic heart failure	Sudden death
Brain	•Constant headaches •Stroke •Neurological damages (memory loss, dementia) •Disability (paralysis)	Sudden death
Kidney	•Renovascular dysfunction, •Chronic kidney failure, •End stage renal diseases (ESDR)	Death
Eyes	Hypertensive retinopathy	Blindness
Vascular system	•Atherosclerosis •Arterial resistance •Aneurysm •Embolus and thrombo-embolus •All the above	Brain, heart, kidney, eyes damages Death

Table 3. End organs damages related to hypertension

always affordable for the majority of the population, especially in developing countries, since managing hypertension represents a lifelong financial investment. Henceforth, research is now turning to alternative and complementary medicine. Many reports support the concept that natural or dietary supplementation can be used to develop effective, safe, simple and inexpensive antihypertensive treatment [6, 28]. As a result, many researches are currently directed towards a search for useful bioactive compounds in medicinal plants as a new strategy for the treatment and management of hypertension [5, 8, 49, 76].

2.6. Alternative therapeutic approach to hypertension

Deeper exploration of phytochemicals found in medicinal plants is used as an approach to discover potential prophylactic and therapeutic agents in cardio protection [7-9]. Medicinal plants can be used to develop effective, safe, simple and inexpensive antihypertensive treatment since they are reputed for their excellent health-enhancing bioactive micronutrients, their cost-effectiveness and their widespread bioavailability [7, 77-78]. As a result, research is currently directed towards discovering useful bioactive compounds in medicinal plants that could be used as new strategies for treatment and management of hypertension [5, 8, 49, 76].

3. *Parkia biglobosa*

3.1. Brief description

Parkia biglobosa, also called the African Locust Bean tree is a multipurpose tree indigenous to the tropical regions of West Africa. *Parkia biglobosa* belongs to the family Mimosaceae (Leguminosae - Mimosoideae) [79-evidences. Therefore, studies of the]. *Parkia biglobosa* is a widespread savannah tree used for nutritional and medicinal purposes [7, 81, 71]. The matured tree can grow up to 30 m in height with a crown large of low branches. The bark is thick and fissured with a grey to brown colour. The leaves are alternate, dark green and bipinnate. The leaves are about 8-30 mm x 1.5-8 mm in size with 13-60 pairs of leaflets held on a long rachis [82].

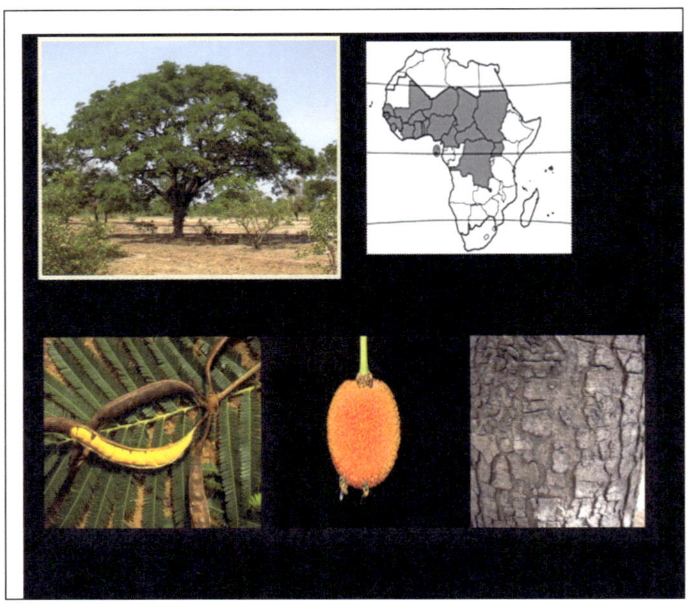

Figure 1. *Parkia biglobosa* [83]

The analysis of the phytochemicals present in *Parkia biglobosa* revealed the presence of alkaloid, flavonoids, tannins, saponins, cardiac glycosides, sterols, resins and terpenes (Table 4) [80, 84-85].

3.2. Potential health benefits of *Parkia biglobosa*

For a long time, native populations of West Africa have been using different parts of *Parkia biglobosa* to meet their nutritional and basic health care needs. In different countries, *Parkia biglobosa* has been used as a multipurpose plant in the therapy of a variety of diseases including

	Plant	*Parkia biglobosa*			*REFERENCES*
	Extracts (W,P,C,M)	**Leaf extracts**	**Bark extracts**	**Root extracts**	
Bioactive components	Saponins	+	+	+	[85, 86, 87]
	Cardiac Glycosides	+	+	+	[85, 87]
	Tannins	+	+	+	[85, 86, 87]
	Flavonoids (Anthocyanins, flavonones, coumarins, catechins)	+	+	+	[85, 86, 87]
	Alkaloids	-	+	+	[85, 87]
	Resins	+	+	+	[85]
	Carbohydrates	+	+	+	[85]
	Sterols and Terpenoids	+	+	+	[86, 87, 88]

Abbreviations: W: water, P: petroleum ester, C: Chloroform, M: Methanol, +: Present, - : Absent.

Table 4. Brief summary of the bioactive components in *Parkia biglobosa*

hypertension. A summary of traditional medicine practices from different West African countries is illustrated in Table 5.

The fact that repetitive information was obtained from traditional healers and population from diverse regions and countries indicated the need to scientifically authenticate these folkloric evidence. Therefore, studies of the extracts of *Parkia biglobosa* have been conducted and experimental and clinical data are now recognizing the health benefits attributed to *Parkia biglobosa* in its diverse parts. *Parkia biglobosa* bark extracts have been identified to have significant anti-inflammatory, analgesic, antibacterial and anti-helminthic activities. For example, the analgesic and anti-inflammatory property of *Parkia biglobosa* bark extract in the management of toothache has been demonstrated [102]. The anti-venom activity of the bark extract against snake bites has also been reported [103]. In 2007, some clinical investigations described the antibacterial properties of *Parkia biglobosa* bark and root extracts against *Staphylococcus aureus, Pseudomonas aeruginosa, Klebsiella pneumoniae, Escherichia coli, Shigella dysenteriae* responsible for urinary tract and digestive system infections [84, 86, 104]. Additionally, *Parkia biglobosa* stem bark has been attributed anti-microbial effects against *Bacillus subtilitis* and was recommended as a natural preservative against pharmacological contaminations [85]. *Parkia biglobosa* leaf extract were described to exhibit anti-plasmodial activity against malaria [105]. Recently, antioxidant, anti-carcinogenic and anti-trypanosomic activities of the plant have been acknowledged [78, 97, 106-107].

3.3. Potential benefits of *Parkia biglobosa* in the treatment of hypertension and CVD

Previous investigations have indicated the hypotensive potential of *Parkia biglobosa* extracts. For example, it was reported that a methanolic seed extract decreased blood pressure in the

Countries	Used Parts	Traditional medicine practice	References
Benin	All parts	Treatment of digestive system diseases (diarrhoea, dysentery, abdominal pain) Treatment of diseases of the cardiovascular system Treatment of injuries and burns Treatment of infectious diseases (shingles, malaria, abscesses, yellow fever, scabies, measles, chicken-pox, oedema, jaundice) Treatment of paediatric pathologies Treatment of symptoms and syndromes: malaise, tiredness, headaches, hip pain, ache, rheumatism, elephantiasis, onset of paralysis	[89]
Burkina Faso	Fermented seeds, leaves, stem bark	Treatment of oral infections: Gingivitis, toothache, sores (tongues and lips)	[90]
Ghana	Leaves, stem bark, raw fruit, fermented seed	Treatment of malaria, stomach ache	[77]
Ivory coast	Stem bark	Treatment of malaria	[91]
Mali	Leaves	Wound healing	[92]
	Leaves, stem bark	Treatment of malaria, urinary tract infection and internal wounds of pregnant women	[93]
	Stem bark	Personal health, insect management	[94]
Nigeria (North)	Leaves	Treatment of inflammations	[95]
	Stem bark	Treatment of diarrhoea	[96]
Nigeria (South West)	Stem bark	Treatment of trypanosomiasis, fever, ulcer, wound healing	[78, 97]
	Roots	Treatment of hypertension, infertility, stomach ache, sore eye, anti-poison	[98, 99]
	Leaves	Treatment of stroke, leprosy, skin lesion, eye infections	[99]
Nigeria (South East)	Stem bark	Treatment of hypertension	[7]
Togo	Roots	Treatment of haemorrhoids, Diarrhoea	[100]
	Stem bark	Cardioprotection	[101]

Table 5. West African folkloric use of *Parkia biglobosa* for the treatment of diseases

rat [10], an aqueous bark extract decreased blood pressure in rabbits [12] a hydroalcoholic bark extract of *Parkia biglobosa* caused vasorelaxation [13] and a methanolic leaf extract demonstrated hypotensive activities [14]. Hypercholesterolemia and hypertriglyceridemia are known risk factors associated with hypertension and CVD. The anti-hyperlipidaemia effect of the aqueous and methanolic extracts of *Parkia biglobosa* has been described to reduce hypercholesterolemia and hypertriglyceridemia in diabetic rats [11]. Therefore, *Parkia biglobosa* could offer protection against the development of coronary heart diseases in diabetics [11]. Recently, another study on the methanolic leaf extract of Parkia biglobosa also confirmed protection against doxorubicin-induced cardiotoxicity in rats [87]. In this study, scientists proposed that protection was offered through the antioxidant content and anti-inflammatory properties of the plant extract. Alternatively, it was proposed that protection against cardiotoxicity might have originated from the potential synergistic interactions among the plant phytochemicals. In fact, *Parkia biglobosa* has a rich composition of secondary metabolites which have been individually reported to possess excellent cardiovascular properties, namely:

- saponins (a vast group of glycosides) recently known for providing cardioprotective effects in experimental model [108],
- cardiac glycosides (group of steroidal glycosides) reported to act as cardiotonic agent [109],
- tannic acid (typical product containing hydrolysable tannins) known for its ability to reduce serum cholesterol and triglycerides [110-111],
- triterpenoids such as lupeol known to display antioxidant, anti-hypercholesterolemic and cardioprotective activities [112-113],
- catechins (flavan-3-ol compounds) reported to reduce atherosclerotic plaques formation in animal models [114],
- epicatechins known to reduce the risk of stroke and heart failure [115-116].

Furthermore, it was also reported that a leaf extract of *Parkia biglobosa* is a strong inducer of endothelium-dependent relaxations involving both NO and EDHF via a redox-sensitive mechanism [117]. Moreover, it was suggested that procyanidins fraction of the leaf extract exerted beneficial effects on the endothelial function by decreasing vascular tone and are the major inducers of the vasorelaxation [117].

In conclusion, many experimental and ethnoparmacological studies gave credence to the health enhancing-potential of *Parkia biglobosa* extracts in the treatment of disease conditions such as high blood pressure and CVD. However, there is still an important shortage of scientific evidence elucidating the exact mechanisms through which *Parkia biglobosa* extracts offer protection against hypertension. Therefore, further studies are warranted in CVD diseased-model in order to identify the main phytoconstituents involved in the hypotensive response. The mechanisms of action through which the plant extract offer protection against cardiotoxicity and hypertension should also be investigated. Furthermore, the indigenous population have not adopted standardised methods (the population continue to use uncontrolled dosages and in most instances, preparations of *Parkia biglobosa* extracts are stored in inappropriate conditions) on the medicinal use of the plant. Therefore, caution and care are still needed to be applied on the folkloric use of *Parkia biglobosa*.

Author details

O.B.L. Alinde*, A.J. Esterhuyse and O.O. Oguntibeju

*Address all correspondence to: alindeb@cput.ac.za, lidwina785@gmail.com

Oxidative Stress Research Centre, Department of Biomedical Sciences, Faculty of Health & Wellness Sciences, Cape Peninsula University of Technology, Bellville, South Africa

References

[1] Mathers C, Stevens G, Mascarenhas M. Global health risks: mortality and burden of disease attributable to selected major risks. World Health Organization; 2009.

[2] World Health Organisation (a). World Health Statistics 2012. World Health Organisation; 2012.

[3] World Health Organisation (b). World Health Statistics 2012: A snapshot of global health. World Health Organisation; 2012.

[4] Pires JE, Sebastião YV, Langa AJ, Nery SV. Hypertension in Northern Angola: prevalence, associated factors, awareness, treatment and control. BMC Public Health 2013; 13(1): 1-10.

[5] Somova L, Shode F, Ramnanan P, Nadar A. Antihypertensive, antiatherosclerotic and antioxidant activity of triterpenoids isolated from *Olea europaea,* subspecies Africana leaves. J Ethnopharmacol 2003; 84(2): 299-305.

[6] Bazzano LA. Dietary intake of fruit and vegetables and risk of diabetes mellitus and cardiovascular diseases. World Health Organisation; 2005.

[7] Gbolade A. Ethnobotanical study of plants used in treating hypertension in Edo State of Nigeria. J Ethnopharmacol 2012; 144: 1-10.

[8] Raji IA, Mugabo P, Obikeze K. Effect of *Tulbaghia violacea* on the blood pressure and heart rate in male spontaneously hypertensive Wistar rats. J Ethnopharmacol 2012; 140(1): 98-106.

[9] Boon C, Ng M, Choo Y, Mok S.. Super, Red Palm and Palm Oleins Improve the Blood Pressure, Heart Size, Aortic Media Thickness and Lipid Profile in Spontaneously Hypertensive Rats. PLoS One 2013; 8(2): e55908.

[10] Assane M, Baba Moussa R, Bassene E, Sere A. Antihypertensive action of *Parkia biglobosa* (Jacq) Benth seeds in the rat. Dakar Med 1993; 38(1): 49-54.

[11] Odetola A, Akinloye O, Egunjobi C, Adekunle W, Ayoola A. Possible antidiabetic and antihyperlipidaemic effect of fermented *Parkia biglobosa* (jacq) extract in alloxan-induced diabetic rats. Clin Exp Pharmacol Physiol 2006; 33(9): 808-812.

[12] Kassi Y, Aka KJ, Abo KJ, Mea A, Bi SAN, Ehile EE. Effet antihypertensif d' un extrait aqueux d' écorce de tronc de *Parkia biglobosa* (mimosaceae) sur la pression artérielle de lapin. Sci. Nat 2008; 5(2): 133-143.

[13] Kane MO, Sarr M, Gueye PM, Ndiaye CAB, Diaw M, Ba A, Sar FB, Sall/Diallo A. Effets relaxants vasculaires d'un extrait hydroalcoolique d'écorce de *Parkia biglobosa* (mimosaceae). Science Lib Editions Mersenne 2009; 2 (090901).

[14] Olaleye TM, Komolafe K, Akindahunsi AA. Effects of methanolic leaf extract of *Parkia biglobosa* on some biochemical indices and hemodynamic parameters in rats. J Chem Pharm Res 2013; 5(1): 213-220.

[15] Chobanian AV, Bakris GL, Black HR, Cushman WC, Green LA, Izzo JL, Jones DW, Materson BJ, Oparil S, Wright JT. Seventh report of the joint national committee on prevention, detection, evaluation, and treatment of high blood pressure. Hypertension 2003; 42(6): 1206-1252.

[16] Olives C, Myerson R, Mokdad AH, Murray CJ, Lim SS. Prevalence, Awareness, Treatment, and Control of Hypertension in United States Counties, 2001–2009. PLoS One 2013; 8(4): e60308.

[17] Wilkins K, Campbell NR, Joffres MR, McAlister FA, Nichol M, Quach S, Johansen HL, Tremblay MS. Blood pressure in Canadian adults. Health Rep 2010; 21(1): 37-46.

[18] Atwood KM, Robitaille CJ, Reimer K, Dai S, Johansen HL, Smith MJ. Comparison of Diagnosed, Self-Reported, and Physically-Measured Hypertension in Canada. Can J Cardiol 2013; 29: 606-612.

[19] Lu X, Shi P, Luo C, Zhou Y, Yu H, Guo C, Wu F. Prevalence of hypertension in overweight and obese children from a large school-based population in Shanghai, China. BMC Public Health 2013; 13(1): 24.

[20] Danielson M & Dammstrom B. The prevalence of secondary and curable hypertension. Acta Med Scand Suppl 1981; 209(1-6): 451-455.

[21] Sinclair AM, Isles CG, Brown I, Cameron H, Murray GD, Robertson JW. Secondary hypertension in a blood pressure clinic. Arch Intern Med 1987; 147(7): 1289-1293.

[22] Anderson Jr GH, Blakeman N, Streeten DH. The effect of age on prevalence of secondary forms of hypertension in 4429 consecutively referred patients. J Hypertens 1994; 12(5): 609-615.

[23] Omura M, Saito J, Yamaguchi K, Kakuta Y, Nishikawa T. Prospective study on the prevalence of secondary hypertension among hypertensive patients visiting a general outpatient clinic in Japan. Hypertens Res 2004; 27(3): 193-202.

[24] Kearney PM, Whelton M, Reynolds K, Muntner P, Whelton PK, He J. Global burden of hypertension: analysis of worldwide data. Lancet 2005; 365(9455): 217-223.

[25] Friese RS, Altshuler AE, Zhang K, Miramontes-Gonzalez JP, Hightower CM, Jirout ML, Salem RM, Gayen JR, Mahapatra NR, Biswas N. MicroRNA-22 and promoter motif polymorphisms at the Chga locus in genetic hypertension: functional and therapeutic implications for gene expression and the pathogenesis of hypertension. Human Molecular Genetic 2013; 22(18): 3624-3640.

[26] Harrison DG. The Mosaic Theory revisited: common molecular mechanisms coordinating diverse organ and cellular events in hypertension. J Am Soc Hypertens 2013; 7(1): 68-74.

[27] Tu W & Pratt JH. A consideration of genetic mechanisms behind the development of hypertension in Blacks. Curr Hypertens Rep 2013; 15: 1-6.

[28] Thompkinson D, Bhavana V, Kanika P. Dietary approaches for management of cardio-vascular health-a review. J Food Sci Technol 2012; doi 10.1007/s13197-012-0661-8.

[29] Majane OH, Vengethasamy L, du Toit EF, Makaula S, Woodiwiss AJ, Norton GR. Dietary-induced obesity hastens the progression from concentric cardiac hypertrophy to pump dysfunction in spontaneously hypertensive rats. Hypertension 2009; 54(6): 1376-1383.

[30] Heesch CM. Reflexes that control cardiovascular function. Am J Physiol 1999; 277: S234–S243.

[31] Brown AM. Receptors under pressure. An update on baroreceptors. Circ Res 1980; 46(1): 1-10.

[32] Parmer RJ, Cervenka JH, Stone RA. Baroreflex sensitivity and heredity in essential hypertension. Circulation 1992; 85(2): 497-503.

[33] Balijepalli C. Blood Pressure Distribution in the German Population. PhD Thesis, University Duisburg-Essen; 2012.

[34] Jordan J, Biaggioni I. Genetic influences on human baroreflex regulation. Autonomic Neuroscience. J Basic Clin Physiol Pharmacol 2012; 172: 23-25.

[35] O'Connor DT. Catecholamine storage vesicle protein expression in genetic hypertension. Blood Press 1999; 8(5-6): 285-295.

[36] Salem RM, Cadman PE, Chen Y, Rao F, Wen G, Hamilton BA, Rana BK, Smith DW, Stridsberg M, Ward HJ. Chromogranin A polymorphisms are associated with hypertensive renal disease. Clin J Am Soc Nephrol 2008; 19(3): 600-614.

[37] O'Connor DT & Bernstein KN. Radioimmunoassay of chromogranin A in plasma as a measure of exocytotic sympathoadrenal activity in normal subjects and patients with pheochromocytoma. N Engl J Med 1984; 311(12): 764-770.

[38] O'Connor DT, Kailasam MT, Kennedy BP, Ziegler MG, Yanaihara N, Parmer RJ. Early decline in the catecholamine release-inhibitory peptide catestatin in humans at genetic risk of hypertension. J Clin Hypertens 2002; 20(7): 1335-1345.

[39] Helle K, Corti A, Metz-Boutigue M, Tota B. The endocrine role for chromogranin A: a prohormone for peptides with regulatory properties. Mol Cell 2007; 64(22): 2863-2886.

[40] Rao F, Wen G, Gayen JR, Das M, Vaingankar SM, Rana BK, Mahata M, Kennedy BP, Salem RM, Stridsberg M. Catecholamine release–inhibitory peptide catestatin (chromogranin a352–372): naturally occurring amino acid variant gly364ser causes profound changes in human autonomic activity and alters risk for hypertension. Circulation 2007; 115(17): 2271-2281.

[41] Fung MM, Salem RM, Mehtani P, Thomas B, Lu CF, Perez B, Rao F, Stridsberg M, Ziegler MG, Mahata SK. Direct vasoactive effects of the chromogranin A (CHGA) peptide catestatin in humans *in vivo*. Clin Exp Hypertens 2010; 32(5): 278-287.

[42] Sharma JN. The kinin system in hypertensive pathophysiology. Inflammopharmacology 2013; 21(1): 1-9.

[43] Douglas R, Ehlers M, Sturrock E. The anti-fibrotic peptide Ac-Sdkp: opportunities for ACE inhibitor design. Clin Exp Pharmacol Physiol 2013; 40(8):535-541.

[44] Bergel D. The static elastic properties of the arterial wall. Physiol J 1961; 156(3): 445-457.

[45] Folkow B. "Structural factor" in primary and secondary hypertension. Hypertension 1990 ; 16(1): 89-101.

[46] Grassi G, Cattaneo BM, Seravalle G, Lanfranchi A, Mancia G. Baroreflex control of sympathetic nerve activity in essential and secondary hypertension. Hypertension 1998; 31(1): 68-72.

[47] Luscher T & Vanhoutte PM. Endothelium-dependent contractions to acetylcholine in the aorta of the spontaneously hypertensive rat. Hypertension 1986; 8(4): 344-348.

[48] Russell V, Allie S, Wiggins T. Increased noradrenergic activity in prefrontal cortex slices of an animal model for attention-deficit hyperactivity disorder-the spontaneously hypertensive rat. Behav Brain Res 2000; 117(1): 69-74.

[49] Fernandez-Musoles R, Salom JB, Martinez-Maqueda D, Lopez-Diez JJ, Recio I, Manzanares P. Antihypertensive effects of lactoferrin hydrolysates: inhibition of angiotensin-and endothelin-converting enzymes. Food Chem 2013; 139: 994-1000.

[50] Tanabe A, Naruse M, Naruse K, Hase M, Yoshimoto T, Tanaka M, Seki T, Demura R, Demura H. Left ventricular hypertrophy is more prominent in patients with primary aldosteronism than in patients with other types of secondary hypertension. Hypertens Res: Hypertens Res 1997; 20(2): 85-90.

[51] Holmlund A, Holm G, Lind L. Severity of periodontal disease and number of remaining teeth are related to the prevalence of myocardial infarction and hypertension in a study based on 4,254 subjects. J Periodontol 2006; 77(7): 1173-1178.

[52] Garg N, Bhatia T, Jaiswal A. Approach to a case of Secondary Hypertension. Clinical Queries: Nephrology 2013; 2: 62-70.

[53] Hamilton CA, Miller WH, Al-Benna S, Brosnan MJ, Drummond RD, McBride MW, Dominiczak AF. Strategies to reduce oxidative stress in cardiovascular disease. Clin Sci 2004; 106(3): 219-234.

[54] Fortuno A, San Jose G, Moreno MU, Diez J, Zalba G. Oxidative stress and vascular remodelling. Exp Physiol 2005; 90(4): 457-462.

[55] Berk BC. Novel approaches to treat oxidative stress and cardiovascular diseases. Trans Am Clin Climatol Assoc 2007; 118: 209-214.

[56] Heistad DD, Wakisaka Y, Miller J, Chu Y, Pena-Silva R. Novel aspects of oxidative stress in cardiovascular diseases. Circulation Journal: Circ J 2009; 73(2): 201-207.

[57] Valko M, Leibfritz D, Moncol J, Cronin MTD, Mazur M, Telser J. Free radicals and antioxidants in normal physiological functions and human disease. Int J Biochem Cell Biol 2007; 39(1): 44-84.

[58] Ceriello A. Possible role of oxidative stress in the pathogenesis of hypertension. Diabetes Care 2008; 31(Supplement 2): S181-S184.

[59] Montezano A & Touyz RM. Reactive oxygen species, vascular Noxs and hypertension: Focus on translational and clinical research. Antioxid Redox Signal 2013; doi: 10.1089/ars.2013.5302.

[60] Vaziri ND, Wang XQ, Oveisi F, Rad B. Induction of oxidative stress by glutathione depletion causes severe hypertension in normal rats. Hypertension 2000; 36(1): 142-146.

[61] Mansego ML, Solar GDM, Alonso MP, Martínez F, Sáez GT, Escudero JCM, Redón J, Chaves FJ. Polymorphisms of antioxidant enzymes, blood pressure and risk of hypertension. J Clin Hypertens 2011; 29(3): 492-500.

[62] Hsueh Y, Lin P, Chen H, Shiue H, Chung C, Tsai C, Huang Y, Chiou H, Chen C. Genetic polymorphisms of oxidative and antioxidant enzymes and arsenic-related hypertension. J Toxicol Environ Health 2005; Part A, 68(17-18): 1471-1484.

[63] Guzik TJ, Hoch NE, Brown KA, McCann LA, Rahman A, Dikalov S, Goronzy J, Weyand C, Harrison DG. Role of the T cell in the genesis of angiotensin II–induced hypertension and vascular dysfunction. J Exp Med 2007; 204(10): 2449-2460.

[64] Cheung BM, Ong KL, Tso AW, Leung RY, Cherny SS, Sham PC, Thomas GN, Lam TH, Lam KS. Relationship of plasma interleukin-6 and its genetic variants with hypertension in Hong Kong Chinese. Am J Hypertens 2011; 24(12): 1331-1337.

[65] Hlebowicz J, Persson M, Gullberg B, Sonestedt E, Wallström P, Drake I, Nilsson J, Hedblad B, Wirfält E. Food patterns, inflammation markers and incidence of cardiovascular disease: the Malmö Diet and Cancer study. J Intern Med 2011; 270(4): 365-376.

[66] Lob HE, Marvar PJ, Guzik TJ, Sharma S, McCann LA, Weyand C, Gordon FJ, Harrison DG. Induction of hypertension and peripheral inflammation by reduction of extracellular superoxide dismutase in the central nervous system. Hypertension 2010; 55(2): 277-283.

[67] McIntyre M, Bohr DF, Dominiczak AF. Endothelial Function in Hypertension The role of superoxide anion. Hypertension 1999; 34(4): 539-545.

[68] Landmesser U, Dikalov S, Price SR, McCann L, Fukai T, Holland SM, Mitch WE, Harrison DG. Oxidation of tetrahydrobiopterin leads to uncoupling of endothelial cell nitric oxide synthase in hypertension. J Clin Invest 2003; 111(8): 1201-1209.

[69] Harrison D, Widder J, Grumbach I, Chen W, Weber M, Searles C. Endothelial mechanotransduction, nitric oxide and vascular inflammation. J Intern Med 2006, 259(4): 351-363.

[70] Harrison DG. Oxidative stress and vascular inflammation. In G. Hoffman, C. Weyand, C. Langford, J. Goronzy (Eds.). Inflammatory diseases of blood vessels (2nd ed.), John Wiley and Sons; 2012. p94-104.

[71] Veliotes DG, Norton GR, Correia RJ, Strijdom H, Badenhorst D, Brooksbank R, Woodiwiss AJ. Impact of aldosterone receptor blockade on the deleterious cardiac effects of adrenergic activation in hypertensive rats. J Cardiovasc Pharmacol 2010; 56(2): 203-211.

[72] Abu-Ghefreh A, Khan I. A role of intestine in hypertension: mechanism of suppression of intestinal Na-H exchanger isoform-3 in spontaneously hypertensive rats. Clin Exp Hypertens 2013; 35(7):543-549.

[73] Quintana-Villamandos B, Delgado-Martos MJ, Sánchez-Hernández JJ, Gómez de Diego JJ, Fernández-Criado Mdel C, Canillas F, Martos-Rodríguez A, Delgado-Baeza E. Early regression of left ventricular hypertrophy after treatment with esmolol in an experimental rat model of primary hypertension. Hypertens Res 2013; 36: 408-413.

[74] Cutler JA. Calcium-channel blockers for hypertension: uncertainty continues. N Engl J Med 1998; 338(10): 679-681.

[75] Blood Pressure Lowering Treatment Trialists'Collaboration. Effects of ACE inhibitors, calcium antagonists, and other blood-pressure-lowering drugs: results of prospectively designed overviews of randomised trials. Lancet 2000; 355(1): 955-964.

[76] Guzman-Uriarte ML, Sánchez-Magaña LM, Angulo-Meza GY, Cuevas-Rodríguez EO, Gutiérrez-Dorado R, Mora-Rochín S, Milán-Carrillo J, Valdez-Ortiz A, Reyes-Moreno C. Solid state bioconversion for producing common bean (*Phaseolus vulgaris*

L.) Functional flour with high antioxidant activity and antihypertensive potential. Food Nutr (Roma) 2013; 4: 480-490.

[77] Asase A, Oteng-Yeboah AA, Odamtten GT, Simmonds MS. Ethnobotanical study of some Ghanaian anti-malarial plants. J Ethnopharmacol 2005; 99(2): 273-279.

[78] Osho I & Lajide L. Prescreening evaluation of some plant extracts used in ethno-veterinary practices as antitrypanosomal agents. J Med Plant Res 2012; 6(11): 2056-2060.

[79] Luckow M & Hopkins HC. A cladistic analysis of *Parkia* (Leguminosae: Mimosoideae). Am J Bot 1995; 82(10): 1300-1320.

[80] Adaramola T, Ariwaodo J, Adeniji K. Distribution, Phytochemistry and Antioxidant Properties of the Genus *Parkia* R. br.(Mimosaceae) in Nigeria. IJPPR 2013; 4(4), 172-178.

[81] Teklehaimanot Z. Exploiting the potential of indigenous agroforestry trees: *Parkia biglobosa a*nd Vitellaria paradoxa in sub-Saharan Africa. Agroforest Syst 2004; 61: 207-220.

[82] World Agroforestry centre. n.d. *Parkia biglobosa.* http://www.worldagroforestry.org/treedb2/speciesprofile.php?Spid=1255. [June 2013].

[83] Sina S & Traoré SA. *Parkia biglobosa* (Jacq.) R.Br. ex G.Don. [Internet] Record from PROTA4U. Oyen, L.P.A. & Lemmens, R.H.M.J. (Editors). PROTA (Plant Resources of Tropical Africa / Ressources végétales de l'Afrique tropicale) 2002, Wageningen, Netherlands. http://www.prota4u.org/search.asp (accessed 23 August 2013).

[84] Ajaiyeoba EO. Phytochemical and antibacterial properties of *Parkia biglobosa* and *Parkia bicolor* leaf extracts. AJBR 2003; 5(3): 125-129.

[85] Udobi C & Onaolapo J. Phytochemical analysis and antibacterial evaluation of the leaf stem bark and root of the African locust bean (*Parkia biglobosa*). J Med Plant Res 2009; 3(5): 338-344.

[86] Millogo-Kone H, Guissou I, Nacoulma O, Traore A. Antimicrobial effects of the stem bark extracts of *Parkia biglobosa* (jacq.) Benth. on Shigellae. Afr J Tradit Complement Altern Med 2008; 4(4): 392-396.

[87] Komolafe K, Akinmoladun AC, Olaleye TM. Methanolic leaf extract of *Parkia biglobosa p*rotects against doxorubicin-induced cardiotoxicity in rats. IJARNP 2013; 6(3): 39-47.

[88] Tala VRS, Candida da Silva V, Rodrigues CM, Nkengfack AE, Campaner dos Santos L, Vilegas W. Characterization of Proanthocyanidins from *Parkia biglobosa* (Jacq.) G. Don.(Fabaceae) by Flow Injection Analysis-Electrospray Ionization Ion Trap Tandem Mass Spectrometry and Liquid Chromatography/Electrospray Ionization Mass Spectrometry. Molecules 2013; 18(3): 2803-2820.

[89] Koura K, Ganglo JC, Assogbadjo AE, Agbangla C. Ethnic differences in use values and use patterns of *Parkia biglobosa* in northern Benin. J Ethnobiol Ethnomed 2011; 7:42.

[90] Tapsoba H, Deschamps J. Use of medicinal plants for the treatment of oral diseases in Burkina faso. J Ethnopharmacol 2006; 104(1):68-78.

[91] Ménan H, Banzouzi J, Hocquette A, Pélissier Y, Blache Y, Koné M, Mallié M, Assi LA, Valentin A. Antiplasmodial activity and cytotoxicity of plants used in West African traditional medicine for the treatment of malaria. J Ethnopharmacol 2006; 105(1): 131-6.

[92] Inngjerdingen K, Nergård CS, Diallo D, Mounkoro PP, Paulsen BS. An ethnopharmacological survey of plants used for wound healing in Dogonland, Mali, West Africa. J Ethnopharmacol 2004; 92(2):233-44.

[93] Nordeng H, Al-Zayadi W, Diallo D, Ballo N, Paulsen BS. Traditional medicine practitioners' knowledge and views on treatment of pregnant women in three regions of Mali. J Ethnobiol Ethnomed 2013; 9(1):67.

[94] Lehman AD, Dunkel FV, Klein RA, Ouattara S, Diallo D, Gamby KT, N'Diaye M. Insect management products from Malian traditional medicine-Establishing systematic criteria for their identification. J Ethnopharmacol 2007; 110(2):235-249.

[95] Abubakar M, Musa A, Ahmed A, Hussaini I. The perception and practice of traditional medicine in the treatment of cancers and inflammations by the Hausa and Fulani tribes of northern Nigeria. J Ethnopharmacol 2007; 111(3):625-629.

[96] Agunu A, Yusuf S, Andrew GO, Zezi AU, Abdurahman EM. Evaluation of five medicinal plants used in diarrhoea treatment in Nigeria. J Ethnopharmacol 2005; 101(1): 27-30.

[97] Adetutu A, Winston MA, Corcoran O, Chimezie F. Antibacterial activity and in vitro cytotoxicity of extracts and fractions of *Parkia biglobosa* (Jacq.) Benth stem bark and *Ageratum conyzoides* Linn. leaves. Environ Toxicol Pharmacol 2012; 34: 478-483.

[98] Lawal I, Uzokwe N, Igboanugo A, Adio A, Awosan E, Nwogwugwu J, Faloye B, Olatunji B, Adesoga A. Ethno medicinal information on collation and identification of some medicinal plants in research institutes of South-West Nigeria. AJPP 2010; 4(1): 1-7.

[99] Erakhrumen A, Ogunsanwo O, Ajewole O. Assessment of some other traditional uses of accepted agroforestry fuelwood species in Akinyele and Ido local government areas, Oyo state, Nigeria. IJSF 2010; 3(1):47-65.

[100] Tchacondo T, Karou SD, Batawila K, Agban A, Ouro-Bang'na K, Anani KT, Gbeassor M, de Souza C. Herbal remedies and their adverse effects in tem tribe traditional medicine in Togo. Afr J Tradit Complement Altern Med 2011; 8(1):45-60.

[101] Adi K, Metowogo K, Mouzou A, Lawson-Evi P, Eklu-Gadegbeku K, Agbonon A, Lamboni C, Essien K, Aklikokou K, Gbeassor M. Evaluation of cardioprotective effects of *Parkia biglobosa* (jacq. benth) Mimosaceae stem bark. J App Pharm Sci 2013; 3(02):060-4.

[102] Kouadio F, Kanko C, Juge M, Grimaud N, Jean A, N'guessan Y, Petit J. Analgesic and antiinflammatory activities of an extract from *Parkia biglobosa* used in traditional medicine in the Ivory Coast. Phytother Res 2000; 14(8): 635-637.

[103] Asuzu I & Harvey A. The antisnake venom activities of *Parkia biglobosa* (Mimosaceae) stem bark extract. Toxicon 2003; 42(7): 763-768.

[104] El-Mahmood A & Ameh J. In vitro antibacterial activity of *Parkia biglobosa* (Jacq.) root bark extract against some microorganisms associated with urinary tract infections. Afr J Biotechnol 2007; 6(11): 1272-1275.

[105] Builders M, Wannang N, Aguiyi J. Antiplasmodial activities of *Parkia biglobosa* leaves: *In vivo* and *In vitro* studies. Ann Biol Res 2011; 2(4): 8-20.

[106] Lamien-Meda A, Lamien CE, Compaoré MM, Meda RN, Kiendrebeogo M, Zeba B, Millogo JF, Nacoulma OG. Polyphenol content and antioxidant activity of fourteen wild edible fruits from Burkina Faso. Molecules 2008; 13(3): 581-594.

[107] Nwaehujor C, Ezeigbo I, Udeh N, Asuzu I. Anti-inflammatory and anti-oxidant activities of the methanolic extracts of the stalk of *Parkia biglobosa* (JACQ.) BENTH. Hygeia J D Med 2011; 8: 34-40.

[108] Xu H, Yu X, Qu S, Chen Y, Wang Z, Sui D. *In vivo* and *in vitro* cardioprotective effects of *Panax quinquefolium* 20 (S)-protopanaxadiol saponins (PQDS), isolated from *Panax quinquefolium*. Die Pharmazie-An Int J Pharm Sci 2013; 68(4): 287-292.

[109] Xie J, Dial LD, Shapiro JI. Na/K-ATPase signaling and the tradeoff between natriuresis and cardiac fibrosis.In cardiomyopathies, Milei, J. (Ed.) InTech, DOI: 10.5772/54722; 2013.

[110] Zou B, Li C, Chen J, Dong X, Zhang Y, Du J. High molecular weight persimmon tannin is a potent hypolipidemic in high-cholesterol diet fed rats. Food Res Int 2012; 48(2): 970-977.

[111] Fan H, Wu D, Tian W, Ma X. Inhibitory effects of tannic acid on fatty acid synthase and 3T3-L1 preadipocyte. BBA- Molecular and Cell Biology of Lipids 2013; 1831(7): 1260-1266.

[112] Sudharsan P, Mythili Y, Selvakumar E, Varalakshmi P. Cardioprotective effect of pentacyclic triterpene, lupeol and its ester on cyclophosphamide-induced oxidative stress. Hum Exp Toxicol 2005; 24(6): 313-318.

http://dx.doi.org/10.5772/57229

[113] Sudhahar V, Kumar SA, Sudharsan PT, Varalakshmi P. Protective effect of lupeol and its ester on cardiac abnormalities in experimental hypercholesterolemia. Vascul Pharmacol 2007, 46(6): 412-418.

[114] Miura, Y., Chiba, T., Tomita, I., Koizumi, H., Miura, S., Umegaki, K., Hara, Y. & Ikeda, M. 2001. Tea catechins prevent the development of atherosclerosis in apoprotein E–deficient mice. J Nutr, 131(1): 27-32.

[115] Shah, Z.A., Li, R., Ahmad, A.S., Kensler, T.W., Yamamoto, M., Biswal, S. & Doré, S. 2010. The flavanol (−)-epicatechin prevents stroke damage through the Nrf2/HO1 pathway. J Cereb Blood Flow Metab, 30(12): 1951-1961.

[116] Flammer, A.J., Sudano, I., Wolfrum, M., Thomas, R., Enseleit, F., Périat, D., Kaiser, P., Hirt, A., Hermann, M. & Serafini, M. 2012. Cardiovascular effects of flavanol-rich chocolate in patients with heart failure. Eur Heart J, 33(17): 2172-2180.

[117] Tokoudagba, J., Auger, C., Bréant, L., N'Gom, S., Chabert, P., Idris-Khodja, N., Gbaguidi, F., Gbenou, J., Moudachirou, M., Lobstein, A. 2010. Procyanidin-rich fractions from *Parkia biglobosa* (Mimosaceae) leaves cause redox-sensitive endothelium-dependent relaxation involving NO and EDHF in porcine coronary artery. J Ethnopharmacol, 132(1): 246-250.